# THE NON-THROMBOTIC ROLE OF PLATELETS IN HEALTH AND DISEASE

Edited by **Steve Kerrigan** and **Niamh Moran**

**The Non-Thrombotic Role of Platelets in Health and Disease**
http://dx.doi.org/10.5772/58357
Edited by Steve Kerrigan and Niamh Moran

**Contributors**

Niamh Moran, Dermot Cox, Alex Balduino, Paul F. Bray, Douglass A. Drelich, Christian Humpel, Voahanginirina Randriamboavonjy, Brian O'Sullivan, Steve W. W. Kerrigan, Alexander Brill, John Hartwig, Maryam AlObaidly

**Published by InTech**

Janeza Trdine 9, 51000 Rijeka, Croatia



**Publishing Process Manager** Iva Simcic

**Technical Editor** InTech DTP team

**Cover** InTech Design team

First published November, 2015

Printed in Croatia

Additional hard copies can be obtained from orders@intechopen.com

The Non-Thrombotic Role of Platelets in Health and Disease, Edited by Steve Kerrigan and Niamh Moran

p. cm.

ISBN 978-953-51-2208-1

For EU product safety concerns:
IN TECH d.o.o., Prolaz Marije Krucifikse Kozulić 3, 51000 Rijeka, Croatia,
info@intechopen.com or visit our website at intechopen.com.

# Meet the editors

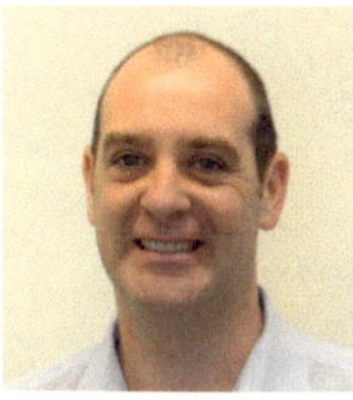

Dr. Steven W. Kerrigan is a pharmacologist with a PhD in Infection of the Cardiovascular System, specifically focusing on characterising platelet-bacterial interactions at the molecular level. Currently, Dr. Kerrigan is the head of the Cardiovascular Infection Group in the Royal College of Surgeons in Ireland and is an associate editor of several international journals specialized in host infection. Dr. Kerrigan has published many papers in high impact journals which make a significant contribution to our understanding of blood borne infection.

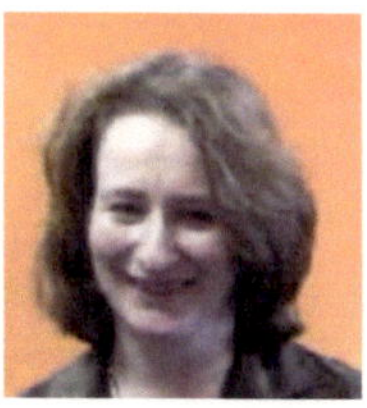

Prof. Niamh Moran is a biochemical pharmacologist who has devoted much of her research career to the understanding of the molecular events underlying platelet activation. She has developed a number of high throughput assays for assessing platelet function that can identify platelet activation in clinical samples. The work of her laboratory has demonstrated independent regulation of platelet activation events in homeostasis and haemostasis, in health and disease.

# Contents

# Preface

Platelets are small anucleate, short lived particle derived from the larger precursor cell, the megakaryocyte. First discovered by Bizzozero in 1882, they were rediscovered in the 1960's after many decades of oblivion. It is now well established that platelets play a key role in thrombosis and haemostasis. However, as our basic knowledge in platelet biology has improved through the years, it is becoming more evident that the role of this small particle of a cell extends beyond that of thrombosis and haemostasis alone. Functional roles for platelets in homeostasis have been identified. Thus, platelets also appear to play a significant role in other elements of bodily homestasis. For example, their quiet capacity to orchestrate events in several processes including pregnancy, infection and immunity, their potential use of platelet biomarkers in psychiatric disorders and finally their ability to transport a plethora of bioactive molecules highlighting their potential uses to enhance wound healing and enable tissue regeneration suggest that we are only beginning to understand the importance of this unique cellular particle.

Currently no single publication specifically focuses on the multiple alternate roles of platelets. The ***Non-Thrombotic Role of Platelets in Health and Disease*** aims to address this.

The book is separated into 4 sections;

Section I. Platelet production and function

Section II. Platelets in inflammation, infection and immunity

Section III. Platelets in various disease states

Section IV. Platelets in tissue regeneration

The authors of each of the 11 chapters are world leaders in their respective fields. While significant advances have been made recently in the nonthromboic role of platelets in health and disease the primary intent of this book is to elevate awareness and enthusiasm in further investigating these new functions.

**ACKNOWLEDGMENTS**

The editors would like to acknowledge financial support from the Health Research Board of Ireland, School of Pharmacy, Molecular and Cellular Therapeutics and the Office of Research and Innovation in the Royal College of Surgeons in Ireland.

**Dr. Steve Kerrigan M.Sc, PhD, C.Biol, FSB**
Senior Lecturer in Pharmacology / Principal Investigator Host Infection Group
RCSI School of Postgraduate Studies / MCT
Royal College of Surgeons, Ireland

**Prof. Niamh Moran PhD**
Principal Investigator, Platelet Biology / Head of School of Postgraduate Studies
RCSI School of Postgraduate Studies / Molecular and Cellular Therapeutics
Royal College of Surgeons, Ireland

Section 1

# Platelet Production and Function

Chapter 1

# Production and Destruction of Platelets

Joseph Jr Italiano and John Hartwig

Additional information is available at the end of the chapter

http://dx.doi.org/10.5772/60678

## 1. Introduction

Platelet counts in blood are controlled by the rates of their production by megakaryocytes and the kinetics of their removal. Alterations in either process can lead to thrombocytopenia (TCP) or thrombocytosis. Under conditions of TCP, the spleen and liver are the sites for accelerated platelet destruction, and in thrombocytosis, the spleen can become a supplemental breeding ground for megakaryocytes, in addition to the bone marrow space. Humans produce and remove $10^{11}$ platelets per day. Senile or damaged platelets are detected as such and are removed from blood. Platelets must also be removed locally at diverse sites where they have discovered vascular damage, attached and become activated to prevent blood leakage. The mechanism of this local removal in the blood vascular system is not well described or understood. The removal of platelets from flowing blood mandates a system that detects changes that accumulate in the platelet surface with age and that responds by binding and removing the platelets when changes reach a critical level. Surface changes must either increase the availability of clearance ligands or remove anti-clearance signals such as CD47 [1]. Changes in the platelet surface that signal for removal include phosphatidylserine upregulation, deglycosylation of membrane glycoproteins, in particular Gp1bα of the vWf receptor, and Ig binding. Diseases that accelerate removal arbitrate their impact at the platelet surface.

This section highlights recent advancements in understanding how platelet lifetimes in blood are regulated and the discovery of a surprising feedback pathway that links platelet removal by hepatocytes in liver to platelet production in the bone marrow.

## 2. Sites and cells that remove senile platelets

Platelet senescence is driven by both an internal proteolytic clock and through external changes that occur on the cell surface as they circulate in blood. Internally, platelets have an apoptotic mechanism that sets limits on the overall platelet lifetime at ~10 days [2]. At the time of birth, each mature platelet has a defined quota of the pro-survival protein Bcl-x that with time degrades, releasing its brake on the activities of Bak and Bax that subsequently induce mitochondrial lysis, cytochrome C release, and the activation of cytoplasmic capases. Capases disassemble the cytoskeleton and lead to the upregulation of phosphatidylserine to the platelet surface. Cells that have phosphatidylserine on their surfaces are avidly recognized and removed by the professional phagocytes, macrophages and immature dendritic cells. Multiple receptors have been identified for phosphatidylserine on phagocytes including CLM-1 or CD300f [3], Tim-4 [4], BaI1 [5], or Stabilin-1 receptor [6].

Platelets express CD47 on their surface. CD47, also called integrin associated protein [7], is a member of the immunoglobulin superfamily that associates with the integrins, $\alpha IIb\beta 3$ and $\alpha v\beta 3$, on platelets. A role for CD47 in maintaining platelets in circulation was first recognized in knockout mice, which have platelets counts reduced by ~20% compared to normal. This highly glycosylated surface protein is recognized by the SIRP$\alpha$ transmembrane protein on phagocytes that contains two immunoreceptor tyrosine-based inhibitory domains in its cytoplasmic domain. Hence, ligation by CD47 transmits anti-phagocytic signals to macrophages, independent of the phagocytic receptor engaged, helping to prevent macrophages for engaging phagocytic pathways involving Fc receptors.

One example where phosphatidylserine exposure can induce macrophages to remove platelets occurs with FlnA null platelets. Mice having megakaryocytes and platelets that lack FlnA are macrothrombocytopenic, with platelet counts reduced by 80-90%, compared to WT mice. FlnA null platelets are unstable because they lack FlnA's actin filament crosslinking activity and its membrane glycoprotein attachment sites, which link the actin cytoskeleton to the plasma membrane. FlnA constitutively binds to the GP1b$\alpha$ chains of the vWF complex, as well as certain $\beta$-integrin chains. The high density of the vWfR-FlnA interaction, ~12,000 per platelet, stabilizes the membrane by attaching it to the underlying actin cytoskeleton. Because the vWfR is linked to the sides of actin filaments it also regulates the topology of the vWf receptor, aligning the receptor in linear arrays on the platelet surface. When studied *in vitro*, FlnA null platelets spontaneously fragment into microparticles that are 100% positive for annexin V binding, which reports flipping of phosphatidylserine to the cell surface. Microparticles from the FlnA null platelets are, however, rarely found in freshly isolated blood, unless macrophages are first ablated in the mice using phagocytic liposomes filled with clodronate, a potent toxin when ingested. This finding demonstrates that macrophages normally clear both FlnA null platelets and microparticles derived from them *in situ*, most likely using phosphatidylserine recognizing receptors [8].

## 3. Sialic acid and platelet circulatory lifetime

Sialic acid terminates the N- and O-linked glycans of all cell surface glycoproteins. Desialylation of platelet glycans was the first recognized mechanism that can target platelets for clearance. In 1975, Greenberg and colleagues [9] showed that desialylation of platelets (and erythrocytes) *in vitro* using neuraminidase resulted in rapid removal upon retransfusion. Subsequently, it was found that sialic acid is lost during platelet storage *in vitro* [10] and as platelets age *in vivo* [11]. Recently, the mechanism that removes sialic acid-depleted platelets has been identified. Studies from 2 independent labs have found that liver hepatocytes, using their asialoglycoprotein receptor (Asgr), remove desialylated platelets as well as certain desialylated plasma proteins.

The Asgr was one of the first receptors to be identified and characterized [12] over 40 years ago. Each surface Asgr is a heterotrimer composed of 2 HL-1 chains and 1 HL-2 chain. Knock out animals lacking in the expression of either chain, therefore, do not have functional Asgr receptors on their hepatocytes. The Asgr is a C-type lectin that recognizes exposed β-galactose, the underlying moiety to which sialic acid is linked in carbohydrate chains. Most glycoproteins have their glycans capped by α2,3-linked sialic acid. Galactose exposure is mediated by sialidases present in blood or released into blood by infectious bacteria. Interestingly and of high clinical impact, the Asgr can also bind to α2,6 linked sialic acid residues on glycoproteins.

Desialylated platelets are recognized and removed by the liver Asgr [13-15]. The specific function of the Asgr in platelet removal has been demonstrated by the following evidences: (1) HepG2 cells bind and ingest desialylated platelets *in vitro*; (2) Mice lacking functional Asgrs ($HL2^{-/-}$) have high platelet counts (increased by 50% over $HL2^{+/+}$) because their platelets circulate for longer lifespans. Platelet circulatory lifetime is lengthened by 35% in the $HL\text{-}2^{-/-}$ animals. Lectin profiling of platelets derived from the $HL2^{-/-}$ mice shows they have higher amounts of exposed β-galactose as expected. Hence, the lengthening of platelet lifetimes in these animals is caused by the loss of the removal system, not because the platelet surface escapes desialylation in the circulation. This finding is expected if the Asgr routinely removes desialylated platelets since the amount of desialylation will increase as the senile platelets continue to circulate; (3) Conversely, $St3gal4^{-/-}$ mice that lack the main sialyltransferase enzyme responsible for the linkage of sialic acid to galactose, have low platelet counts and short platelet circulation lifetimes. Once again, platelets harvested from these null mice have high levels of exposed galactose that bind the RCA I lectin avidly. Circulation times for these platelets can be extended to near normal by transfusion of them into $HL2^{-/-}$ mice. This again demonstrates the central role of the Asgr in recognizing and removing desialylated platelets. (4) Last, platelet desialylation *in vitro* using sialidases or *in situ* following injection of sialidase causes a rapid clearance of platelets from blood in WT mice, but not $HL2^{-/-}$mice, in a process that is not altered by macrophage ablation.

## 4. Feedback between liver and bone marrow

The importance of hepatocyte-platelet interaction extends beyond simple removal, as the recognition and ingestion of platelets by the Asgr generates cytoplasmic signals in hepatocytes that induce the formation and secretion of cytokines to promote marrow and megakaryocyte growth and maturation. In this case, the key cytokine produced in response to platelet ingestion is thrombopoietin [16]. Thus, the hepatocyte-platelet interaction directly feeds back to megakaryocytes in marrow, helping to stimulate platelet production.

## 5. Platelet reactive receptors on macrophages

In addition to its receptors that recognize phosphatidylserine, macrophage surfaces are festooned with receptors that can ingest damaged and/or diseased platelets. One group includes the lectin receptors that recognize carbohydrate alterations in platelet glycoproteins. The phagocytic integrin, $\alpha_M\beta_2$, recognizes and removes chilled and rewarmed platelets that release glycosylases causing β-GlcNAc moieties to expose on N-linked GP1bα glycans. In addition, a second domain on $\alpha_M\beta_2$ recognizes a different portion of GP1bα [17]. Mannose receptors are a second example of a receptor that detects glycan alterations, recognizing underlying mannose moieties exposed by glycosylases [18]. Fcγ receptors remove Ig-coated platelets from blood and when anti-platelet Igs are present their effectiveness leads to thrombocytopenia.

## 6. Diseases causing accelerated platelet clearance by macrophages

Accelerated clearance requires either the accumulation of opsonins on the platelet surface such as Igs and complement or the presence of agents in blood that remove protective molecules. Both types of mechanisms occur.

There are many examples of acquired or induced immune thrombocytopenia that cause platelet removal when anti-platelet Igs are generated, deposited on platelets, and are detected by Fcγ receptors on macrophages. These include congenital and drug or pathogen induced thrombocytopenia. In general, platelet clearance is primarily driven by splenic macrophages, a process that can result in splenomegaly. In many cases, patients having ITP, respond well to anti-Fc antibody treatment.

## 7. Platelet clearance mediated by hepatocytes

Bacterial-derived sialidases, released into blood during sepsis, cause platelet counts to drop precipitously. The target of the blood born bacterial sialidases is sialic acid that caps N-linked glycans on GP1bα, as demonstrated using mice lacking GP1bα [19], which are resistant to clearance induced by pneumococcal sepsis in WT mice. Cleavage of sialic acid on GP1bα exposes underlying galactose moieties that are recognized by the Asgr [13]. Animals lacking a functional Asgr do not accelerate their platelet clearance in response to sepsis.

A related process accounts for the circulation failure of platelets transfused after rewarming from refrigerated storage. Resting platelets contain sialidases that are stored in an internal compartment that can be released by activation [15, 20]. Rewarming from the cold releases a portion of the sialidase activity to the platelet surface and into the storage media, a process that mediates desialylation of the platelet surface glycoproteins. Since the accelerated clearance of chilled and rewarmed platelets is to a large extend ablated in mice lacking the Asgr

http://dx.doi.org/10.5772/60678

(HL-$2^{-/-}$ mice), it is the main receptor that recognizes and removes cold damaged platelets. Ablation of macrophage function in HL-$2^{-/-}$ mice further restores platelet circulation by 15-20%. Hence, macrophages also participate in clearance.

## 8. Accelerated platelet clearance in Wiskott-Aldrich syndrome

Mutation, truncation and/or deletion of WASp, a protein encoded on the X-chromosome and expressed by blood cells, results in a profound lymphocyte dysfunction that severely compromises the immune system. Severe thrombocytopenia (TCP) is also a signature component of the Wiskott-Aldrich syndrome; WAS platelets are small and have shortened circulatory lifetimes. WAS patients produce diverse autoantibodies and WAS platelets collect higher amounts of surface-associated immunoglobulins (Igs) than do normal platelets [21]. Many human WAS patients respond to splenectomy with increased platelet counts, despite the finding that all patients have been found to be refractory to anti-Fcγ antibodies. Unlike ITP, homologous platelets circulate normally in WAS patients strongly suggesting a more complex mechanism for removal that involves receptors other than Fc.

WASp KO mice have been shown to retain the key features of WAS disease, having T and B lymphocyte dysfunction, enlarged spleens, low platelet counts (70% of normal) and shortened platelet survival times in blood. It has been widely believed that platelet clearance is accelerated in these animals because the autoimmune aspect of the disease results in increased Igs bound to the platelets surface that led to recognition by splenic macrophages. However, as in the human conditions, normal platelets, when transfused into WASp KO mice, circulate normally indicating that a simple anti-platelet antibody mediated clearance is not the mechanism. In mice, splenectomy has been shown to be without effect on the clearance rate.

In efforts to identify the mechanism of removal, WASp Null platelets were transfused into mice lacking specific phagocytic receptors. A survey on macrophage receptors failed to reveal any in which the WASp null platelets had enhanced circulatory lifetimes. However, WASp KO platelets were found to circulate normally in Asgr null mice, a finding once again posits the Asgr as a central molecule involved in the recognition and removal of damaged platelets. The surface of WASp KO platelets is, however, not desialylated and lectin binding studies have instead revealed hypersialylation. This sialylation occurs specifically in the 2,6 linkage, not the normal 2,3 linkage. Critically, the Asgr also receptor recognizes this unique sialic linkage, leading to binding and platelet removal. The carrier of this sialic acid turns out to be surface bound Ig and sialylation of its Fc N-linked glycan shifts recognition of the Fc domain from macrophages to the hepatocytes.

Interestingly, the source of the 2,6 sialyltranferase (ST6Gal1) is liver hepatocytes, which make and secrete this enzyme into blood. This blood enzyme is an acute phase reactant protein, upregulated in liver in response to bacterial sepsis, cancer, or inflammation. In this case, platelet ingestion itself, feedbacks to upregulate ST6Gal1 mRNA transcription and translation and this increases by 3-4 fold the blood levels of this enzyme.

## 9. Cause of surface alterations that lead to the deposition of Igs on the WASp KO platelet

The modification(s) in WASp KO platelet surface that leads to Ig production by WASp KO B-lymphocytes and Ig-binding are not known. Since WT platelets do not collect Igs in WASp KO plasma or have accelerated clearance in WASp KO animals, surface alterations are specific for the WASp KO platelets. Because WASp is a protein that interacts with the actin cytoskeleton, it is likely that internal cytoskeletal changes in its absence result in an altered topology of platelet receptors or the expression of the neo-epitope. In general, platelet function in the absence of WASp is near normal although as the precision of assays increase, some differences have now been recognized. Active platelets lack small focal actin assembly sites in the absence of WASp, although spreading and filopodial formation are normal. In resting platelets, failure to express WASp alters the stability of microtubules, increasing their acetylation and slowing their turnover. How these internal changes alter the surface remains for future studies.

## 10. Platelet production

The basic processes involved in megakaryocyte commitment, maturation and platelet formation are well described although many precise details remain to be clarified. Megakaryocytes derive from a renewable population of hematopoietic stem cells that continuously enter the MK/platelet lineage and once committed to produce platelets, live for only a few more weeks before they are converted into hundreds of platelets. Proplatelet and platelet production requires a massive enlargement in MK size that is driven by high levels of mRNA transcription from their amplified polyploid nuclei followed by mRNA translation into platelet essential components. This includes the production of an abundant internal network of membranes called the demarcation membrane system (DMS) that dramatically increases the apparent membrane to surface ratio during proplatelet formation, platelet specific granules, and the synthesis of large amounts of the cytoskeletal machinery that is used to form and fill assembling platelets.

As MKs mature, they develop an extensive network of internal membranes called the DMS that are enriched phosphatidylinositol 4,5 bisphosphate and the vWf receptor [22] and are used as the primary membrane source for proplatelet elongation. Recent studies by Eckly et al [23] have begun to shed some light on DMS formation, describing how the DMS forms and matures. To form the DMS, the plasma membrane of megakaryocytes enfolds at specific sites and a perinuclear pre-DMS is generated. Next, the pre-DMS is expanded into its mature form by material added from golgi-derived vesicles and endoplasmic reticulum-mediated lipid transfer. This structural description is in accordance with the studies on platelet glycosyltransferases, which arrive early in the forming DMS and eventually make their way to the megakaryocyte and platelet surfaces [24]. Only a small number of proteins have been identified thus far to participate in the DMS formation process based on alterations in its structure in certain knockout animals. Gross disruptions of this network are found in megakaryocytes isolated from either filamin A knockout or pacsin2 knockout mice, the latter of which connects GP1bα to the actin cytoskeleton and binds pacsin2, a molecule that deforms membrane. The relationship between the DMS and the platelet open canalicular system (OCS) is not clear. The OCS, like the DMS, is a unique anastomosing network of internal membrane tubes that is connected to the plasma membrane at multiple points. The internal canals of the OCS can be identified because they contain vWfR, and hence can be labeled with anti-GP1bα antibodies (Kahr et al).

To release platelets, megakaryocytes in the marrow space move to and nestle the marrow sinusoids where they project their proplatelet protrusions into the blood flow [25, 26]. Whether all proplatelets are directed to grow specifically into the sinusoids or if only some of the proplatelets elaborated by a MK find their way into the sinusoids is unknown, although living MKs in marrow have been observed to have many proplatelet projections, some of which project into the marrow space while others project into the sinusoids [27]. Studies have demonstrated that proplatelet fragments considerably larger than platelets are released by MKs into blood [26, 27] and that proplatelets can be both found, and can mature into platelets, in blood [28].

The state of our current knowledge of the mechanics of proplatelet production has come primarily from studies on MKs in culture. This work has clarified the essential role of microtubules, which were recognized early as the most prominent structure found within the MK projections [29] and that proplatelet and platelet production were adversely affected by MT poisons [30]. Subsequent gene expression studies established the importance of β1-tubulin, a tubulin isoform specific for MKs, to the maturation of MKs into proplatelet producing machines [31]. More recent studies using gene deleted MKs have begun to reveal the precise roles of specific proteins in proplatelet and platelet production and these are highlighted below.

Signals that initiate proplatelet formation, if present, remain undefined and it remains possible that the program to make platelets starts when the synthesis of cytoskeletal proteins for this process reaches a critical mass. From a mechanical view, centrosome dissolution precedes proplatelet extension, and the release of MTs from these multiple nucleating sites correlates best with the start of proplatelet elaboration. Released MTs first collect as bundles in the MK cortex where they are driven apart by their associated motor protein, dynein. These MT-dynein reactions deform the membrane outward and generate the structural motor of the proplatelet, which is a MT bundle that folds over in the proplatelet tip and runs back into the shafts. Each bundle is composed of many MTs that are continuously growing and shrinking from their ends. Six types of behaviors characterize the elaboration of proplatelets: elongation, branching, pausing, fusions, fragmentations, and retractions. While the average elongation rate for proplatelets over time is ~1 μm/min, extension normally occurs in bursts and pauses. Burst rates greatly exceed the average rates and under flow, and rates of >30 μm/min have been observed. These rates correlate well with the sliding rates of MTs within the bundles. Pauses in proplatelet extension are not caused by a stoppage in MT sliding, which continues at a 1-6 μm/min rate. Sliding reactions in paused proplatelets appear to build tension into the bundle which when released leads to branching and/or fragmentation. This implies that there are regions within the bundles where MTs are crosslinked to increase resistance or they are pushing against resistive structures. Branching is a modified form of extension derived from tension asymmetry where a portion of the MT bundle detaches from the mother bundle and elongates rapidly forming a new tear shaped structure and proplatelet shaft. Retraction, where the sliding could either reverse or all crosslinking derived tension releases, could serve to subfragment the proplatelets.

In addition to playing a crucial role in proplatelet elongation, the microtubules lining the shafts of proplatelets serve a secondary function — tracks for the transport of membrane, organelles, and granules into proplatelets and assembling platelets at proplatelet ends [32]. Individual organelles are sent from the cell body into the proplatelets, where they move bidirectionally until they are captured at proplatelet ends. Immunofluorescence and electron microscopy studies indicate that organelles are in direct contact with microtubules, and actin poisons do not diminish organelle motion. Therefore, movement appears to involve microtubule-based forces. Bidirectional organelle movement is conveyed in part by the bipolar organization of microtubules within the proplatelet, as kinesin-coated beads move bidirectionally over the microtubule arrays of permeabilized proplatelets. Of the two major microtubule motors — kinesin and dynein — only the plus-end-directed kinesin is situated in a pattern similar to organelles and granules, and is likely responsible for transporting these elements along microtubules. It appears that a twofold mechanism of organelle and granule movement occurs in platelet assembly. First, organelles and granules travel along microtubules and, second, the microtubules themselves can slide bidirectionally in relation to other motile filaments to indirectly move organelles along proplatelets in a "piggyback" fashion

Although microtubules and associated motor and regulatory proteins power proplatelet motility, elimination of certain actin cytoskeletal-associated proteins have now been demonstrated to modulate this process. These include a number of actin-associated proteins, membrane contouring proteins, and signaling proteins.

## 11. Influence of actin-associated proteins on thrombopoiesis

Since proplatelets elongate, but do not branch, in the presence of the actin disrupting drug cytochalasin B, it is surprising that the deletion of certain actin associated proteins from the megakaryocyte lineage leads to macrothrombocytopenia. It seems likely that the removal of actin modulating proteins, alters and/or increases filamentous actin (F-actin) and cytoskeletal structure to have a dominant inhibitory effect proplatelet maturation and/or platelet release from proplatelets.

## 12. Actin crosslinking proteins

Three proteins, filamin A (FlnA), actinin 1 (Actn1) and spectrin, that crosslink F-actin using a related F-actin binding site, are critical components of the mature platelet cytoskeleton and regulate proplatelet formation and motility.

**FlnA.** FlnA, an elongated homodimer 160 nm in length, is an essential actin filament cross-linking and scaffolding protein that interacts with multiple platelet proteins including the vWfR, β-integrins, migfilin, Syk, and filGAP, in addition to crosslinking F-actin. Each FlnA subunit has an N-terminal actin-binding domain (ABD) that is followed by 24 Ig-like repeats, the last of which contains the self-association site for molecules. In platelets, FlnA crosslinks the actin filaments posited beneath the plasma membrane into a rigid network and using its 2 Gp1bα binding sites attaches actin filaments to the vWfR. Since there are 12,000 molecules of FlnA per platelet, and 25,000 Gp1bα chains, the amount of FlnA is sufficient to link 95% of the vWfR to actin since each FlnA binds two Gp1bα chains. Loss of this linkage, either by the failure to express stable GP(1bαβ9)$_2$5 complexes on the platelet surface, or by the absence of cyto-plasmic FlnA in conditional mice whose MK/platelet lineage lacks FlnA expression, results in a macrothrombocytopenia in which platelet counts are reduced by 80-90%. Not only does the loss of FlnA result in large platelets, the FlnA-null platelets are extremely fragile, and spontaneously subfragment within blood, resulting in short circulation lifetimes and accelerated removal of the fragments by macrophages. The enlarged platelet phenotype of the FlnA null platelets is very similar to that found in patients having Bernard-Soulier Syndrome, which because they do not express stable surface vWfR, also lack the important FlnA-mediated vWfR-cytoskeletal attachments. Human periventricular heterotopia patients with FlnA mutations and/or truncations have also been found to bleed and have low platelet counts [33-35]. Interestingly, failure to express FlnA in MKs disorganizes the DMS system. Alterations in the DMS in the absence of FlnA may involve its lipid-deforming partner, pacsin2 (see below). Proplatelet elaboration is accelerated in FlnA null MKs *in vitro*. Hence, FlnA imposes restraints on the timing of platelet production.

**Actn1.** Actinin dimers are short rods, 40 nm in length, built from an antiparallel, side-to-side alignment of its subunits. Each subunit chain has an NT ABD followed by 4 α-helical repeats, related in structure to those in spectrin, and last, an EF hand motif. In nonmuscle cells, binding of the actinin isoforms that are expressed (Actn1 and Actn4) to F-actin are regulated by calcium although the muscle isoforms have lost this sensitivity. Human patients with macrothrombocytopenia have been identified that express mutant actn1 molecules having sequence changes within their NT actin binding site [36]. Since these actn1 mutants reduce the proplatelet formation and cause MKs to elaborate thick proplatelets when expressed in mouse MKs, it is believed actinin function can alter the MK to proplatelet transition. Actn1 is expressed in platelets at levels equivalent to FlnA [37].

**Spectrin.** Platelets, like erythrocytes, have a planar membrane skeleton that laminates the plasma membrane and is linked to the underlying actin cytoskeleton. This skeleton is composed of twisted and elongated spectrin tetramers that interconnect by binding to the barbed ends of actin filaments, a interaction that is promoted by β-adducin, a molecule that binds to both spectrin, near its ABD, and the barbed filament end of an actin filament [38]. Tetramers are assembled from heterodimers; α,β dimers are 100 nm in length, are bipolar and side-to-side constructs, in which the β-chain donates the actin binding domain on one end (NT of the b-chain), with the self-association domain posited on the other end. Head-to-head binding of dimers forms tetramers, a process that is dynamic and can be disrupted using small fragments of β-chain C-Terminal to compete for this binding site. When such negative dominant fragments are expressed into MK cultures, proplatelet elaboration is blocked. Similarly, the exposure of permeabilized proplatelets with this small C-Terminal protein construct results in blebbing and swelling, and ultimately complete loss of cytoskeletal integrity.

**Myosin 2A and Rho/ROCK.** MYH9 gene disorders (myosin 2a) cause May-Hegglin and the related Epstein, Fechtner, Sebastian, and Alport syndromes in humans, all of which have thrombocytopenia. However, the myosin 2A story is complex. Gene inactivation studies in mice have shown that loss of myosin 2a protein expression in MKs accelerates the production of large platelets, while MYH9 gene mutations in humans have dominant negative effects and reduce platelet production. The most severe mutations that effect platelet counts, posit within the myosin head motor domain, while mutations in the tail domain, allow somewhat higher, but still abnormal platelet counts. The general consensus on these myosin-mediated defects are that myosin activity is necessary to constrain proplatelet formation in MKs as they mature and that inactivation of myosin thus plays a role in initiating proplatelet elaboration. In addition, since myosin activity is regulated by MLC phosphorylation, modification of pathways that regulate either the kinases or phosphatase activities that are directed toward myosin can lead to phenotypes similar to those found for myosin mutant or loss of function.

Platelet specific RhoA deficiency causes macrothrombocytopenia with platelet counts reduced by ~50% from normal. The $RhoA^{-/-}$ platelets have many functional defects that cause animals to readily bleed, but they have normal lifetimes in blood [39]. One pathway by which RhoA deficiency may affect MK maturation and platelet formation is through ROCK modulation of myosin 2a activity in MKs. RhoA activates ROCK, inhibiting myosin LC phosphatase and hence leading to increased myosin LC phosphorylation. This activity is thought to restrain proplatelet elaboration and thus RhoA deficiency to release this brake, causing premature proplatelet formation and leading to enlarged and dysfunctional platelets.

| Protein | Megakaryocyte phenotype | Proplatelet phenotype | Platelet phenotype | Clearance Phenotype | References |
|---|---|---|---|---|---|
| GP1ba KO | | | Large, fragile | | [19] |
| Filamin A KO | Accelerated proplatelet elaboration, altered DMS | Accelerated | 10-20% of normal: Large, fragile | | [8] |
| Actinin 1 ABD mutants | Decreased proplatelet number, increased proplatelet thickness | Reduced, thickened | Large | | [36] |

| Protein | Megakaryocyte phenotype | Proplatelet phenotype | Platelet phenotype | Clearance Phenotype | References |
|---|---|---|---|---|---|
| Nonmuscle myosin HC IIA KO | | Increased, formation accelerated | Heterogenous, Reduced by 70% | Normal | [41] |
| Dynamin 2 KO | | Reduced, thickened | 20% of normal, size highly variable | | |
| CIP4 KO | | Reduced | | | [42] |
| Pacsin 2 KO | | | Normal | | |
| WASp or WIP KO | | Accelerated | Slightly small | Accelerated | [43] |
| β1-tubulin | Compensate by upregulating β2 and β5-tubulin | Proplatelet formation blocked | Amorphic, reduced by 70-75% | | [44] |
| Rab27b | | | | | [45] |
| Cofilin-1 | | | Large | | [46] |
| ADF | normal | | 90% of normal, size normal | | [46] |
| ADF/Cofilin1 | Numbers increased 3X; DMS and cytoplasmic structure altered | decreased | 5% of normal count; sizes variable, amorphic | | [46] |
| Actin interacting protein (Aip1/Wdr1) | Defective megakaryo-poiesis: small, DMS abnormalities | | 20% of normal: large | Normal | [40] |
| Profilin 1 | | | Large, size variable | | [47] |
| RhoA | | | 50% of normal, large -125% | Slight increase in turnover rate | [39] |
| Spectrin | | Proplatelets disrupted by dimer-dimer self-association inhibitor | | | [48] |
| Tmod3 | Altered DMS | Enlarged tips | Large, decreased count | | [49] |

**Table 1.** Effect of Mouse KOs on Platelet Production and/or Platelet Clearance.

**Cofilin-1/ADF and Aip1 (Wdr1].** Cofilin-1 and ADF are highly homologous protein isoforms in the ADF/cofilin family that accelerate actin turnover in cells. The third member of this family, m-cofilin or cofilin-2, is expressed only in muscle tissue. Cofilin/ADF bind along the sides of actin filaments, preferentially targeting ADP-subunits, and thereby, recognize the old portions of filaments. Binding induces a twist in the filament, causing its severing. Exposure of low affinity filament ends following the severing event, promotes dissociation from these ends, and this stimulates actin filament turnover in cells. Conditional mice lacking cofilin-1 have been produced. When cofilin-1 is specifically deleted form the MK/platelet lineage, large platelets result and platelet counts are mildly reduced (60-80% of normal). $ADF^{-/-}$ mice, on the other hand, have near normal platelet counts and normal platelet function. However, when ADF-/- mice are crossed with the mice carrying the floxed cofilin-1 allele, platelet production in the DKO offspring is severely diminished. The morphologies of the released platelets are highly variable, as the normal discoid space is distorted by their dense fillings of actin filaments. In agreement with these mouse studies, proplatelets are sparse on the double knockout MKs in vitro.

Cofilin is regulated by Aip1, a protein that binds and enhances filament severing /actin depolymerization activity. The importance of this protein to platelet production has been demonstrated [40]. N-ethyl-N-nitrosourea mutagenesis generated mice with profound thrombocytopenia, bleeding, and enlarged, amorphic platelets contain a gene mutation that was mapped to Wdr1 gene. The high degree of similarity to the phenotype of in the ADF/cofilin double knockout, strongly suggests both proteins are in the same thrombogenesis effector pathway.

**Profilin1A and Wasp/Wip.** Profilin is a small protein that promotes filament assembly. It binds ADP-monomers, converting them to ATP-monomers, which are permitted to only interact with the high affinity end of actin filaments (barbed end with respect to myosin S1 binding). Mice whose MKs/platelets specifically lack profilin 1 have macrothrombocytopenia with counts reduced by 40-50%. Platelet turnover is accelerated and the mature platelets have only a sparse internal actin cytoskeleton. Surprisingly, although their actin cytoskeleton is disrupted, profilin null platelets have a robust MT cytoskeleton with a thickened MT coil and more stable hyper-acetylated microtubules.

In certain ways, the profilin 1 KO phenotype is similar to the behavior of platelets in Wiskott-Aldrich syndrome, or in WASp or WIP KO mice. WASp is a signaling protein promotes actin assembly system, binding to Arp2/3 when activated by binding of GTP-cdc42. However, the bulk of studies performed on human WAS platelets or platelets derived from KO mice revealed normal and ever hyper-function for the WASp null platelets. Human patients have low platelet counts that are caused by accelerated platelet clearance, a process that lowers the platelet count in the Wasp/Wip KO mice. Recently studies have shown the MT ring in platelets from WAS patients to be hyper-acetylated, like the profilin 1 KO platelets. However, in the WAS syndrome, platelets in the circulation are small, not large, as is found in the Profilin null animals.

http://dx.doi.org/10.5772/60678

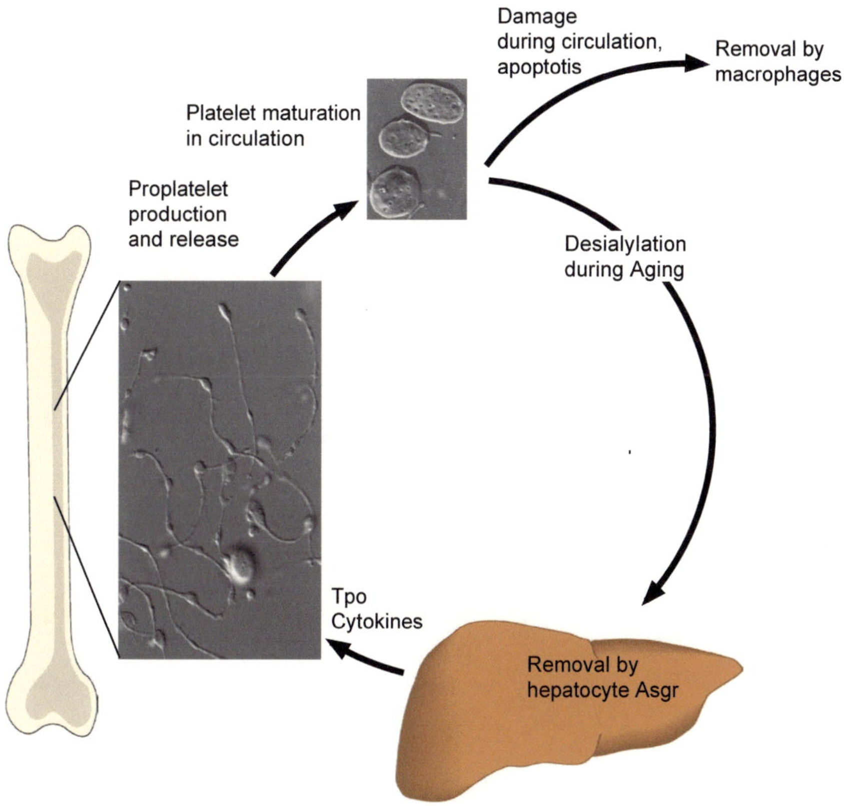


**Figure 1. Life cycle of the platelet.** Megakaryocytes in the bone marrow release proplatelets into the blood where they mature into platelets. If damaged, platelets are detected and removed by splenic macrophages and liver Kupffer cells. As platelets age in the circulation they become desialylated. The fate of desialylated platelets differs from that of acutely damaged platelets. Desialylated platelets are recognized and are removed from the blood in the liver sinusoids by liver hepatocytes using their Asgr. Platelet ingestion by hepatocytes stimulates them to produce TPO and release it into the blood.

**CIP4/Pacsin2/Dynamin.** Membrane deforming proteins that use F-BAR domains curve membranes, or GTP as an energy source to bud vesicles from membranes, are necessary for normal MK maturation and platelet release.

**CIP4.** CIP4 is a F-Bar containing, Cdc42 interacting and WASp binding protein. CIP4$^{-/-}$ mice have a mild thrombocytopenia with a 25% decrease in platelet counts. MK numbers and ploidy are normal in the KO mice but isolated MKs from these mice are less effective in producing proplatelets in culture.

**Pacsin 2.** Pacsin 2, the only family member expressed in mouse platelets, is a FlnA partner that has an F-BAR and SH3 domain that bindings dynamin and N-WASp. Pacsin2 plays an important role in organizing internal membranes in platelets and megakaryocytes. In platelets, it locates at the entrances of the OCS. In MKs it is dispersed throughout the internal anastomosing network of DMS membranes. FlnA binding is important for its functions as the distribution of pascin2 and the arrangement of internal membranes is grossly altered in FlnA null MKS.

**Dynamin.** Dynamins are a family of three cytoplasmic mechanochemical proteins (DNM1-3) that regulate membrane dynamics with actin during such processes as cytokinesis, budding of transport vesicles, phagocytosis, and cell motility. Dynamin 2 and 3 are upregulated as MKs mature and iRNA knockdown of DNM3 has been reported to interfere with maturation and proplatelet production *in vitro*. Specific inactivation of the DNM2 gene in mice MKs/platelets profoundly diminishes platelet production and function.

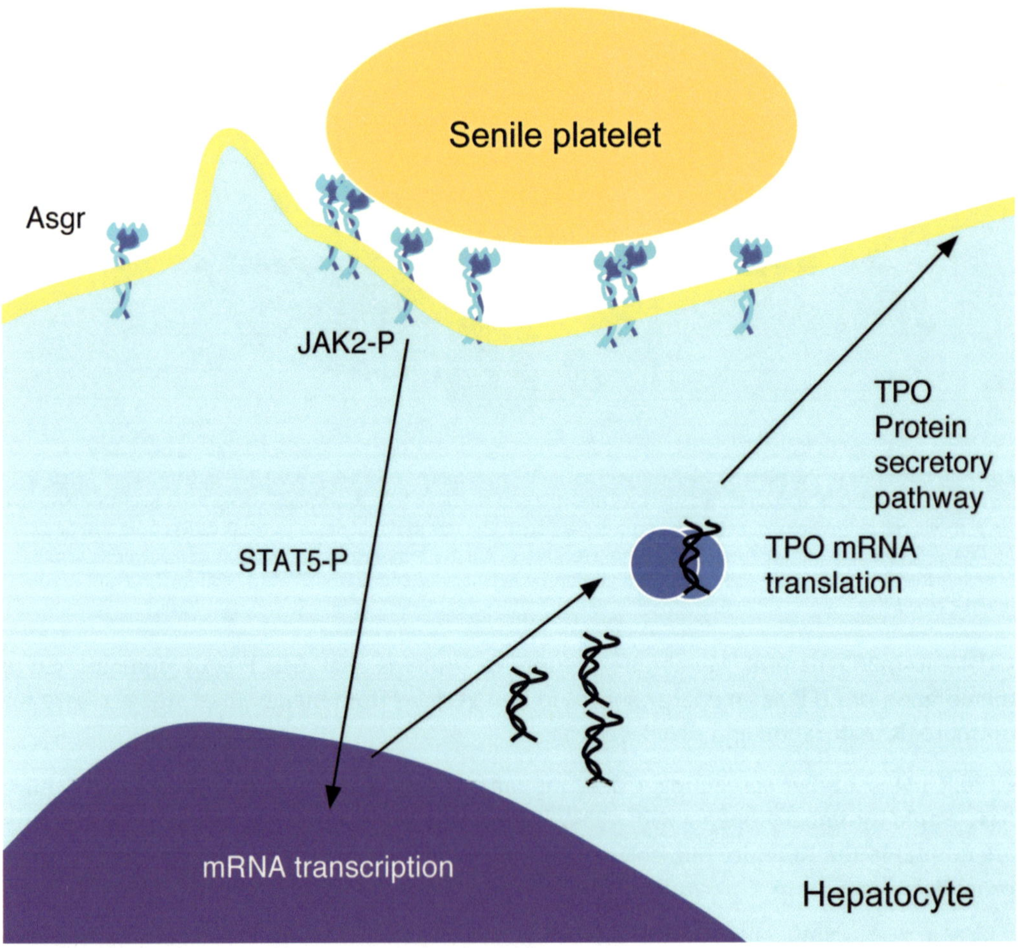


**Figure 2. Platelet ingestion stimulates TPO signaling to the bone marrow.** As platelets are detected and removed by the Asgr, the Jak-STAT pathway is activated. This leads to TPO mRNA transcription and translation, increasing blood TPO levels.

http://dx.doi.org/10.5772/60678

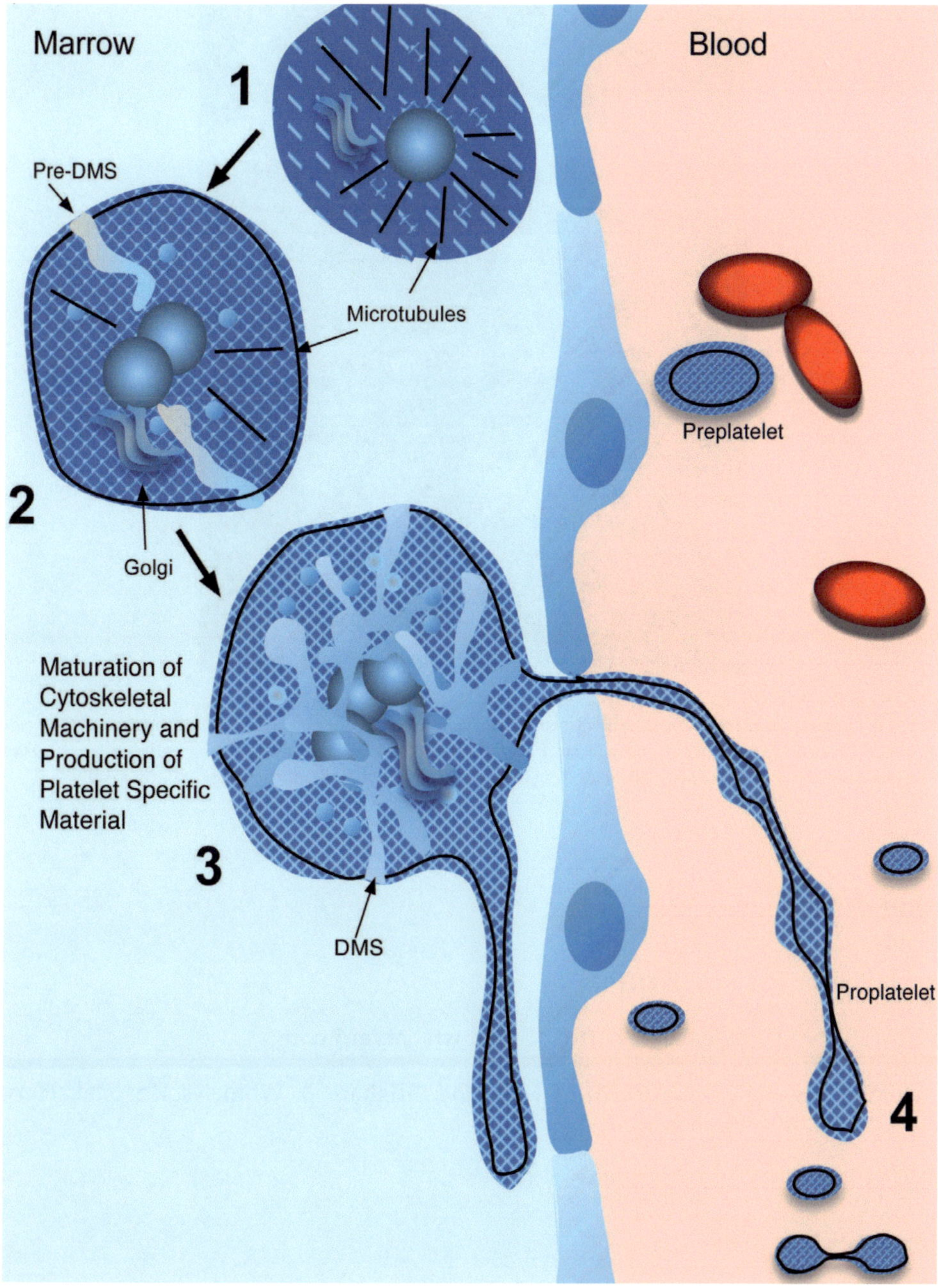


**Figure 3. Steps in MK maturation and proplatelet release.** (1) Immature MK. Microtubules radiate outward from centrosomes and DMS has not developed. (2) Ploidy increases, the pre-DMS begins to form, the centrosomes dissolve, and the released microtubules move out to the cell cortex and form bundles. (3) Ploidy increases to 8-16n, the DMS and platelet specific granules are produced, the cytoplasm has become enriched in cytoskeletal proteins, and the sliding of the MT within the bundles has begun. Sliding elongates proplatelets into the venous sinusoids and they are released into blood. (4) Platelets mature from proplatelets and preplatelets that release into blood.

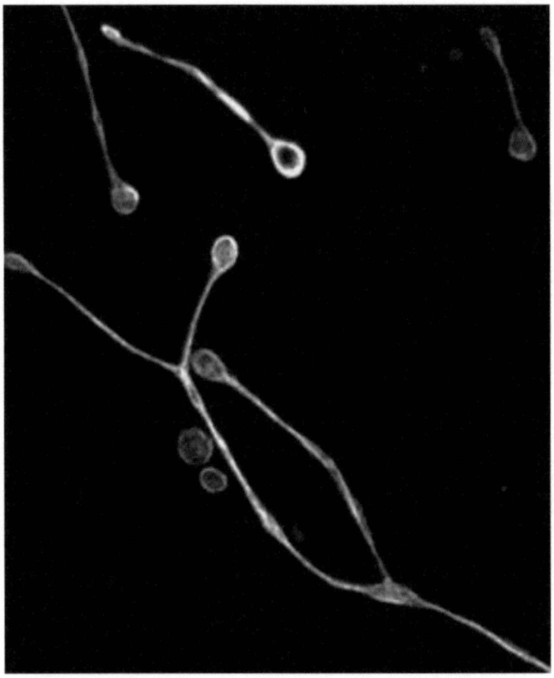

**Figure 4. Localization of microtubules within proplatelets.** Immunofluorescence studies on murine megakaryocytes grown in culture and labeled with β1-tubulin antibodies indicate that microtubules line the entire length of proplatelets. The hallmark features of proplatelets, including the tip, swellings, shafts and branch points are visible.

## Author details

Joseph Jr Italiano and John Hartwig*

*Address all correspondence to: hartwig@rics.bwh.harvard.edu

Hematology Division, Department of Medicine, Brigham & Women's Hospital, Harvard Medical School, Boston, MA, USA

## References

[1] M. Olsson, P. Bruhns, W. Frazier, J. Ravetch, P.-A. Olderborg, Platelet homeostasis is regulated by platelet expression of CD47 under normal conditions and in passive immune thrombocytopenia. *Blood* 105, 3577 (2005).

[2] K. Mason *et al.*, Programmed anuclear cell death delimits platelet life span. *Cell* 128, 1173 (2007).

[3] L. Tian *et al.*, p85a recruitment by the CD300f phosphatidylserine receptor mediates apoptotic cell clearance required for autoimmunity suppression. *Nature Comm.*, (2014).

[4] M. Miyanishi *et al.*, Identification of Tim4 as a phosphatidylserine receptor. *Nature* 450, 435 (2007).

[5] D. Park *et al.*, BAI1 is an engulfment receptor for apoptotic cells upstream of the LMO/Dock180/Rac module. *Nature* 450, 192 (2007).

[6] S.-Y. Park *et al.*, Rapid cell corpse clearance by stabilin-2, a membrane phosphatidylserine receptor. *Cell Death Differ.* 15, 192 (2008).

[7] E. Brown, W. Frazier, Integrin-assocated protein (CD47) and its ligands. *Trends Cell Biol.* 11, 130 (2001).

[8] A. Jurak Begonja, K. M. Hoffmeister, J. H. Hartwig, H. Falet, FlnA-null megakaryocytes prematurely release large and fragile platelets that circulate poorly. *Blood* 118, 2285 (2011).

[9] J. Greenberg, M. Packham, J. Cazenave, H. Reimers, J. Mustard, Effects on platelet function of removal of platelet sialic acid by neuraminidase. *Lab Invest.* 32, 476 (1975).

[10] G. Soslau, J. Giles, The loss of sialic acid and its prevention in stored human platelets. *Thromb. Res.* 26, 443 (1982).

[11] M. Steiner, S. Vancura, Asymmetirical loss of sialic acid from membrane glycoproteins during platelet aging. *Thromb. Res.* 40, 465 (1985).

[12] G. Ashwell, A. Morell, The role of surface carbohydrates in the hepatic recognition and transport of circulating glycoproteins. *Adv. Enzymol. Relat. Areas Mol. Biol.* 41, 99 (1974).

[13] P. Grewal *et al.*, Inducing host protection in pneumococcal sepsis by preactivation of the Ashwell-Morell receptor. *Proc. Nat.. Acad. Sci, USA* 110, 20218 (2013).

[14] P. Grewal *et al.*, The Ashwell receptor mitigates the lethal coagulopathy of sepsis. *Nature Med.* 14, 648 (2008).

[15] V. Rumjantseva *et al.*, Dual roles for hepatic lectin receptors in the clearance of chilled platelets. *Nat Med* 15, 1273 (Nov, 2009).

[16] R. Grozovsky, A. Begonja, J. Hartwig, H. Falet, K. Hoffmeister, The Ashwell-Morell receptor regulates hepatic thrombopoietin production via JAK2-STAT3 signaling. *Nat.Med* In press, (2014).

[17] D. Simon *et al.*, Platelet glycoprotein Ib$\alpha$ is a counterrecptor for the leukocyte integrin mac-1 (CD11b/CD18). *J. Exp. Med.* 192, 193 (2000).

[18] R. Ezekowitz, K. Sastry, P. Bailly, A. Warner, Molecular characterization of the human macrophage mannose receptor: demonstration of multiple carbohydrate-recog-

nition domains and phagocytosis of yeasts in Cos-1 cells. *J. Exp. Med.* 172, 1785 (1990).

[19] J. Ware, S. Russell, Z. Ruggeri, Generation and rescue of a murine model of platelet dysfunction: the Bernard-Soulier syndrome. *Proc. Natl. Acad. Sci., USA* 97, 2803 (2000).

[20] A. L. Sorensen *et al.*, Role of sialic acid for platelet life span: exposure of beta-galactose results in the rapid clearance of platelets from the circulation by asialoglycoprotein receptor-expressing liver macrophages and hepatocytes. *Blood* 114, 1645 (Aug 20, 2009).

[21] L. Corash, B. Shafer, R. Blasese, Platelet-associated immunoglobulin, platelet size, and the effect of splenectomy in the Wiskott-Aldrich syndrome. *Blood* 65, 1439 (1985).

[22] H. Schulze *et al.*, Characterization of the megakaryocyte demarcation membrane system and its role in thrombopoiesis. *Blood* 107, 3868 (2006).

[23] F. Pertuy *et al.*, Myosin IIA is critical for organelle distribution and F-actin organiztion in megakaryocytes and platelets. *Blood* 123, 1261 (2014).

[24] H. H. Wandall *et al.*, The origin and function of platelet glycosyltransferases. *Blood* 120, 626 (Jul 19, 2012).

[25] J. Radley, Ultrastructural aspects of platelet production. *Megakaryocyte Development and Function*, 387 (1986).

[26] O. Behnke, A. Forer, From megakaryocytes to platelets: platelet morphogenesis takes place in the bloodstream. *European J. Hematology* 60, 3 (1998).

[27] T. Junt *et al.*, Direct visualization of thrombopoiesis in the bone marrow of living mice. *Science* 317, 1767 (2007).

[28] J. N. Thon *et al.*, Cytoskeletal mechanics of proplatelet maturation and platelet release. *J Cell Biol* 191, 861 (Nov 15, 2010).

[29] R. Leven, Megakaryocyte motility and platelet formation. *Scanning microscopy* 1, 1701 (1987).

[30] F. Tablin, M. Castro, R. Leven, Blood platelet formation in vitro. The role of the cytoskeleton in megakaryocyte fragmentation. *J. Cell Sci.* 97, 59 (1990).

[31] Y. Chang *et al.*, Proplatelet formation is regulated by the rho/ROCK pathway. *Blood* 109, 4229 (2007).

[32] S. R. Patel *et al.*, Differential roles of microtubule assembly and sliding in proplatelet formation by megakaryocytes. *Blood* 106, 4076 (Dec 15, 2005).

[33] S. Feng, X. Lu, J. Reséndiz, M. Kroll, Pathological shear stress directly regulates platelet aIIbb3 signaling. *Am. J. Cell Physiol.* 291, C1346 (2006).

[34] Y. Feng, C. Walsh, The many faces of filamin: a versatile molecular scaffold for cell motility and signalling. *Nature Cell Biol.* 6, 1034 (2004).

[35] J. W. Fox *et al.*, Mutations in filamin 1 prevent migration of cerebral cortical neurons in human periventricular heterotopia. *Neuron* 21, 1315 (1998).

[36] S. Kunishima *et al.*, ACTN1 mutations cause congenital macrothrombocytopenia. *Am. J. Human Gen.* 92, 431 (2013).

[37] S. Rosenberg, A. Stracher, K. Burridge, Isolation and characterization of a calcium-sensitive $\alpha$-actinin-like protein from human platelet cytoskeletons. *J. Biol. Chem.* 256, 12986 (1981).

[38] K. Barkalow, J. Italiano Jr, Y. Matsuoka, V. Bennett, J. Hartwig, a-Adducin dissociates from F-actin filaments and spectrin during platelet activation. *J. Cell Biol.* 161, 557 (2003).

[39] I. Pleines *et al.*, Megakaryocyte-specific RhoA deficiency causes macrothrombocytopenia and defective platelet activation in hemostasis and thrombosis. *Blood* 119, 1054 (2012).

[40] B. Kile *et al.*, Mutations in the cofilin partner Aip1/Wdr1 cause autoinflammatory disease and macrothrombocytopenia. *Blood* 110, 2371 (2007).

[41] S. Kunishima *et al.*, Mutations in the NMMHC-A gene cause autosomal dominant macrothrombocytopenia with leukocyte inclusions (May-Hegglin anomaly/Sebastian syndrome). *Blood* 97, 1147 (2001).

[42] Y. Chen *et al.*, Loss of the F-BAR protein CIP4 reduces platelet production by impairing membrane-cytoskeleton remodeling. *Blood* 122, (2013).

[43] S. Sabri *et al.*, Deficiency in the Wiskott-Aldrich protein induces premature proplatelet formation and platelet production in the bond marrow compartment. *Blood* 108, 134 (2006).

[44] H. Schwer *et al.*, A lineage-restricted and divergent b tubulin isoform is essential for the biogenesis, structure and function of mammalian blood platelets. *Curr. Biol.* 11, 579 (2001).

[45] S. Tiwari *et al.*, A role for Rab27b in NF-E2-dependent pathways of platelet formation. *Blood* 102, 3970 (2003).

[46] Bender M *et al.*, ADF/n-cofilin-dependent actin turnover determines platelet formation and sizing. *Blood* 116, 1767 (2010).

[47] M. Bender *et al.*, Microtubule sliding drives proplatelet elongation andis dependent on cytoplasmic dynein. *Blood* In Press, (2014).

[48] S. Patel-Hett *et al.*, The spectrin-based membrane skeleton stabilizes mouse megakaryocyte membrane systems and is essential for proplatelet and platelet formation. *B*lood 118, 1641 (Aug 11, 2011).

[49] A. Sui et al., Tmod3 participates in platelet formation and sizing in mouse fetal liver FASEB J 28, 278.9 (2014).

Chapter 2

# The Traditional Role of Platelets in Hemostasis

Douglass A. Drelich and Paul F. Bray

Additional information is available at the end of the chapter

http://dx.doi.org/10.5772/60595

## 1. Introduction

Hemostatic balance is central to health maintenance. Hemostasis must be initiated rapidly to prevent excessive blood loss. However, it must be tightly controlled to prevent over exuberant thrombus formation with resultant pathologic occlusion of arterial or venous vascular beds. Platelets are central to this hemostatic balance via primary hemostasis, support of coagulation, and even anti-fibrinolytic effects. Quantitative and qualitative platelet disorders have classically focused on hemorrhagic and thrombotic diseases, the severity of which can range from mild to life-threatening. Recent advances have demonstrated that platelets have functions beyond their traditional hemostatic role such as supporting vascular integrity, angiogenesis, immune function, tumor metastases, etc. These "non-traditional" functions of platelet will be discussed in other chapters. In this chapter we present a brief review of the traditional roles of platelets in hemostasis and thrombosis.

## 2. Structure

Platelets have many unique structural features that facilitate their contributions to thrombus formation. The cell membrane of platelets consists of a phospholipid bilayer embedded with cholesterol, glycoproteins, and glycolipids. Platelet membranes are asymmetrically organized. Negatively charged phospholipids in resting platelets are preferentially present on the inner leaflet, most notably phosphatidylserine.[1] The platelet membrane is rich in a variety of glycoproteins (GPs) that bind agonists to activate platelets and that serve primarily adhesive functions (Table 1). Transmembrane glycoproteins may distribute preferentially to cholesterol-rich microdomains, called "lipid rafts."[2]

| Platelet Surface Receptors for Adhesive Proteins | | | |
|---|---|---|---|
| **GP designation** | **Integrin designation** | **Other names** | **Primary ligands** |
| GPIa-IIa | $\alpha_2\beta_1$ | VLA-2 | Collagen |
| GPIb-V-IX | n/a | CD42 | Von Willebrand Factor |
| GPIc-IIa | $\alpha_5\beta_1$ | VLA-5 | Fibronectin |
| GPIIb-IIIa | $\alpha_{IIb}\beta_3$ | CD61 (β subunit), CD41 | Fibrinogen (and several others) |
| GPIV | n/a | GPIIIB, CD36 | Collagen |

**Table 1.** Platelet Surface Adhesion Proteins

Resting platelets in circulation have a stable discoid shape that is maintained by a circumferential coil of microtubules and a membrane cytoskeleton composed of actin, spectrin and other proteins.[3] The platelet plasma membrane is contiguous with the open canalicular system (OCS), a complex series of connecting tunnels that are open to the extracellular space. In addition to supplying membrane surface area to the spreading platelet, the canalicular system provides a potential route for the release of granule contents critical for delivery of the numerous vasoactive elements present in platelet granules. This also serves as a storage site for glycoproteins that are receptors for adhesive molecules. While the OCS is contiguous with the extracellular space, the dense tubular system is a closed channel network analogous to the sarcoplasmic reticulum as a site where calcium can be sequestered. Release of calcium from this system is a critical step in platelet activation.

Platelets have three different types of granules (Table 2). Dense granules contain adenine nucleotides (e.g., ADP and ATP), calcium, bioactive amines (e.g., serotonin and histamine) and polyphosphates. α-granules are rich in larger adhesive proteins.

| |
|---|
| **Dense granules** |
| ADP |
| ATP |
| Calcium |
| Serotonin |
| **α-granules** |
| Platelet factor 4 (PF4) |
| von Willebrand Factor |
| Fibrinogen |
| Fibronectin |
| Factor V |
| Factor XI |
| Protein S |
| PAI-1 |

**Table 2.** Platelet Granule Contents important for hemostasis

http://dx.doi.org/10.5772/60595

## 3. Thrombopoiesis

In the healthy state, platelets have an average lifespan of 8-9 days. This requires an active production mechanism. Bone marrow megakaryocytes produce approximately $10^{11}$ platelets daily. Each individual magakaryocyte can produce between 1000 and 3000 platelets.[4] Most of the molecules present in the mature platelet are produced by the megakaryocyte, but some such as fibrinogen and immunogloulin, are endocytosed from the surrounding plasma milieu. Megakaryocytes produce platelets by extending long projections. Cytoplasm in the developing platelets largely resembles that of the megakaryocyte. However, certain contents, particularly granules, appear to be moved into the developing proplatelets by an active transport mechanism.[5]

Several cytokines effect the development of platelets. IL-3, GM-CSF, and stem cell factor all appear important in maintaining the health and proliferation of megakaryocytes. However, the key regulator of platelet formation is thrombopoietin (TPO). TPO is a 50-70 kDa protein that has homology to erythropoietin.[6] TPO interacts with its key receptor c-Mpl, leading to dimerization initiating a signal transduction cascade through JAK, STAT, and MAPK pathways. TPO is made in the liver and to a lesser extent the kidney.

## 4. Platelet-mediated hemostasis

During both normal in vivo hemostasis and pathologic thrombus formation, numerous physiologic responses occur simultaneously, such as vasoconstriction, platelet plug formation and coagulation. Platelet thrombus formation itself involves a set of unique molecular responses and signaling pathways that also occur simultaneously. From a discussion point of view, this complexity makes it convenient to arbitrarily compartmentalize these processes.

### 4.1. Tethering and firm attachment

Platelet plug formation is initiated by exposure to a break in the endothelial lining of blood vessels. This has two important sequelae. The first is the loss of a variety of inhibitors of platelet function. The intact endothelium produces nitric oxide and prostacyclin both of which are inhibitors of platelet function, and the loss of endothelium leads to the loss of CD39 which in its intact state breaks down adenosine diphosphate (ADP), an activator of platelets. Exposure of subendothelial elements also allows the initial recruitment of platelets from the circulation via interactions between adhesive glycoproteins on the platelet surface and subendothelial proteins. [7]

Von Willebrand Factor (VWF) is critical for platelet-mediated thrombus formation in vessels with high shear rates and high shear stress. VWF is a multimeric protein that ranges in molecular weight from 0.5 daltons (dimers) to greater than 20 million daltons (multimers).[8] The hemostatic efficacy of VWF is directly proportional to its size with the largest molecules being the most prothrombotic. Subendothelial VWF is derived from plasma VWF that binds collagen after vessel injury and the abluminal secretion from endothelial cells. VWF circulates as a globular protein but undergoes conformational changes when exposed to high shear stress conditions. This unfolding exposes binding domains that allow the large von Willebrand multimers to form a bridge between subendothelial collagen and circulating platelets. The von Willebrand protein contains multiple functional domains including binding domains for both collagen and platelet GPIb$\alpha$.

The initial binding of VWF to the platelets is mediated by interaction between the A1 domain of VWF with the GPIb$\alpha$ subunit of the GPIb-V-IX complex.[9] GPIb$\alpha$ has an N-terminal segment comprised of two $\beta$-loops flanking a leucine-rich repeat segment. GPIX is a small, single chain polypeptide. The exact contribution of this peptide to the function of the complex is not well understood. This bridging mediates a rapid but reversible platelet adhesion that allows for rolling of platelets along the damaged endothelium. Occupation of this complex by VWF also leads to platelet signaling responses, including rearrangement of the cytoskeleton, increase in intracellular calcium, and granule release. The reduced platelet velocity mediated by the VWF-GPIb$\alpha$ interaction, coupled with activation of integrin $\alpha_2\beta_1$ enables stable, irreversible interactions to form between collagen and platelet integrin $\alpha_2\beta_1$.

### 4.2. Activation

Once platelets are captured from the circulation, activation steps lead to numerous changes in the platelets. These include conformational changes, rapid calcium influx, degranulation, thromboxane production, etc. The changes are induced by numerous agonists interacting with specific receptors on the platelet plasma membrane.

With increasingly sophisticated technologies for assessing platelet function and thrombus formation in vivo and under flow condition, there is an enhanced appreciation of the heterogeneity of platelets in a developing thrombus. Thus, there appears to be diverse microenvironments such that regions near the vessel wall may contain degranulated and irreversibly activated platelets, while the luminal region may have minimally activated and reversible adhered platelets that may or may not undergo thrombus stabilization.[10, 14]

As noted above, exposure of subendothelial collagen begins the initial tethering process. Once platelets are engaged in rolling on this matrix they have the opportunity to interact with GPVI, which is the major platelet collagen signaling receptor.[15] GPVI is a type 1 transmembrane protein belonging to the Ig superfamily. It associates with an Fc receptor $\gamma$-chain which serves as the signal transducing unit. Engagement of repetitive motifs on collagen by multiple GPVI molecules leads to crosslinking of GPVI dimers and phosphorylation of the FcR$\gamma$ chain immunoreceptor tyrosine-based activation motifs (ITAMs). This initiates a Syk-dependent signaling cascade finally resulting in activation of phospholipase C$\gamma$2 (PLC$\gamma$2) and phosphoinositide-3 kinase (PI3K) that generates inositol-1,4,5-trisphosphate (IP3). IP3 induces calcium mobilization, degranulation and integrin $\alpha_{IIb}\beta_3$ activation. Activated $\alpha_{IIb}\beta_3$ binds fibrinogen and VWF, leading to platelet aggregation.

The exposure of subendothelial collagen also exposes extravascular tissue factor, initiating coagulation and thrombin generation. This cascade is enhanced by PS exposure on activated platelet and endothelial cell membranes. Thrombin is a potent activator of platelets. Human platelets express two thrombin-activated G protein coupled receptors (GPCRs), PAR1 and PAR4.[16, 17] PAR activation occurs when a protease, such as thrombin, binds and cleaves the amino-terminus of the receptor. Binding of the new amino-terminus to the second extracellular loop of the PAR induces conformational changes in transmembrane domains enabling activation of G proteins.[18, 20] PAR1 and PAR4 activation lead to activation of $G\alpha q$, which activates PLCβ. PLCβ hydrolyzes phosphatidylinositol-4,5-bisphosphate (PIP2) to generate diacylglycerol (DAG) and IP3, leading to PKC activation and increased calcium mobilization, respectively.[21] In platelets, these pathways work in concert to activate the integrin $\alpha IIb\beta 3$ resulting in aggregation. PAR1 has a higher affinity for thrombin, and calcium transiently rises sharply after PAR1 activation followed by a relatively fast return to baseline levels. In contrast, PAR4 induces a more gradual and sustained rise in calcium and accounts for the majority of intracellular calcium flux.[22, 23] These platelet PAR1 and PAR4 kinetic signaling differences are reminiscent of the initiation and propagation phases of coagulation, where there is a burst of thrombin generation (quickly shut off by tissue factor pathway inhibitor [TFPI]) followed by a sustained and quantitatively greater production of thrombin by the intrinsic pathway.

| **Receptor** | **Agonist** |
|---|---|
| GPVI | Collagen |
| PAR4, PAR1 | Thrombin |
| $P2Y_{12}$, $P2Y_1$ | ADP |
| $\alpha_{2a}$ | Epinephrine |
| TPα, TPβ | TXA2 |

**Table 3.** Important Platelet Receptors and Agonists

There are two important amplification pathways in platelet activation.[24] The first is through the release of ADP from dense granule secretion. ADP is a potent platelet agonist that, when added to in vitro platelets, leads to $TXA_2$ production, phosphorylation of a number of proteins, increased cytosolic $Ca^{++}$, shape change, aggregation, and secretion. This pathway is required for maximal platelet aggregation induced by other agonists. Platelets have two ADP receptors, $P2Y_1$ and $P2Y_{12}$, and both are GPCRs. $P2Y_{12}$ activates $G\alpha i$, which promotes aggregation by inhibiting cyclic AMP (cAMP) formation. $P2Y_{12}$ mediated activation of protein kinase A leads to VASP phorphorylation. $P2Y_{12}$ is inhibited by the thienopyridines, commonly used anti-platelet agents that have benefit in the management of ischemic vascular disease. $P2Y_1$ appears to be necessary, but not sufficient to induce full platelet aggregation. Platelets from $P2Y_1$ knockout mice cannot change shape or aggregate to ADP but cAMP is still decreased in those platelets due to its effect on $P2Y_{12}$. $P2Y_1$ activates $G\alpha q$ with subsequent calcium mobilization.

The second feedback amplification pathway involves the metabolism of arachidonic acid (AA) to thromboxane A2 (TXA2).[24] A number of agonists stimulate the release of arachidonic acid from the stores in the plasma membrane, in particular phosphatidylcholine and phosphatidylethanolamine. Phospholipase A2 (PLA2) is the most important enzyme in the release of AA from those phospholipids. PLA2 can be activated by rising cytosolic calcium levels though there also appear to be calcium independent mechanisms. Released AA is then metabolized by cycloxegenase 1 (COX-1) to Prostaglandin G2 which subsequently is converted to Prostaglandin H2. Thromboxane synthase then produces TXA2. Aspirin irreversibly acetylates COX and also has benefit in preventing arterial ischemic syndromes. TXA2 diffuses out of platelets and binds to prostanoid GPCR family receptors, notably TP$\alpha$ and TP$\beta$, which also activate platelets via Gq.

Epinephrine activates platelets through adrenergic $\alpha_{2a}$ GPCRs that couple with G$\alpha$i family members to inhibit adenylyl cyclase leading to decreased cAMP and increased intracellular calcium concentration. It appears that epinephrine synergizes with other agonists, particularly ADP. It is unclear if epinephrine can lead to full aggregation by itself in vitro, although there are reports of families with mild bleeding disorders due to defects in epinephrine-induced platelet aggregation.

### 4.3. Shape change

The most dramatic observable change to platelets as they undergo activation is the change from their discoid form to a spread form with many filopodia. Agonists, such as thrombin and TXA2, activate GPCRs coupled to G$\alpha$12/13, which signal through RhoA –ROCK and myosin to reorganize the actin cytoskeleton and produce shape change.[24] Platelets contain large amounts of actin in both the globular (G-actin) and multimeric filamentous (F-actin) forms. Following activation; the proportion of F-actin increases from 40-50% to 70-80%. In an organized process, actin filaments from the resting platelet are cleaved into smaller fragments. These then form the beginnings of new, longer actin filaments. This process is regulated, in part, by increase phosphatidylinositol-4,5-biphosphate ($PIP_2$). Simultaneous to the changes in actin, myosin is phosphorylated by myosin light chain kinase activated by the calcium-calmodulin complex. This leads to association with F-actin as well as binding the complex to the membrane via interaction with the GPIb-IX complex. In resting platelets, filamin acts to stabilize the actin framework underlying the membrane and limits the movement of the GPIb. Increasing cytoplasmic $Ca^{++}$ concentrations activate calpain cleaving the actin binding protein leading to release from the GPIb complex. The outcome of this complex series of reactions is the centralization of actin into thick, fibrous masses associated with phosphorylated myosin filaments.

### 4.4. Degranulation

The above-mentioned agonists all induce platelet exocytosis of granules.[25] **S**oluble **N**-ethylmaleimide-sensitive factor **a**ttachment protein **re**ceptors or SNAREs mediate this delivery.[26] This includes t-SNAREs (target receptors), v-SNAREs (vesicle associated membrane receptors), and soluble components such as N-ethylmaleimide-sensitive fusion proteins (NSF) and NSF attachment protein. Reorganization of the cytoskeleton in conjunction with the SNARE machinery facilitates exocytosis of these granules, which contain a large variety of mediators important to the hemostatic and other roles of platelets.

http://dx.doi.org/10.5772/60595

**Dense Granules**. There are approximately three to eight dense granules per platelet. These are 20 to 30 nm in size and are electron dense due to the high calcium content. Dense granules also have high concentrations of serotonin, ADP, and ATP. ADP is an important platelet activator and this concentration of ADP in the dense granules and its delivery to developing thrombi by degranulation is an important amplification step in activating other platelets localized by adhesive molecules.

**$\alpha$-Granules**. There are 50 to 80 $\alpha$–granules per platelet. They are much larger than dense granules at approximately 200 nm in diameter. Upon platelet activation, $\alpha$ granules fuse with the plasma membrane, releasing their cargo, substantively increasing the total platelet membrane surface area. $\alpha$-granule membranes are rich in important adhesive integral membrane proteins, like GPIb-IX and $\alpha_{IIb}\beta_3$, which enhance adhesive properties. $\alpha$-granule cargo includes adhesive proteins and coagulation factors like fibrinogen and VWF, representing an important amplification feature of platelet thrombus growth. Fibrinogen is present in concentrations greater than that of plasma. Notably, megakaryocytes do not appear to synthesize fibrinogen, and it is endocytosed via $\alpha_{IIb}\beta_3$. Patients lacking $\alpha_{IIb}\beta_3$ also lack $\alpha$-granule fibrinogen. $\alpha$-granule VWF has high molecular weight, which is the most efficient form for hemostasis. Platelets $\alpha$-granules also contribute substantial amounts of coagulation Factor V and Factor XI, as well as thrombospondin-1 which is important for platelet activation via signaling through CD47. $\alpha$-granules contain a number of antifibrinolytic molecules including $\alpha_2$-antiplasmin and plasminogen activator inhibitor (PAI-1).

Proteomic studies indicate $\alpha$-granules contain more than 300 different soluble proteins.[27] Many of the non-hemostatic and systemic effects of circulating platelets are mediated by these molecules, and include chemokines (e.g., PF4, β-TG, MCP-, RANTES and others), antimicrobial proteins (thymosin-β4 and thrombocidins), immune modulators (complement, factor H, IgG), growth factors (PDGF, TGF β and others) and pro-angiogenic (VGF, FGF) and anti-angiogenic (endostatin, angiostatin) factors.

### 4.5. Aggregation

Platelets contain ≈80,000 αIIbβ3 (GPIIb-IIIa) complexes, the most abundant plasma membrane GP.[28] In the resting platelet, αIIbβ3 exists primarily in a low affinity conformation that is not able to bind its major ligands, which are fibrinogen, VWF, fibronectin and thrombospondin-1. The final common pathway of platelet activation leads to integrin activation to a high affinity state.[29] This is referred to as inside-out signaling. The high affinity conformation binds fibrinogen (or other adhesive ligands), and the bound fibrinogen serves as a bridge to other platelets, resulting in an expanding platelet aggregate. The importance of $\alpha_{IIb}\beta_3$ in platelet function and normal hemostasis is underscored by the moderately severe bleeding seen in patients with Glanzmann thrombasthenia, an inherited disorder caused by absent or dysfunctional αIIbβ3.

αIIbβ3 is the prototypic member of the integrin family of heterodimeric integral membrane adhesion receptors. This receptor consists of 18 $\alpha$ subunits that associate noncovalently with 8 β subunits. αIIb is expressed only in megakaryocytes and platelets, and localizes to the plasma membrane, OCS, and $\alpha$-granules. β3 has a broad tissue distribution. Platelets also express the αvβ3 vitronectin receptor in low abundance. Crystalization of the extracellular domain of αvβ3 and the head domain of αIIbβ3 have provided detailed structural information about these integrins.[30, 32]

Talin is an abundant cytoskeletal protein that links integrins to the actin cytoskeleton. The agonist-induced rise in intracellular calcium results in binding of the talin head domain to the cytoplasmic domain of integrin β3. This interaction leads to an unclasping of the intracellular and transmembrane components of the $\alpha_{IIb}$ and $\beta_3$ molecules, causing spreading of the two proteins and exposure of the ligand binding site. The precise molecular details by which talin is enabled to bind β3 are unclear, but efficient integrin activation likely involves (1) the guanine nucleotide exchange factor CalDAG-GEFI, (2) activation of the small GTPase Rap1, (3) kindlin-3 binding to the β3 cytoplasmic tail, and (4) calpain cleavage of talin.

## 5. Role in coagulation

Platelets contribute substantially to thrombin generation, which further induces additional platelet activation. In addition, platelet thrombus stabilization requires local fibrin generation that depends on thrombin generation. When platelets are stimulated by strong agonists, the negatively charged phospholipids on the inner leaflet of the platelet plasma membrane are "flipped" to the outer leaflet. This reorganization may be mediated by the calcium activated scramblase TMEM16F.[33] Translocation of negatively charged phospholipids forms a stage upon which coagulation reactions occur. The formation of the "tenase" complex that converts Factor X to activated Factor X requires phospholipid. The development of the prothrombinase complex also requires negatively charged phospholipid as the surface upon which the complex assembles.

Activation of platelets by strong agonists also leads to the development and shedding of platelet microparticles. These have a high density of negatively charged phospholipids and are thus able to support the formation of the "tenase" and prothrombinase complex as noted above. They also contain coagulation Factor Va with which to support the formation of thrombin as well as supplying arachidonic acid which can contribute to further formation of TXA2.

Platelets α-granule release also provides coagulation factors V, XI and XIII. Factor V may be particularly important as platelet Factor V is modified in a manner rendering it more resistant to cleavage by activated protein C.

## 6. Platelets in pathologic thrombosis

Pathologic studies show that venous thrombi are platelet-poor, while arterial thrombi are platelet-rich. In addition, although anti-platelet therapy is known to have benefit in preventing recurrent venous thrombi, the benefits appear to be greater for myocardial infarction and stroke. These pathologic and clinical observations are consistent with the known effect of shear stress on platelet thrombus formation. The effects of higher shear stress are clear for VWF. VWF adopts a folder globular structure under a low shear environment, obscuring the domains that mediate binding to platelets. In contrast, the mechanical effects induced by high shear unfolds VWF and exposes the GPIbα A1-binding domain of VWF. In addition, high shear rates are able to activate platelets directly.[34] In summary, platelets make a modest contribution to venous thrombosis and a more substantive contribution to arterial thrombosis. However, the fundamental molecular mechanisms of platelet thrombus formation appear to be similar in health and disease.

## Author details

Douglass A. Drelich and Paul F. Bray*

*Address all correspondence to: paul.bray@jefferson.edu

The Division of Hematology and The Cardeza Foundation for Hematologic Research, Department of Medicine, Sidney Kimmel Medical College, Thomas Jefferson University, Philadelphia, PA, USA

## References

[1] Marcus AJ, Ullman HL, Safier LB. Lipid composition of subcellular particles of human blood platelets. *J. Lipid Res.* 1969;10:108-114

[2] Gousset K, Wolkers WF, Tsvetkova NM, Oliver AE, Field CL, Walker NJ, Crowe JH, Tablin F. Evidence for a physiological role for membrane rafts in human platelets. *J. Cell. Physiol.* 2002;190:117-128

[3] White JG. Platelet structure. In: Michelson AD, ed. *Platelets*. Elsevier; 2013:117-144.

[4] Harker LA, Roskos LK, Marzec UM, Carter RA, Cherry JK, Sundell B, Cheung EN, Terry D, Sheridan W. Effects of megakaryocyte growth and development factor on platelet production, platelet life span, and platelet function in healthy human volunteers. *Blood*. 2000;95:2514-2522

[5] Italiano JE, Jr., Patel-Hett S, Hartwig JH. Mechanics of proplatelet elaboration. *J Thromb Haemost*. 2007;5 Suppl 1:18-23

[6] Kaushansky K, Lok S, Holly RD, Broudy VC, Lin N, Bailey MC, Forstrom JW, Buddle MM, Oort PJ, Hagen FS, et al. Promotion of megakaryocyte progenitor expansion and differentiation by the c-mpl ligand thrombopoietin. *Nature*. 1994;369:568-571

[7] Chen J, Lopez JA. Interactions of platelets with subendothelium and endothelium. *Microcirculation*. 2005;12:235-246

[8] Sadler JE. Von willebrand factor assembly and secretion. *J Thromb Haemost*. 2009;7 Suppl 1:24-27

[9] Lopez JA, Dong JF. Structure and function of the glycoprotein ib-ix-v complex. *Curr Opin Hematol*. 1997;4:323-329

[10] Ivanciu L, Krishnaswamy S, Camire RM. New insights into the spatiotemporal localization of prothrombinase in vivo. *Blood*. 2014;124:1705-1714

[11] Welsh JD, Stalker TJ, Voronov R, Muthard RW, Tomaiuolo M, Diamond SL, Brass LF. A systems approach to hemostasis: 1. The interdependence of thrombus architecture and agonist movements in the gaps between platelets. *Blood*. 2014;124:1808-1815

[12] Tomaiuolo M, Stalker TJ, Welsh JD, Diamond SL, Sinno T, Brass LF. A systems approach to hemostasis: 2. Computational analysis of molecular transport in the thrombus microenvironment. *Blood*. 2014;124:1816-1823

[13] Stalker TJ, Welsh JD, Tomaiuolo M, Wu J, Colace TV, Diamond SL, Brass LF. A systems approach to hemostasis: 3. Thrombus consolidation regulates intrathrombus solute transport and local thrombin activity. *Blood*. 2014;124:1824-1831

[14] Welsh JD, Colace TV, Muthard RW, Stalker TJ, Brass LF, Diamond SL. Platelet-targeting sensor reveals thrombin gradients within blood clots forming in microfluidic assays and in mouse. *J Thromb Haemost*. 2012;10:2344-2353

[15] Nieswandt B, Watson SP. Platelet-collagen interaction: Is gpvi the central receptor? *Blood*. 2003;102:449-461

[16] Coughlin SR. Thrombin signalling and protease-activated receptors. *Nature*. 2000;407:258-264

[17] Jamieson GA. Pathophysiology of platelet thrombin receptors. *Thromb. Haemostasis*. 1997;78:242-246

[18] Gether U, Kobilka BK. G protein-coupled receptors. Ii. Mechanism of agonist activation. *J. Biol. Chem*. 1998;273:17979-17982

[19] Palczewski K, Kumasaka T, Hori T, Behnke CA, Motoshima H, Fox BA, Le Trong I, Teller DC, Okada T, Stenkamp RE, Yamamoto M, Miyano M. Crystal structure of rhodopsin: A g protein-coupled receptor. *Science*. 2000;289:739-745

[20] Stitham J, Stojanovic A, Ross LA, Blount AC, Jr., Hwa J. Clusters of transmembrane residues are critical for human prostacyclin receptor activation. *Biochemistry*. 2004;43:8974-8986

[21] Abrams CS, Brass,L.F. Platelet signal transduction. In: Coleman RW, Marder, V.J., Clowes, A.W., George, J.N., Goldharber, S.Z., ed. *Hemostasis and thrombosis*. Philadelphia, PA: Lippincott Williams & Wilkins; 2006:617-629.

[22] Covic L, Gresser AL, Kuliopulos A. Biphasic kinetics of activation and signaling for par1 and par4 thrombin receptors in platelets. *Biochemistry*. 2000;39:5458-5467

[23] Holinstat M, Voss B, Bilodeau ML, McLaughlin JN, Cleator J, Hamm HE. Par4, but not par1, signals human platelet aggregation via ca2+ mobilization and synergistic p2y12 receptor activation. *J. Biol. Chem.* 2006;281:26665-26674

[24] Brass LF, Newman, D.K., Wannermacher K.M., Zhu, L., Stalker, T.J. Signal transduction during platelet plug formation. In: Michelson AD, ed. *Platelets*. Elsevier; 2013:367-398.

[25] Flaumenhaft R. Platelet secretion. In: Michelson AD, ed. *Platelets*. Elsevier; 2013:343-366.

[26] Lemons PP, Chen D, Bernstein AM, Bennett MK, Whiteheart SW. Regulated secretion in platelets: Identification of elements of the platelet exocytosis machinery. *Blood*. 1997;90:1490-1500

[27] Coppinger JA, Cagney G, Toomey S, Kislinger T, Belton O, McRedmond JP, Cahill DJ, Emili A, Fitzgerald DJ, Maguire PB. Characterization of the proteins released from activated platelets leads to localization of novel platelet proteins in human atherosclerotic lesions. *Blood*. 2004;103:2096-2104

[28] Coller BS, Shattil SJ. The gpiib/iiia (integrin alphaiibbeta3) odyssey: A technology-driven saga of a receptor with twists, turns, and even a bend. *Blood*. 2008;112:3011-3025

[29] Arnaout MA, Goodman SL, Xiong JP. Structure and mechanics of integrin-based cell adhesion. *Curr. Opin. Cell Biol.* 2007;19:495-507

[30] Xiong JP, Stehle T, Diefenbach B, Zhang R, Dunker R, Scott DL, Joachimiak A, Goodman SL, Arnaout MA. Crystal structure of the extracellular segment of integrin alpha vbeta3. *Science*. 2001;294:339-345

[31] Xiong JP, Stehle T, Zhang R, Joachimiak A, Frech M, Goodman SL, Arnaout MA. Crystal structure of the extracellular segment of integrin alpha vbeta3 in complex with an arg-gly-asp ligand. *Science*. 2002;296:151-155

[32] Xiao T, Takagi J, Coller BS, Wang JH, Springer TA. Structural basis for allostery in integrins and binding to fibrinogen-mimetic therapeutics. *Nature*. 2004;432:59-67

[33] Suzuki J, Umeda M, Sims PJ, Nagata S. Calcium-dependent phospholipid scrambling by tmem16f. *Nature*. 2010;468:834-838

[34] Holme PA, Orvim U, Hamers MJ, Solum NO, Brosstad FR, Barstad RM, Sakariassen KS. Shear-induced platelet activation and platelet microparticle formation at blood flow conditions as in arteries with a severe stenosis. Arterioscler. Thromb. Vasc. Biol. 1997;17:646-653

Section 2

# The Role of Platelets in Inflammation, Infection and Immunity

Chapter 3

# Role of Platelets in Inflammation

Mònica Arman, Holly Payne,
Tatyana Ponomaryov and Alexander Brill

Additional information is available at the end of the chapter

http://dx.doi.org/10. 5772/60536

## 1. Introduction

### 1. 1. Inflammation

Inflammation is a complex of responses of the innate immune system to pathological stimuli such as microbes, pathogens or damage-associated molecular patterns (DAMPs). Local inflammation includes the following classical symptoms: *dolor* (pain), *calor* (heat), *rubor* (redness), *tumor* (swelling) and *functio laesa* (loss of function). Systemic inflammation occurs in different contexts like massive trauma, chronic disease, or as a response to an infection, in which case it is designated as sepsis. Clinical responses during systemic inflammation (systemic inflammatory response syndrome, SIRS) include altered body temperature, elevated pulse rate, elevated respiratory rate, abnormal white blood cell count and other symptoms. [1] The inflammatory response includes (but is not limited to) recruitment of immune cells, such as neutrophils and monocytes, by the vessel wall, followed by their extravasation to tissues. Although inflammation involves multiple mechanisms beyond this process (e. g. , involving complement and kinin systems as well as changes in vascular tonus), we will concentrate herein on the platelet role in vascular endothelial activation and interactions with leukocytes, with a special focus on *in vivo* data.

## 2. Platelet-derived mediators regulating inflammation

Platelets have multiple roles beyond hemostasis and thrombosis and were described as inflammatory cells several decades ago. [2] Platelets contain a number of inflammatory peptide and protein mediators, some of which they retain the capability of synthesizing *de novo*, whereas others are stored and secreted from granules (dense granules, $\alpha$-granules or lysosomes). [3] The release of these cytokines and chemokines, as well as eicosanoids, upon activation enables platelets to recruit leukocytes to the site of inflammation or injury. The table below lists some of the platelet-derived inflammatory mediators:

| Molecule | Family | Location |
|---|---|---|
| IL-1β | Cytokine | Synthesized |
| Thromboxane A2 | Eicosanoid | Synthesized |
| PF4/CXCL4 | Chemokine | α- granules |
| β-thromboglobulin (CXCL7/ NAP-2) | Chemokine | α- granules |
| RANTES (CCL5) | Chemokine | α- granules |
| CD40L | Cytokine | α- granules |
| PDGF | Growth factor | α- granules |
| TGF-β | Growth factor | α- granules |
| TNF-α | Cytokine | α- granules |
| IL-1α | Cytokine | α- granules |
| GRO-α (CXCL1) | Cytokine | α- granules |
| ENA-78 (CXCL5) | Cytokine | α- granules |
| SDF-1 (CXCL12) | Cytokine | α- granules |
| MIP-1α (CCL3) | Chemokine | α- granules |
| MCP-3 (CCL7) | Chemokine | α- granules |
| NAP-2 (CXCL7) | Chemokine | α- granules |
| TARC (CCL17) | Chemokine | α- granules |
| Interleukin-8 (CXCL8) | Chemokine | α- granules |
| Polyphosphates | Phosphates | Dense granules |
| ATP | Nucleotide | Dense granules |
| Serotonin | Monoamine | Dense granules |
| Glutamate | Amino Acid | Dense granules |

**Table 1.** Inflammatory mediators synthesized by and stored in platelets

Platelet α-granules contain large proteins, many of which are involved in regulation of the inflammatory response. [4, 5] Among them, Platelet Factor 4 (PF4) is the most abundant protein secreted by activated platelets (accounting for ~25% of α-granule content). [6] It functions as a chemoattractant for monocytes. PF4 accelerates atherogenesis by causing vascular inflammation and promoting retention of lipoproteins in the vascular wall, which contributes to atherosclerosis. PF4 prevents full interaction of LDL with its receptor, causing lipoproteins to be retained on the cell surface rather than being catabolized. [7]

Platelet-originating thromboxane A2 (TxA2), which is made *de novo* from arachidonic acid upon activation, induces platelet activation and aggregation. [8] This may form a positive feedback loop facilitating further release of stored cytokines.

Platelet-derived IL-1$\alpha$ has been shown to mediate cerebral inflammation *in vivo*. [9] IL-1$\alpha$ secreted from platelets promotes expression of the adhesion molecules ICAM-1 and VCAM-1 on endothelial cells. It also accelerates transendothelial migration of neutrophils and contributes to chronic inflammatory diseases, such as multiple sclerosis. [9] Platelet IL-1$\alpha$ and IL-1β have proinflammatory roles in rheumatoid arthritis; it has been shown that platelet depletion attenuates the disease in mice. [10]

Besides storage, platelets can also synthesize biologically active proteins. For example, thrombin activation results in synthesis of pro-IL-1β. [11] Interestingly, synthesis of pro-IL-1β was inhibited by neutralization of the beta-3 integrin, which implies that direct anti-platelet therapy could have an anti-inflammatory effect. Platelets contain the splicing machinery allowing for cytokine mRNA maturation. [12] IL-1β potentiates its own synthesis in platelets by an autocrine loop, and its production by activated platelets occurs *in vivo*, where it accumulates in thrombus in the ferric chloride-treated carotid artery. [13] This represents a link connecting sterile thrombotic process with formation of proinflammatory milieu. IL-1β from platelets causes both up-regulation of endothelial adhesion receptors and release of proinflammatory IL-6 and IL-8 from endothelial cells. IL-1β is also responsible for activation of NF-κB in endothelial cells, which is required for transcription of inflammatory genes MCP-1 and ICAM-1. [7]

Platelet derived growth factor (PDGF) is able to chemoattract monocytes and eosinophils. [4] The chemokine RANTES (Regulated on Activation, Normal T Cell Expressed and Secreted) recruits monocytes to the inflamed endothelium in a P-selectin-dependent fashion. [14] RANTES plays a role in many inflammatory disorders including asthma, atherosclerosis and delayed-type hypersensitivity reactions. [15]

Among other platelet-derived chemokines, Macrophage Inflammatory Protein (MIP)-1$\alpha$ induces leukocyte chemotaxis *in vivo*. [8, 16] MIP-1$\alpha$ is a chemoattractant for monocytes, macrophages, T-cells and neutrophils and is involved in transendothelial migration at sites of inflammation. [17] MIP-1$\alpha$ is required for a normal inflammatory response to certain types of viruses. MIP-1$\alpha$-null mice develop a reduced inflammatory response to influenza virus and coxsackievirus-induced myocarditis. [17]

Platelets store large amounts of the pro-inflammatory molecule CD40 ligand (CD40L). Interaction of CD40L with CD40 on endothelial cells and macrophages causes release of IL-8 and MCP-1, which attract neutrophils and monocytes. [18] Similarly to IL-1β, CD40L induces adhesion receptor expression on endothelium and release of chemokines thus mediating leukocyte recruitment.

Platelets contain Polyphosphate (polyP) in their dense granules. [19] Proinflammatory and procoagulant functions of polyP have recently been demonstrated. [20] PolyP, released upon platelet stimulation, binds to factor XII activating the FXII-driven contact activation system. The resulting release of the inflammatory mediator bradykinin culminates in the accumulation of neutrophils and increased vascular permeability through binding its receptor BR2. Targeting polyP, for example, with phosphatases may be of potential therapeutic benefit for treating such diseases as rheumatoid arthritis and atherosclerosis. [20] However, the role of polyP in activating the contact phase system has recently been questioned. [21]

Thus, platelets store and release a substantial repertoire of inflammatory mediators. These molecules may contribute to multiple inflammation-related diseases, which make platelets important players in the field of inflammation.

## 3. Platelet-endothelium interactions

Under physiological (non-inflammatory) conditions, production of platelet inhibitors (such as prostacyclin and nitric oxide) by endothelial cells limits platelet interaction with intact endothelium. Adhesion of activated platelets to intact Human Umbilical Vein Endothelial Cells (HUVEC) was demonstrated *in vitro*. [22] Mechanisms of this involved $\alpha_{IIb}\beta_3$ integrin (glycoprotein (GP) IIb/IIIa) on platelets, ICAM-1 and $\alpha_v\beta_3$ integrin on the endothelium and von Willebrand Factor (VWF), fibrinogen and fibronectin as bridging molecules. Platelet GPIb$\alpha$, which is constitutively expressed and does not require activation, was reported to be a receptor to endothelial P-selectin. [23] There is a report demonstrating that platelets contain P-selectin glycoprotein ligand (PSGL)-1 (although 25-100-fold fewer than leukocytes). [24] Blocking PSGL-1 down-regulates the number of rolling and captured platelets on stimulated venule endothelium suggesting that this route can also be implicated in platelet-vessel wall interaction under inflammatory conditions. Integrin $\alpha_v\beta_3$, a vitronectin receptor on the endothelial cells, was shown to participate in platelet recruitment to stimulated endothelium. [25]

*In vivo*, platelets do not spontaneously interact with intact endothelium in murine mesenteric venules. [26] Stimulation of murine vessels with Weibel-Palade body secretagogues calcium ionophore or histamine results in rapid platelet adhesion followed by rolling, peaking 1 min after stimulation. This "stop-and-go" platelet translocation on stimulated endothelium was absent in VWF-null mice. Cleavage of GPIb$\alpha$ from platelet surface also prevented platelet binding to the vessel wall. Therefore, interaction of platelets with activated endothelium *in vivo* is mediated by binding of platelet GPIb$\alpha$ to endothelium-expressed VWF. [26]

Another pathway of platelet binding to the vascular wall involves the glycoprotein VI (GPVI), a major platelet receptor for collagen. This route is most important in platelet interactions with atherosclerotic plaques. Inhibition of GPVI by infusion of GPVI-Fc, a dimeric soluble form of GPVI fused with human Fc fragment, to ApoE$^{-/-}$ mice decreased transient platelet interactions with atherosclerotic artery wall by about half. [27] Long-term administration of a GPVI-blocking antibody also improved endothelial function and prevented propagation of atherosclerosis. [27] GPVI binds activated endothelium through vitronectin and improves cardiac function in a mouse model of heart ischemia-reperfusion by reducing inflammation in the infarcted myocardium. [28] Infusion of soluble GPVI-Fc in either ischemia or reperfusion phase substantially decreased infarct size.

In a model of cerebral ischemia-reperfusion, platelet tumbling on and adhesion to the brain vascular endothelium has been demonstrated. [29] This was specific to veins and no platelet-vessel wall interactions were observed in arteries of different diameter. This interaction was almost entirely dependent on P-selectin as administration of anti-P-selectin antibody abolished it. Neutralization of $\alpha_{IIb}\beta_3$ had certain inhibitory effect too, though less manifested than blocking P-selectin. Rolling and adhesion of platelets was reported also during reperfusion period after retinal ischemia. This process was dependent on endothelial P-selectin, and the time course of P-selectin *de novo* synthesis in the endothelium corresponded to the kinetics of platelet-endothelial interactions. [30]

Platelet adhesion to endothelium of atherosclerotic plaques can also be mediated by the glycoprotein $\alpha_{IIb}$. [31] Platelet adhesion to the atherosclerotic plaque in apo$E^{-/-}$ $\alpha_{IIb}$-double deficient mice was virtually abolished as compared with apo$E^{-/-}$ $\alpha_{IIb}^{+/+}$ controls. Formation of atherosclerotic lesions was reduced in the absence of $\alpha_{IIb}$. Platelet-vessel wall interactions through $\alpha_{IIb}$ are also implicated in the pathogenesis of such thromboinflammatory disease as ischemic stroke as shown in a model of cerebral ischemia-reperfusion in mice. The exact mechanism of $\alpha_{IIb}$ involvement in interactions with inflamed but non-denuded endothelium remains to be clarified. It is known that ischemia promotes fibrinogen deposition on the vessel wall, which leads to platelets recruitment. [32] Local hypoxia and pro-inflammatory shift (like generation of reactive oxygen species (ROS)) result in VWF expression on the endothelium mediating platelet accrual. [33, 34] Thus, two major ligands for $\alpha_{IIb}\beta_3$, fibrinogen and VWF, can appear on the endothelial surface during inflammation and recruit platelets via this integrin.

Platelet accumulation in lung and cerebral vasculature was described in a murine model of malaria[35] as well as in patients. [36] Platelets might damage endothelium and support leukocyte accumulation in the brain vessels thus promoting cerebral inflammation as a part of malaria pathogenesis. [37] Platelet depletion protects mice from disease progression. [38] The role of platelets in malaria may be complex depending on the stage of the disease: platelets could attenuate parasite growth at the early stages whereas at later stages platelets support disease-related inflammation. [39]

Activated platelets can be found in circulation in patients with various inflammatory diseases, such as sepsis, cerebrovascular ischemia and diabetes. [40-42] Besides posing a danger for excessive thrombosis, circulating activated platelets confer a proinflammatory signal. Activated platelets infused into mice stimulate release of Weibel-Palade body constituents and form complexes with leukocytes, leading to elevated recruitment of leukocytes to the vessel wall. [43] Thrombin-activated platelets accumulate at the atherosclerotic carotid artery wall. This process is dramatically inhibited when platelets lack CD40L. [44]

Interaction of platelets with endothelium mediates accumulation of monocytes and deposition of proinflammatory cytokines (e.g. , RANTES) at the vessel wall (Figure 1). It was directly demonstrated in mice using repeated infusions of activated platelets or bone marrow transplantation techniques, that platelets promote the development of larger atherosclerotic plaques. [45, 46] This effect is predominantly mediated by platelet P-selectin.

Thus, platelets bind to the activated/inflamed vascular wall by a set of receptors including P-selectin, glycoproteins Ib$\alpha$, $\alpha_{IIb}$ and VI as well as CD40L. Activated platelets are able to induce a pro-inflammatory shift in the endothelium. Platelet-mediated endothelial activation plays a role in the development of various diseases that have an inflammatory component in their pathogenesis.

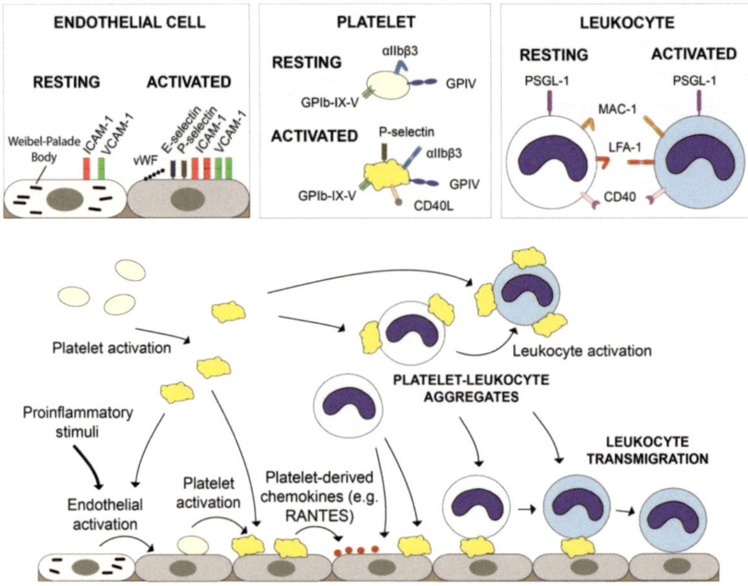


**Figure 1.** Platelet cross-talk with endothelium and leukocytes.

## 4. Platelet-leukocyte interactions

Under physiological conditions, platelets and leukocytes do not bind to each other. Such interaction becomes possible in prothrombotic or proinflammatory state with increased number of blood platelet-leukocyte aggregates (PLA) (Figure 1) observed in such diseases as diabetes mellitus, stroke and others. [47-49]

Binding of platelets to leukocytes can mediate recruitment of the latter to the vessel wall and render leukocytes more prothrombotic promoting synthesis of tissue factor by monocytes. [50] This interaction starts by binding of P-selectin on activated platelets to PSGL-1 on leukocytes initiating a signaling cascade inside leukocytes, which leads to activation of integrins, in particular, Mac-1 and LFA-1 on leukocyte membrane. [51-53] Mac1 can bind platelet receptor GPIb$\alpha$ directly or $\alpha_{IIb}\beta_3$ through fibrinogen bound to the integrin on platelets. [54, 55] Platelet-leukocyte binding is an active process as pre-activation of leukocytes potentiates this interaction whereas tyrosine kinase inhibitors down-regulate it. Full activation of the integrins triggers outside-in signaling regulating multiple leukocyte functions such as transmigration, production of ROS and phagocytosis. [56] Platelet-mediated activation of Mac-1 can lead to sequestration and activation of coagulation Factor X resulting in thrombin generation. [57]

http://dx.doi.org/10.5772/60536

This phenomenon suggests that platelet-leukocyte interaction triggers also the coagulation cascade.

*In vivo,* interactions between platelets and leukocytes occur in various thrombo-inflammatory conditions. For example, blood stasis in the carotid artery induces P-selectin-dependent accumulation of leukocytes surrounded by platelets in the vicinity of the vessel wall. [58] Platelet depletion almost completely abrogates leukocyte recruitment suggesting that development of the inflammatory response in this model is platelet-dependent. Platelet P-selectin is implicated in recruiting leukocytes not only to the inflammation site but also in pure thrombosis. Thrombi in ferric chloride-challenged carotid arteries of P-selectin-deficient mice contained less leukocytes than in control animals. [59] This confirms the central role of P-selectin in platelet interactions with leukocytes.

Formation of platelet-leukocyte rosettes *in vivo* depends on platelet activation. It has been reported that plasma level of circulating PLA more specifically reflects platelet activation than platelet P-selectin expression. [60] Resting platelets infused into mice do not associate with leukocytes. [61] Intravenous injection of collagen together with $\alpha_{IIb}\beta_3$ antagonist to prevent formation of platelet aggregates, results in rapid development of platelet-leukocyte conjugates. These conjugates roll on the vascular wall both in C57BL/6 and aged ApoE-deficient mice prone to atherosclerosis. In both cases, this rolling was mediated by P-selectin. Binding of activated platelets to leukocytes supported leukocyte recruitment by the endothelium through VCAM-1, and elevated leukocyte interactions with vessel wall in inflammation and atherosclerosis. [45] Infusion of activated P-selectin positive but not P-selectin deficient platelets elevated monocyte binding to atherosclerotic endothelium in mice. Formation of PLA resulted in deposition of chemokines, such as RANTES and PF4, on the endothelium thus supporting development of atherosclerosis. Besides leukocytes, activated platelets mediate lymphocyte homing in peripheral lymph nodes. [62] Again, all these phenomena were dependent on platelet surface P-selectin.

Cell activation in leukocyte-platelet interaction is bi-directional, i. e., not only platelets activate leukocytes but also vice versa. [56] In particular, various leukocyte-derived molecules can activate platelets and promote platelet-mediated fibrin deposition. Activated platelets stimulate neutrophils to release their chromatin designated as Neutrophil Extracellular Traps (NETs), [63] at least in part by presenting High Mobility Group Box 1 (HMGB1). [64] NETs can recruit and activate platelets. [65] Histones, an integral part of NETs, directly activate platelets and induce platelet aggregation. [66]

In conclusion, platelets interact with both endothelium and leukocytes mediating accumulation of the latter at the inflammatory site, thus supporting the central step in the inflammatory response.

## 5. Platelet Toll-like receptors

Toll-like receptors (TLRs) are a family of innate immunity pattern-recognition receptors that trigger inflammation in response to microbial products or products of inflamed tissues. TLRs function as front-line sensors of infection, as they recognize conserved structures in pathogens designated as pathogen-associated molecular patterns (PAMPs). [67] TLRs can also sense DAMPs, released by activated or necrotic host cells and upregulated following tissue damage. [68] Human and murine platelets express TLR2, TLR4, TLR7 and TLR9. [69-76] TLR6 has been detected in human platelets. [69] Expression of TLR1 has been reported in one[69] but not in another[77] study.

**Platelet TLR2**. Pam3CSK4, a synthetic agonist of the TLR2/1 complex, triggers platelet activation including integrin $\alpha_{IIb}\beta_3$ transition to an active state, aggregation, alpha- and dense granule release and CD40L expression. [78-80] These responses are inhibited in TLR2-deficient murine platelets and in human platelets by pretreatment with TLR2-blocking antibody. [79] Pam3CSK4 also triggers formation of platelet–neutrophil aggregates (PNA). [79, 80]

In periodontitis, a chronic inflammatory disease of the supportive dental tissues, the gram-negative periodontopathogens directly induce TLR2- and TLR4-dependent surface expression of CD40L in human platelets. [81] *In vivo* challenge with live *Porphyromonas gingivalis* induced formation of PNA in wild-type but not TLR2-deficient mice. [79] *Ex vivo* experiments showed that platelet TLR2 mediated formation of PNA and enhanced phagocytosis of periodonto-pathogens. [81]

Human cytomegalovirus (HCMV), a widespread pathogen that correlates with various diseases including atherosclerosis, binds TLR2-positive platelet subpopulation. This results in platelet degranulation, release of proinflammatory CD40L and IL-1β and proangiogenic vascular endothelial–derived growth factor (VEGF). Murine CMV activates wild-type but not TLR2-deficient mouse platelets. HCMV-activated platelets bind to and activate neutrophils, supporting their adhesion and transmigration through endothelial monolayers. [82] In an *in vivo* model, CMV increased the number of PLA and plasma VEGF levels and demonstrated a trend to enhance neutrophil extravasation in a TLR2-dependent fashion. [82]

**Platelet TLR4**. Platelet activation with thrombin causes increase of TLR4 surface expression in one [83] but not another [72] study. Lipopolysaccharide (LPS), a cell wall component of gram-negative bacteria, is a natural ligand for TLR4. *In vitro*, some studies have reported no [77, 84] or even inhibitory effect[85] of LPS on platelet aggregation whereas others have shown that LPS can potentiate platelet aggregation induced by low doses of other agonists. [86, 87] *In vivo*, intravenous injection of LPS in mice induces formation of platelet aggregates mainly in lung and liver microvasculature. [88, 89] Platelet TLR4 mediated microvascular LPS-induced thrombosis in murine cremaster muscle venules. [84, 90]

LPS present on platelets and leukocytes from patients with hemolytic uremic syndrome (HUS) caused PLA formation. [91] LPS binds human platelets through a complex of TLR4 and CD62, leading to platelet activation. The specificity of LPS binding to platelet TLR4 was confirmed *in vivo* using TLR4 deficient mice. [92]

Platelet TLR4 contributes to LPS-induced thrombocytopenia *in vivo*. [71, 72] In one study, LPS induced thrombocytopenia in wild-type but not TLR4-deficient mice. [71] TLR4-positive but not TLR4-negative platelets accumulated in the murine lungs in response to LPS in a neutro-phil-dependent fashion. In another study, LPS produced thrombocytopenia and increased

http://dx.doi.org/10.5772/60536

serum levels of TNFα in LPS-sensitive mice but not in mice carrying mutated TLR4. [72] LPS-induced TNFα production in LPS-sensitive mice was reduced by platelet depletion and could be restored by platelet transfusion. [72]

In mouse endotoxemia, TLR4-positive but not TLR4-negative platelets accumulate in the lungs. [71] LPS induces platelet binding to sequestered neutrophils primarily in the liver sinusoids and pulmonary capillaries leading to formation of NETs, [93] which are able to trap and kill microbes. [63]

**Platelet TLR7**. A recent study showed that platelet TLR7 mediates platelet activation in response to the single stranded RNA encephalomyocarditis virus (EMCV). [74] This interaction led to platelet granule release, P-selectin surface expression, and increase in PNA, both in mouse and human blood, but did not induce platelet aggregation. There were, however, implications to the host immune response and survival. TLR7 expressed on platelets is implicated in protection against EMCV-induced mortality. Transfusion of TLR7-positive platelets into TLR7-null mice prolonged survival after infection with EMCV whereas transfusion of platelets lacking TLR7 into wild-type mice did not affect the survival rate. [74]

**Platelet TLR9**. In platelets, TLR9 is located in intracellular compartments. [75] TLR9 responds to carboxy(alkylpyrrole) protein adducts, an altered-self ligand generated in oxidative stress, in both human and mouse platelets. This interaction results in aggregation *in vitro* and thrombosis *in vivo*. [76] Physiological platelet agonists synergize with TLR9 ligands by increasing TLR9 expression on the platelet membrane. [76]

## 6. Platelets in sepsis

Sepsis is an uncontrolled systemic reaction to an infection. It can progress into severe sepsis with multiple organ dysfunction and cognitive impairment. Septic shock, in which patients suffer vascular collapse and often are irresponsive to fluid resuscitation and vasopressor therapy, is often the terminal event of severe sepsis. [1] Sepsis is a complex process presenting with multiple pathogenic features, such as dysregulation of the immune and coagulation systems, thrombosis, disruption of endothelial barrier function, increased vascular permeability, microvascular sequestration, tissue damage, etc. [94] This complexity is likely to be responsible for the failure to find new treatments for sepsis, [95] and for the lack of good animal models. [96, 97]

Platelets are both cellular effectors and cellular targets in the pathophysiology of sepsis. Regardless of the initiating events in sepsis, platelets play an important role in the development of multiple organ failure via their haemostatic and thrombotic potential, resulting in thrombotic microangiopathy and disseminated intravascular coagulation. [98, 99, 100] Evidence for an important role of platelets is provided by clinical studies and animal model data demonstrating beneficial effect of antiplatelet agents in sepsis (reviewed in [101]).

Sepsis is frequently accompanied by thrombocytopenia, which is closely associated with disease severity and mortality rate. [98, 99] Multiple mechanisms may contribute to thrombocytopenia in sepsis: disseminated intravascular coagulation with peripheral consumption and destruction of platelets, impaired thrombopoiesis, direct activation by bacteria or their products, phagocytosis, etc. [102-104] Thrombocytopenia is also detected after injection of LPS in mice (a common model for sepsis) [88, 89] through a TLR4-dependent mechanism. [71, 72]

Alterations in circulating platelets occur in septic patients. CD62P expression was elevated in septic platelets in some studies[105, 106] but not in the others[107, 108] Other platelet activation markers found in sepsis include membrane expression of thrombospondin (TSP)[109, 110] and CD63, [106] elevated soluble CD40L level[108] and an increase in beta-thromboglobulin and the beta-thromboglobulin-to-PF4 ratio. [111] Increased VEGF release by agonist-stimulated platelets from septic samples has been reported. [107] Moreover, triggering receptor expressed on myeloid cells (TREM)-like transcript-1 (TLT-1), secreted upon platelet activation, is found in the plasma of patients with sepsis in levels that correlate with disseminated intravascular coagulation. [112, 113]. Animal studies suggest that TLT-1 dampens inflammation and augments platelet aggregation, reducing local hemorrhage. [112] Furthermore, soluble TLT-1 increases platelet adherence to the endothelium[114] and is involved in the regulation of inflammation in the course of sepsis by suppressing leukocyte activation and affecting platelet-neutrophil crosstalk. [115]

An *in vitro* study showed that platelets from septic patients are hyper-adhesive to cultured endothelium. [110] Alterations in platelet aggregation [107, 116] and increase in PLA level, which both might contribute to inflammation and vascular injury, have also been found in sepsis. [105, 109]

Changes in platelet transcriptome have also been reported in sepsis. [117] Expression of spliced tissue factor mRNA in platelets from septic subjects was associated with tissue factor-dependent procoagulant activity. [118] This may be one of the mechanisms by which platelets contribute to microvascular thrombosis in sepsis. [119, 118]

It is likely that different platelet-activating pathways cooperate during sepsis. Platelets are activated by some (but not all) bacteria or their products, and by NETs. [65, 103, 104] This could have beneficial roles in fighting infection (i. e. , pathogen capture within thrombus, pathogen killing, etc). However, uncontrolled thrombus formation in response to bacteria or NETs could have detrimental effects in sepsis. Other processes, such as imbalance between plasma level of high molecular weight VWF and its cleavage protease ADAMTS-13, imbalanced coagulation, systemic endothelial activation, and leukocyte activation, might contribute to potentiating platelet activation in sepsis. [99, 100]

## 7. Platelets and neurovascular inflammation

The central nervous system (CNS) is an immune-privileged site, separated from blood by the blood brain barrier (BBB). Under pathological conditions, BBB may be disrupted. This lets cells from blood into the cerebral tissue and facilitates innate and adaptive immune responses in the CNS. [120, 121]

Platelets are present in the inflamed CNS microvasculature in mice and are capable of activating brain endothelial cells via IL-1$\alpha$ release. Platelets, as inflammatory cells, participate in neural diseases associated with pathogen-induced and sterile inflammation. [122-124]

Sterile neurovascular inflammation accompanies such neural disorders as stroke, multiple sclerosis, and Alzheimer's disease (summarized in [125]). Ischemic stroke elicits a strong inflammatory response. [126] Inhibition of platelet adhesion to the injured vessel wall by blocking surface receptors GPIb$\alpha$ or GPVI protected mice from ischemic injury, implying that platelets are involved in stroke-related cerebral inflammation. [127] The lack of ADAMTS13, an enzyme cleaving VWF rendering it less proadhesive, promoted brain damage whereas infusion of ADAMTS13 ameliorated the defect, [128] further suggesting that platelet adhesion is an important pathogenetic step in ischemic stroke.

Interestingly, limiting platelet aggregation with $\alpha_{IIb}\beta_3$ inhibitors did not protect from stroke in mice[127] and humans. [129] Altogether there are several candidates on the platelet surface or inside platelet granules, including GPIb, GPVI, and VWF that could be potential targets for stroke treatment through reducing thrombo-inflammation without inducing bleeding complications[126, 130-133]

Neuronal loss is accompanied by BBB breakdown and vascular inflammation in age-related **Alzheimer's disease** (AD). [134] Platelet function in AD is altered, and platelet activation state (determined by plasma soluble GPVI levels) is considered a potential biomarker for the disease progression. [135-138] Platelets contain substantial amounts of amyloid precursor protein[139] and various forms of tau protein that could have diagnostic value as biomarkers and/or play a role in disease pathogenesis. [140]

**Multiple sclerosis** (MS) is a devastating T-cell mediated autoimmune neuroinflammatory disease. [141] High levels of platelet activation markers (surface expression of P-selectin) and increased plasma content of platelet-derived microparticles (PMP) were detected in MS patients. [142] Chronic lesions of MS patients contain tissue factor, as has been demonstrated by proteomics approach, [143] and elevated levels of platelet-specific $\alpha_{IIb}$ and $\beta_3$ transcripts were detected by microarray. [144] These findings are in concert with platelet presence in human MS lesions and in the murine brain in experimental autoimmune encephalomyelitis (EAE), rodent model of MS. [145] Platelet depletion as well as blocking GPIb$\alpha$ or $\alpha_{IIb}\beta_3$ by antibody Fab fragments in the inflammatory rather than immunization phase of the disease resulted in decreased EAE severity. Intravital microscopy revealed that platelets directly contributed to leukocyte rolling and adhesion to endothelium of the inflamed postcapillary venules via GPIb-Mac-1 interaction. [145]

Platelet activation in neuroinflammation may result from direct recognition of specific structures of damaged tissue. For instance, massive platelet activation and degranulation was induced upon systemic administration in mice of sialated glycosphingolipids (gangliosides), components of astroglial and neuronal lipid rafts of BBB. The cerebral gangliosides GT1b and GQ1b are specifically recognized by platelets with P-selectin playing the central role. [146]

The pathogenesis of **migraine**, the third most frequent disease worldwide, [147] involves sterile inflammation and hypersensitization of pain pathways. [148] Spontaneous platelet activation and aggregation in migraine patients have been known for years [149, 150] and expression of platelet receptors to fibrinogen and serotonin are altered in migraine patients. [151] PLA accumulating in the blood of patients with migraine[152] may link severe headaches and stroke. [152, 153] Preliminary observations suggest that antiplatelet therapies may be effective to reduce the severity of migraine. [154]

## 8. Platelets in allergic inflammation

Allergic diseases include a variety of conditions (atopic dermatitis, asthma, etc) that are caused by immune responses to environmental antigens. The hallmarks of allergy are the activation of $T_H2$ lymphocytes and the production of allergen-specific IgE antibodies, with the latter causing excessive activation of mast cells, eosinophils and basophils. This may become fatal when hypersensitivity results in systemic response designated as anaphylaxis. In chronic allergic inflammation, large numbers of immune cells accumulate at the affected site, causing substantial tissue damage. [155] The link between platelet activation and allergy has been studied for many years. [156, 157]

Independent studies report elevated plasma levels of platelet activation blood markers (β-thromboglobulin (β-TG), PF4, P-selectin, and PMPs) in patients with atopic dermatitis (AD) and psoriasis. [158-160] as well as in a mouse model of AD. [161] Plasma β-TG and PF4 may be markers for the severity of AD and psoriasis. [158]

In AD, it is possible that platelets contribute to an itch–scratch–hemorrhage cycle via release of pruritogenic factors such as histamine, 5-HT, acid proteases, IL-1β, TGF-β, PAF, and prostaglandin E2. [157]

While studies on platelet activation markers in asthmatic patients are inconclusive likely due to differences in experimental design, [162-167] the role of platelets in lung allergic inflammation has been established in mouse models. [168-171] There is a significant association between activation of platelets and eosinophils in the airways of individuals with asthma. [164] Moreover, circulating PLA are detected in the blood of allergen-challenged asthmatic patients and mice. [168] Platelets are essential for leukocyte recruitment to human and murine lungs in allergic inflammation [168, 170] and to the skin in chronic hapten-induced dermatitis, another mouse model of AD. [172] PLA circulate in the blood of asthmatic patients and in allergen-challenged mice. [165, 168] In all cases, the role of platelets was P-selectin-dependent.

Platelets express functional low (FcεRII) and high affinity (FcεRI) receptors for IgE at low level [173-175] Murine platelets can chemotactically respond to the sensitizing allergen via FcεR *in vitro* and *in vivo*, with platelet influx preceding the influx of leukocytes. [171] Upon engagement of IgE receptors, platelets release a variety of biologically active mediators[175, 176] including RANTES, a potent eosinophil chemoattractant. [177] IgE is stored in platelet $\alpha$-granules and released upon activation, which may potentially amplify the allergic response. [178]

Multiple products released by activated platelets are able to exacerbate the allergic response, e. g. , thromboxanes, histamine, and serotonin. [179, 180, 181] PAF is a potent mediator of allergic inflammation that is both released by and activates immune and inflammatory cells, including platelets [55, 182, 183]. In mice, platelets, and not mast cells, are the main source of serotonin released during allergic inflammatory response. [184] Besides allergic mediators platelets also contain substances limiting inflammation, for example, lipoxins, produced during platelet-leukocyte interactions. [185-188]

In asthma, platelets have been found to actively participate in most of its main features, including bronchial hyperresponsiveness, bronchoconstriction, airway inflammation and airway remodelling. [169, 189]

In conclusion, delineation of platelet contribution to the allergic response may be beneficial in developing more effective therapies, [190] as well as diagnostic and prognostic tools to evaluate efficacy of treatment of various allergic diseases. [191]

## 9. Concluding remarks

Platelets are important players in the development of inflammation. They store multiple inflammatory molecules that, upon release, chemoattract key innate immune cells leukocytes and stimulate endothelium. Platelets interact with leukocytes and support their interaction with vessel wall and egression to tissues. Platelets play a pivotal role in various inflammation-related diseases and targeting platelets could be a promising approach to manipulate the inflammatory response.

## Author details

Mònica Arman, Holly Payne, Tatyana Ponomaryov and Alexander Brill*

*Address all correspondence to: a. brill@bham. ac. uk

Centre for Cardiovascular Sciences, Institute of Biomedical Research, School of Clinical and Experimental Medicine, College of Medical and Dental Sciences, University of Birmingham, Birmingham, UK

## References

[1] Levy MM, Fink MP, Marshall JC, et al. 2001 SCCM/ESICM/ACCP/ATS/SIS International Sepsis Definitions Conference. *Crit Care Med*. 2003;31(4):1250-1256.

[2] Page CP. Platelets as inflammatory cells. *Immunopharmacology*. 1989;17(1):51-59.

[3] Shi G, Morrell CN. Platelets as initiators and mediators of inflammation at the vessel wall. *Thromb Res*. 2011;127(5):387-390.

[4] Boehlen F, Clemetson KJ. Platelet chemokines and their receptors: what is their relevance to platelet storage and transfusion practice? *Transfus Med*. 2001;11(6):403-417.

[5] Smyth SS, McEver RP, Weyrich AS, et al. Platelet functions beyond hemostasis. *J Thromb Haemost*. 2009;7(11):1759-1766.

[6] Lambert MP, Rauova L, Bailey M, Sola-Visner MC, Kowalska MA, Poncz M. Platelet factor 4 is a negative autocrine in vivo regulator of megakaryopoiesis: clinical and therapeutic implications. *Blood*. 2007;110(4):1153-1160.

[7] Gawaz M, Langer H, May AE. Platelets in inflammation and atherogenesis. *J Clin Invest*. 2005;115(12):3378-3384.

[8] Gear AR, Camerini D. Platelet chemokines and chemokine receptors: linking hemostasis, inflammation, and host defense. *Microcirculation*. 2003;10(3-4):335-350.

[9] Thornton P, McColl BW, Greenhalgh A, Denes A, Allan SM, Rothwell NJ. Platelet interleukin-1alpha drives cerebrovascular inflammation. *Blood*. 2010;115(17):3632-3639.

[10] Boilard E, Nigrovic PA, Larabee K, et al. Platelets amplify inflammation in arthritis via collagen-dependent microparticle production. *Science*. 2010;327(5965):580-583.

[11] Lindemann S, Tolley ND, Dixon DA, et al. Activated platelets mediate inflammatory signaling by regulated interleukin 1beta synthesis. *J Cell Biol*. 2001;154(3):485-490.

[12] Denis MM, Tolley ND, Bunting M, et al. Escaping the nuclear confines: signal-dependent pre-mRNA splicing in anucleate platelets. *Cell*. 2005;122(3):379-391.

[13] Brown GT, Narayanan P, Li W, Silverstein RL, McIntyre TM. Lipopolysaccharide stimulates platelets through an IL-1beta autocrine loop. *J Immunol*. 2013;191(10): 5196-5203.

[14] Schober A, Manka D, von Hundelshausen P, et al. Deposition of platelet RANTES triggering monocyte recruitment requires P-selectin and is involved in neointima formation after arterial injury. *Circulation*. 2002;106(12):1523-1529.

[15] Appay V, Rowland-Jones SL. RANTES: a versatile and controversial chemokine. *Trends Immunol*. 2001;22(2):83-87.

[16] Cook DN. The role of MIP-1 alpha in inflammation and hematopoiesis. *J Leukoc Biol*. 1996;59(1):61-66.

[17] Lentzsch S, Gries M, Janz M, Bargou R, Dorken B, Mapara MY. Macrophage inflammatory protein 1-alpha (MIP-1 alpha) triggers migration and signaling cascades mediating survival and proliferation in multiple myeloma (MM) cells. *Blood*. 2003;101(9):3568-3573.

[18] Henn V, Slupsky JR, Grafe M, et al. CD40 ligand on activated platelets triggers an inflammatory reaction of endothelial cells. *Nature*. 1998;391(6667):591-594.

[19] Ruiz FA, Lea CR, Oldfield E, Docampo R. Human platelet dense granules contain polyphosphate and are similar to acidocalcisomes of bacteria and unicellular eukaryotes. *J Biol Chem*. 2004;279(43):44250-44257.

[20] Muller F, Mutch NJ, Schenk WA, et al. Platelet polyphosphates are proinflammatory and procoagulant mediators in vivo. *Cell*. 2009;139(6):1143-1156.

[21] Faxalv L, Boknas N, Strom JO, et al. Putting polyphosphates to the test: evidence against platelet-induced activation of factor XII. *Blood*. 2013;122(23):3818-3824.

[22] Bombeli T, Schwartz BR, Harlan JM. Adhesion of activated platelets to endothelial cells: evidence for a GPIIbIIIa-dependent bridging mechanism and novel roles for endothelial intercellular adhesion molecule 1 (ICAM-1), alphavbeta3 integrin, and GPIbalpha. *J Exp Med*. 1998;187(3):329-339.

[23] Romo GM, Dong JF, Schade AJ, et al. The glycoprotein Ib-IX-V complex is a platelet counterreceptor for P-selectin. *J Exp Med*. 1999;190(6):803-814.

[24] Frenette PS, Denis CV, Weiss L, et al. P-Selectin glycoprotein ligand 1 (PSGL-1) is expressed on platelets and can mediate platelet-endothelial interactions in vivo. *J Exp Med*. 2000;191(8):1413-1422.

[25] Gawaz M, Neumann FJ, Dickfeld T, et al. Vitronectin receptor (alpha(v)beta3) mediates platelet adhesion to the luminal aspect of endothelial cells: implications for reperfusion in acute myocardial infarction. *Circulation*. 1997;96(6):1809-1818.

[26] Andre P, Denis CV, Ware J, et al. Platelets adhere to and translocate on von Willebrand factor presented by endothelium in stimulated veins. *Blood*. 2000;96(10): 3322-3328.

[27] Bultmann A, Li Z, Wagner S, et al. Impact of glycoprotein VI and platelet adhesion on atherosclerosis--a possible role of fibronectin. *J Mol Cell Cardiol*. 2010;49(3):532-542.

[28] Schonberger T, Ziegler M, Borst O, et al. The dimeric platelet collagen receptor GPVI-Fc reduces platelet adhesion to activated endothelium and preserves myocardial function after transient ischemia in mice. *Am J Physiol Cell Physiol*. 2012;303(7):C757-766.

[29] Ishikawa M, Cooper D, Arumugam TV, Zhang JH, Nanda A, Granger DN. Platelet-leukocyte-endothelial cell interactions after middle cerebral artery occlusion and reperfusion. *J Cereb Blood Flow Metab*. 2004;24(8):907-915.

[30] Nishijima K, Kiryu J, Tsujikawa A, et al. In vivo evaluation of platelet--endothelial interactions after transient retinal ischemia. *Invest Ophthalmol Vis Sci*. 2001;42(9): 2102-2109.

[31] Massberg S, Schurzinger K, Lorenz M, et al. Platelet adhesion via glycoprotein IIb integrin is critical for atheroprogression and focal cerebral ischemia: an in vivo study in mice lacking glycoprotein IIb. *Circulation*. 2005;112(8):1180-1188.

[32] Massberg S, Enders G, Matos FC, et al. Fibrinogen deposition at the postischemic vessel wall promotes platelet adhesion during ischemia-reperfusion in vivo. *Blood*. 1999;94(11):3829-3838.

[33] Brill A, Fuchs TA, Chauhan AK, et al. von Willebrand factor-mediated platelet adhesion is critical for deep vein thrombosis in mouse models. *Blood*. 2011;117(4): 1400-1407.

[34] Nishimura S, Manabe I, Nagasaki M, et al. In vivo imaging visualizes discoid platelet aggregations without endothelium disruption and implicates contribution of inflammatory cytokine and integrin signaling. *Blood*. 2012;119(8):e45-56.

[35] Grau GE, Tacchini-Cottier F, Vesin C, et al. TNF-induced microvascular pathology: active role for platelets and importance of the LFA-1/ICAM-1 interaction. *Eur Cytokine Netw*. 1993;4(6):415-419.

[36] Grau GE, Mackenzie CD, Carr RA, et al. Platelet accumulation in brain microvessels in fatal pediatric cerebral malaria. *J Infect Dis*. 2003;187(3):461-466.

[37] Faille D, El-Assaad F, Alessi MC, Fusai T, Combes V, Grau GE. Platelet-endothelial cell interactions in cerebral malaria: the end of a cordial understanding. *Thromb Haemost*. 2009;102(6):1093-1102.

[38] van der Heyde HC, Gramaglia I, Sun G, Woods C. Platelet depletion by anti-CD41 (alphaIIb) mAb injection early but not late in the course of disease protects against Plasmodium berghei pathogenesis by altering the levels of pathogenic cytokines. *Blood*. 2005;105(5):1956-1963.

[39] Aggrey AA, Srivastava K, Ture S, Field DJ, Morrell CN. Platelet induction of the acute-phase response is protective in murine experimental cerebral malaria. *J Immunol*. 2013;190(9):4685-4691.

[40] Ogura H, Kawasaki T, Tanaka H, et al. Activated platelets enhance microparticle formation and platelet-leukocyte interaction in severe trauma and sepsis. *J Trauma*. 2001;50(5):801-809.

[41] Grau AJ, Ruf A, Vogt A, et al. Increased fraction of circulating activated platelets in acute and previous cerebrovascular ischemia. *Thromb Haemost*. 1998;80(2):298-301.

[42] Nomura S, Shouzu A, Omoto S, Nishikawa M, Fukuhara S. Significance of chemokines and activated platelets in patients with diabetes. *Clin Exp Immunol*. 2000;121(3): 437-443.

[43] Dole VS, Bergmeier W, Mitchell HA, Eichenberger SC, Wagner DD. Activated platelets induce Weibel-Palade-body secretion and leukocyte rolling in vivo: role of P-selectin. *Blood*. 2005;106(7):2334-2339.

[44] Lievens D, Zernecke A, Seijkens T, et al. Platelet CD40L mediates thrombotic and inflammatory processes in atherosclerosis. *Blood*. 2010;116(20):4317-4327.

[45] Huo Y, Schober A, Forlow SB, et al. Circulating activated platelets exacerbate atherosclerosis in mice deficient in apolipoprotein E. *Nat Med*. 2003;9(1):61-67.

[46] Burger PC, Wagner DD. Platelet P-selectin facilitates atherosclerotic lesion development. *Blood*. 2003;101(7):2661-2666.

[47] Elalamy I, Chakroun T, Gerotziafas GT, et al. Circulating platelet-leukocyte aggregates: a marker of microvascular injury in diabetic patients. *Thromb Res*. 2008;121(6): 843-848.

[48] Turgut B, Turgut N, Celik Y, Tekgunduz E, Pamuk GE, Demir M. Differences in platelet-leukocyte aggregates among subtypes of acute cerebral ischemia. *J Neurol Sci*. 2011;305(1-2):126-130.

[49] de Abreu AV, Rondina MT, Weyrich AS, Zimmerman GA. Inflammation. *In: Platelets, 3d edition*. 2012.

[50] Lindmark E, Tenno T, Siegbahn A. Role of platelet P-selectin and CD40 ligand in the induction of monocytic tissue factor expression. *Arterioscler Thromb Vasc Biol*. 2000;20(10):2322-2328.

[51] Wang HB, Wang JT, Zhang L, et al. P-selectin primes leukocyte integrin activation during inflammation. *Nat Immunol*. 2007;8(8):882-892.

[52] Evangelista V, Manarini S, Rotondo S, et al. Platelet/polymorphonuclear leukocyte interaction in dynamic conditions: evidence of adhesion cascade and cross talk between P-selectin and the beta 2 integrin CD11b/CD18. *Blood*. 1996;88(11):4183-4194.

[53] Evangelista V, Manarini S, Sideri R, et al. Platelet/polymorphonuclear leukocyte interaction: P-selectin triggers protein-tyrosine phosphorylation-dependent CD11b/ CD18 adhesion: role of PSGL-1 as a signaling molecule. *Blood*. 1999;93(3):876-885.

[54] Simon DI, Chen Z, Xu H, et al. Platelet glycoprotein ibalpha is a counterreceptor for the leukocyte integrin Mac-1 (CD11b/CD18). *J Exp Med*. 2000;192(2):193-204.

[55] Weber C, Springer TA. Neutrophil accumulation on activated, surface-adherent platelets in flow is mediated by interaction of Mac-1 with fibrinogen bound to alphaIIb-beta3 and stimulated by platelet-activating factor. *J Clin Invest*. 1997;100(8):2085-2093.

[56] Ghasemzadeh M, Hosseini E. Platelet-leukocyte crosstalk: Linking proinflammatory responses to procoagulant state. *Thromb Res*. 2013;131(3):191-197.

[57] Plescia J, Altieri DC. Activation of Mac-1 (CD11b/CD18)-bound factor X by released cathepsin G defines an alternative pathway of leucocyte initiation of coagulation. *Biochem J*. 1996;319 (Pt 3):873-879.

[58] Kawasaki T, Dewerchin M, Lijnen HR, Vreys I, Vermylen J, Hoylaerts MF. Mouse carotid artery ligation induces platelet-leukocyte-dependent luminal fibrin, required for neointima development. *Circ Res*. 2001;88(2):159-166.

[59] Yokoyama S, Ikeda H, Haramaki N, Yasukawa H, Murohara T, Imaizumi T. Platelet P-selectin plays an important role in arterial thrombogenesis by forming large stable platelet-leukocyte aggregates. *J Am Coll Cardiol*. 2005;45(8):1280-1286.

[60] Michelson AD, Barnard MR, Krueger LA, Valeri CR, Furman MI. Circulating monocyte-platelet aggregates are a more sensitive marker of in vivo platelet activation than platelet surface P-selectin: studies in baboons, human coronary intervention, and human acute myocardial infarction. *Circulation*. 2001;104(13):1533-1537.

[61] Appeldoorn CC, Bonnefoy A, Lutters BC, et al. Gallic acid antagonizes P-selectin-mediated platelet-leukocyte interactions: implications for the French paradox. *Circulation*. 2005;111(1):106-112.

[62] Diacovo TG, Puri KD, Warnock RA, Springer TA, von Andrian UH. Platelet-mediated lymphocyte delivery to high endothelial venules. *Science*. 1996;273(5272):252-255.

[63] Brinkmann V, Reichard U, Goosmann C, et al. Neutrophil extracellular traps kill bacteria. *Science*. 2004;303(5663):1532-1535.

[64] Maugeri N, Campana L, Gavina M, et al. Activated platelets present High Mobility Group Box 1 to neutrophils, inducing autophagy and promoting the extrusion of neutrophil extracellular traps. *J Thromb Haemost*. 2014.

[65] Fuchs TA, Brill A, Duerschmied D, et al. Extracellular DNA traps promote thrombosis. *Proc Natl Acad Sci U S A*. 2010;107(36):15880-15885.

[66] Fuchs TA, Bhandari AA, Wagner DD. Histones induce rapid and profound thrombocytopenia in mice. *Blood*. 2011;118(13):3708-3714.

[67] Kawai T, Akira S. Toll-like receptors and their crosstalk with other innate receptors in infection and immunity. *Immunity*. 2011;34(5):637-650.

[68] Piccinini AM, Midwood KS. DAMPening inflammation by modulating TLR signalling. *Mediators Inflamm*. 2010;2010.

[69] Shiraki R, Inoue N, Kawasaki S, et al. Expression of Toll-like receptors on human platelets. *Thromb Res*. 2004;113(6):379-385.

[70] Cognasse F, Hamzeh H, Chavarin P, Acquart S, Genin C, Garraud O. Evidence of Toll-like receptor molecules on human platelets. *Immunol Cell Biol*. 2005;83(2):196-198.

[71] Andonegui G, Kerfoot SM, McNagny K, Ebbert KV, Patel KD, Kubes P. Platelets express functional Toll-like receptor-4. *Blood*. 2005;106(7):2417-2423.

[72] Aslam R, Speck ER, Kim M, et al. Platelet Toll-like receptor expression modulates lipopolysaccharide-induced thrombocytopenia and tumor necrosis factor-alpha production in vivo. *Blood*. 2006;107(2):637-641.

[73] Beaulieu LM, Freedman JE. The role of inflammation in regulating platelet production and function: Toll-like receptors in platelets and megakaryocytes. *Thromb Res*. 2010;125(3):205-209.

[74] Koupenova M, Vitseva O, Mackay CR, et al. Platelet-TLR7 mediates host survival and platelet count during viral infection in the absence of platelet-dependent thrombosis. *Blood*. 2014.

[75] Thon JN, Peters CG, Machlus KR, et al. T granules in human platelets function in TLR9 organization and signaling. *J Cell Biol*. 2012;198(4):561-574.

[76] Panigrahi S, Ma Y, Hong L, et al. Engagement of platelet toll-like receptor 9 by novel endogenous ligands promotes platelet hyperreactivity and thrombosis. *Circ Res*. 2013;112(1):103-112.

[77] Ward JR, Bingle L, Judge HM, et al. Agonists of toll-like receptor (TLR)2 and TLR4 are unable to modulate platelet activation by adenosine diphosphate and platelet activating factor. *Thromb Haemost*. 2005;94(4):831-838.

[78] Kalvegren H, Skoglund C, Helldahl C, Lerm M, Grenegard M, Bengtsson T. Toll-like receptor 2 stimulation of platelets is mediated by purinergic P2X1-dependent Ca2+ mobilisation, cyclooxygenase and purinergic P2Y1 and P2Y12 receptor activation. *Thromb Haemost*. 2010;103(2):398-407.

[79] Blair P, Rex S, Vitseva O, et al. Stimulation of Toll-like receptor 2 in human platelets induces a thromboinflammatory response through activation of phosphoinositide 3-kinase. *Circ Res*. 2009;104(3):346-354.

[80] Rivadeneyra L, Carestia A, Etulain J, et al. Regulation of platelet responses triggered by Toll-like receptor 2 and 4 ligands is another non-genomic role of nuclear factor-kappaB. *Thromb Res*. 2014;133(2):235-243.

[81] Assinger A, Laky M, Badrnya S, Esfandeyari A, Volf I. Periodontopathogens induce expression of CD40L on human platelets via TLR2 and TLR4. *Thromb Res*. 2012;130(3):e73-78.

[82] Assinger A, Kral JB, Yaiw KC, et al. Human cytomegalovirus-platelet interaction triggers toll-like receptor 2-dependent proinflammatory and proangiogenic responses. *Arterioscler Thromb Vasc Biol*. 2014;34(4):801-809.

[83] Tsai JC, Lin YW, Huang CY, et al. The role of calpain-myosin 9-Rab7b pathway in mediating the expression of Toll-like receptor 4 in platelets: a novel mechanism involved in alpha-granules trafficking. *PLoS One*. 2014;9(1):e85833.

[84] Rumbaut RE, Bellera RV, Randhawa JK, et al. Endotoxin enhances microvascular thrombosis in mouse cremaster venules via a TLR4-dependent, neutrophil-independent mechanism. *Am J Physiol Heart Circ Physiol*. 2006;290(4):H1671-1679.

[85] Hashimoto K, Jayachandran M, Owen WG, Miller VM. Aggregation and microparticle production through toll-like receptor 4 activation in platelets from recently menopausal women. *J Cardiovasc Pharmacol*. 2009;54(1):57-62.

[86] Zhang G, Han J, Welch EJ, et al. Lipopolysaccharide stimulates platelet secretion and potentiates platelet aggregation via TLR4/MyD88 and the cGMP-dependent protein kinase pathway. *J Immunol*. 2009;182(12):7997-8004.

[87] Montrucchio G, Bosco O, Del Sorbo L, et al. Mechanisms of the priming effect of low doses of lipopoly-saccharides on leukocyte-dependent platelet aggregation in whole blood. *Thromb Haemost*. 2003;90(5):872-881.

[88] Endo Y, Shibazaki M, Nakamura M, Takada H. Contrasting effects of lipopolysaccharides (endotoxins) from oral black-pigmented bacteria and Enterobacteriaceae on platelets, a major source of serotonin, and on histamine-forming enzyme in mice. *J Infect Dis*. 1997;175(6):1404-1412.

[89] Shibazaki M, Kawabata Y, Yokochi T, Nishida A, Takada H, Endo Y. Complement-dependent accumulation and degradation of platelets in the lung and liver induced by injection of lipopolysaccharides. *Infect Immun*. 1999;67(10):5186-5191.

[90] Stark RJ, Aghakasiri N, Rumbaut RE. Platelet-derived Toll-like receptor 4 (Tlr-4) is sufficient to promote microvascular thrombosis in endotoxemia. *PLoS One*. 2012;7(7):e41254.

[91] Stahl AL, Sartz L, Nelsson A, Bekassy ZD, Karpman D. Shiga toxin and lipopolysaccharide induce platelet-leukocyte aggregates and tissue factor release, a thrombotic mechanism in hemolytic uremic syndrome. *PLoS One*. 2009;4(9):e6990.

[92] Stahl AL, Svensson M, Morgelin M, et al. Lipopolysaccharide from enterohemorrhagic Escherichia coli binds to platelets through TLR4 and CD62 and is detected on circulating platelets in patients with hemolytic uremic syndrome. *Blood*. 2006;108(1): 167-176.

[93] Clark SR, Ma AC, Tavener SA, et al. Platelet TLR4 activates neutrophil extracellular traps to ensnare bacteria in septic blood. *Nat Med*. 2007;13(4):463-469.

[94] Angus DC, van der Poll T. Severe sepsis and septic shock. *N Engl J Med*. 2013;369(9): 840-851.

[95] Marshall JC. Why have clinical trials in sepsis failed? *Trends Mol Med*. 2014;20(4): 195-203.

[96] Buras JA, Holzmann B, Sitkovsky M. Animal models of sepsis: setting the stage. *Nat Rev Drug Discov*. 2005;4(10):854-865.

[97] Seok J, Warren HS, Cuenca AG, et al. Genomic responses in mouse models poorly mimic human inflammatory diseases. *Proc Natl Acad Sci U S A*. 2013;110(9):3507-3512.

[98] Vincent JL, Yagushi A, Pradier O. Platelet function in sepsis. *Crit Care Med*. 2002;30(5 Suppl):S313-317.

[99] Katz JN, Kolappa KP, Becker RC. Beyond thrombosis: the versatile platelet in critical illness. *Chest*. 2011;139(3):658-668.

[100] Semeraro N, Ammollo CT, Semeraro F, Colucci M. Sepsis, thrombosis and organ dysfunction. *Thromb Res*. 2012;129(3):290-295.

[101] Akinosoglou K, Alexopoulos D. Use of antiplatelet agents in sepsis: a glimpse into the future. *Thromb Res*. 2014;133(2):131-138.

[102] Warkentin TE, Aird WC, Rand JH. Platelet-endothelial interactions: sepsis, HIT, and antiphospholipid syndrome. *Hematology Am Soc Hematol Educ Program*. 2003:497-519.

[103] Cox D, Kerrigan SW, Watson SP. Platelets and the innate immune system: mechanisms of bacterial-induced platelet activation. *J Thromb Haemost*. 2011;9(6):1097-1107.

[104] Semple JW, Italiano JE, Jr. , Freedman J. Platelets and the immune continuum. *Nat Rev Immunol*. 2011;11(4):264-274.

[105] Russwurm S, Vickers J, Meier-Hellmann A, et al. Platelet and leukocyte activation correlate with the severity of septic organ dysfunction. *Shock*. 2002;17(4):263-268.

[106] Salat A, Bodingbauer G, Boehm D, et al. Changes of platelet surface antigens in patients suffering from abdominal septic shock. *Thromb Res*. 1999;95(6):289-294.

[107] Yaguchi A, Lobo FL, Vincent JL, Pradier O. Platelet function in sepsis. *J Thromb Haemost*. 2004;2(12):2096-2102.

[108] Inwald DP, Faust SN, Lister P, et al. Platelet and soluble CD40L in meningococcal sepsis. *Intensive Care Med*. 2006;32(9):1432-1437.

[109] Gawaz M, Fateh-Moghadam S, Pilz G, Gurland HJ, Werdan K. Platelet activation and interaction with leucocytes in patients with sepsis or multiple organ failure. *Eur J Clin Invest*. 1995;25(11):843-851.

[110] Gawaz M, Dickfeld T, Bogner C, Fateh-Moghadam S, Neumann FJ. Platelet function in septic multiple organ dysfunction syndrome. *Intensive Care Med*. 1997;23(4): 379-385.

[111] Mavrommatis AC, Theodoridis T, Orfanidou A, Roussos C, Christopoulou-Kokkinou V, Zakynthinos S. Coagulation system and platelets are fully activated in uncomplicated sepsis. *Crit Care Med.* 2000;28(2):451-457.

[112] Washington AV, Gibot S, Acevedo I, et al. TREM-like transcript-1 protects against inflammation-associated hemorrhage by facilitating platelet aggregation in mice and humans. *J Clin Invest.* 2009;119(6):1489-1501.

[113] Esponda O, Morales J, Aguilar A, Gomez M, Washington AV. Clinical studies support a role for trem-like transcript-1 during the progression of sepsis. *Bol Asoc Med P R.* 2010;102(3):59-61.

[114] Morales J, Villa K, Gattis J, et al. Soluble TLT-1 modulates platelet-endothelial cell interactions and actin polymerization. *Blood Coagul Fibrinolysis.* 2010;21(3):229-236.

[115] Derive M, Bouazza Y, Sennoun N, et al. Soluble TREM-like transcript-1 regulates leukocyte activation and controls microbial sepsis. *J Immunol.* 2012;188(11):5585-5592.

[116] Boldt J, Menges T, Wollbruck M, Sonneborn S, Hempelmann G. Platelet function in critically ill patients. *Chest.* 1994;106(3):899-903.

[117] Freishtat RJ, Natale J, Benton AS, et al. Sepsis alters the megakaryocyte-platelet transcriptional axis resulting in granzyme B-mediated lymphotoxicity. *Am J Respir Crit Care Med.* 2009;179(6):467-473.

[118] Rondina MT, Schwertz H, Harris ES, et al. The septic milieu triggers expression of spliced tissue factor mRNA in human platelets. *J Thromb Haemost.* 2011;9(4):748-758.

[119] Schwertz H, Tolley ND, Foulks JM, et al. Signal-dependent splicing of tissue factor pre-mRNA modulates the thrombogenicity of human platelets. *J Exp Med.* 2006;203(11):2433-2440.

[120] Kaur C, Ling EA. Blood brain barrier in hypoxic-ischemic conditions. *Curr Neurovasc Res.* 2008;5(1):71-81.

[121] Zlokovic BV. The blood-brain barrier in health and chronic neurodegenerative disorders. *Neuron.* 2008;57(2):178-201.

[122] Langer HF, Chavakis T. Platelets and neurovascular inflammation. *Thromb Haemost.* 2013;110(5):888-893.

[123] Behari M, Shrivastava M. Role of platelets in neurodegenerative diseases: a universal pathophysiology. *Int J Neurosci.* 2013;123(5):287-299.

[124] Horstman LL, Jy W, Ahn YS, et al. Role of platelets in neuroinflammation: a wide-angle perspective. *J Neuroinflammation.* 2010;7:10.

[125] Amor S, Peferoen LA, Vogel DY, et al. Inflammation in neurodegenerative diseases--an update. *Immunology.* 2014;142(2):151-166.

[126] Nieswandt B, Kleinschnitz C, Stoll G. Ischaemic stroke: a thrombo-inflammatory disease? *J Physiol*. 2011;589(Pt 17):4115-4123.

[127] Kleinschnitz C, Pozgajova M, Pham M, Bendszus M, Nieswandt B, Stoll G. Targeting platelets in acute experimental stroke: impact of glycoprotein Ib, VI, and IIb/IIIa blockade on infarct size, functional outcome, and intracranial bleeding. *Circulation*. 2007;115(17):2323-2330.

[128] Zhao BQ, Chauhan AK, Canault M, et al. von Willebrand factor-cleaving protease ADAMTS13 reduces ischemic brain injury in experimental stroke. *Blood*. 2009;114(15):3329-3334.

[129] Adams HP, Jr. , Effron MB, Torner J, et al. Emergency administration of abciximab for treatment of patients with acute ischemic stroke: results of an international phase III trial: Abciximab in Emergency Treatment of Stroke Trial (AbESTT-II). *Stroke*. 2008;39(1):87-99.

[130] Stoll G, Kleinschnitz C, Nieswandt B. Molecular mechanisms of thrombus formation in ischemic stroke: novel insights and targets for treatment. *Blood*. 2008;112(9): 3555-3562.

[131] De Meyer SF, Stoll G, Wagner DD, Kleinschnitz C. von Willebrand factor: an emerging target in stroke therapy. *Stroke*. 2012;43(2):599-606.

[132] Goebel S, Li Z, Vogelmann J, et al. The GPVI-Fc fusion protein Revacept improves cerebral infarct volume and functional outcome in stroke. *PLoS One*. 2013;8(7):e66960.

[133] Belayev L, Eady TN, Khoutorova L, et al. Superior Neuroprotective Efficacy of LAU-0901, a Novel Platelet-Activating Factor Antagonist, in Experimental Stroke. *Transl Stroke Res*. 2012;3(1):154-163.

[134] Sardi F, Fassina L, Venturini L, et al. Alzheimer's disease, autoimmunity and inflammation. The good, the bad and the ugly. *Autoimmun Rev*. 2011;11(2):149-153.

[135] de Silva HA, Aronson JK, Grahame-Smith DG, Jobst KA, Smith AD. Abnormal function of potassium channels in platelets of patients with Alzheimer's disease. *Lancet*. 1998;352(9140):1590-1593.

[136] Laske C, Leyhe T, Stransky E, et al. Association of platelet-derived soluble glycoprotein VI in plasma with Alzheimer's disease. *J Psychiatr Res*. 2008;42(9):746-751.

[137] Stellos K, Panagiota V, Kogel A, Leyhe T, Gawaz M, Laske C. Predictive value of platelet activation for the rate of cognitive decline in Alzheimer's disease patients. *J Cereb Blood Flow Metab*. 2010;30(11):1817-1820.

[138] Catricala S, Torti M, Ricevuti G. Alzheimer disease and platelets: how's that relevant. *Immun Ageing*. 2012;9(1):20.

[139] Di Luca M, Pastorino L, Bianchetti A, et al. Differential level of platelet amyloid beta precursor protein isoforms: an early marker for Alzheimer disease. *Arch Neurol.* 1998;55(9):1195-1200.

[140] Neumann K, Farias G, Slachevsky A, Perez P, Maccioni RB. Human platelets tau: a potential peripheral marker for Alzheimer's disease. *J Alzheimers Dis.* 2011;25(1): 103-109.

[141] Hernandez-Pedro NY, Espinosa-Ramirez G, de la Cruz VP, Pineda B, Sotelo J. Initial immunopathogenesis of multiple sclerosis: innate immune response. *Clin Dev Immunol.* 2013;2013:413465.

[142] Sheremata WA, Jy W, Horstman LL, Ahn YS, Alexander JS, Minagar A. Evidence of platelet activation in multiple sclerosis. *J Neuroinflammation.* 2008;5:27.

[143] Han MH, Hwang SI, Roy DB, et al. Proteomic analysis of active multiple sclerosis lesions reveals therapeutic targets. *Nature.* 2008;451(7182):1076-1081.

[144] Lock C, Hermans G, Pedotti R, et al. Gene-microarray analysis of multiple sclerosis lesions yields new targets validated in autoimmune encephalomyelitis. *Nat Med.* 2002;8(5):500-508.

[145] Langer HF, Choi EY, Zhou H, et al. Platelets contribute to the pathogenesis of experimental autoimmune encephalomyelitis. *Circ Res.* 2012;110(9):1202-1210.

[146] Sotnikov I, Veremeyko T, Starossom SC, Barteneva N, Weiner HL, Ponomarev ED. Platelets recognize brain-specific glycolipid structures, respond to neurovascular damage and promote neuroinflammation. *PLoS One.* 2013;8(3):e58979.

[147] Vos T, Flaxman AD, Naghavi M, et al. Years lived with disability (YLDs) for 1160 sequelae of 289 diseases and injuries 1990-2010: a systematic analysis for the Global Burden of Disease Study 2010. *Lancet.* 2012;380(9859):2163-2196.

[148] Danese E, Montagnana M, Lippi G. Platelets and migraine. *Thromb Res.* 2014;134(1): 17-22.

[149] Couch JR, Hassanein RS. Platelet aggregability in migraine. *Neurology.* 1977;27(9): 843-848.

[150] D'Andrea G, Cananzi AR, Toldo M, Ferro-Milone F. Platelet activation and migraine: a study with flunarizine. *Headache.* 1986;26(7):339-342.

[151] Govitrapong P, Limthavon C, Srikiatkhachorn A. 5-HT2 serotonin receptor on blood platelet of migraine patients. *Headache.* 1992;32(10):480-484.

[152] Zeller JA, Frahm K, Baron R, Stingele R, Deuschl G. Platelet-leukocyte interaction and platelet activation in migraine: a link to ischemic stroke? *J Neurol Neurosurg Psychiatry.* 2004;75(7):984-987.

[153] Jamieson DG, Cheng NT, Skliut M. Headache and acute stroke. *Curr Pain Headache Rep*. 2014;18(9):444.

[154] Wilmshurst PT, Nightingale S, Walsh KP, Morrison WL. Clopidogrel reduces migraine with aura after transcatheter closure of persistent foramen ovale and atrial septal defects. *Heart*. 2005;91(9):1173-1175.

[155] Galli SJ, Tsai M, Piliponsky AM. The development of allergic inflammation. *Nature*. 2008;454(7203):445-454.

[156] Kasperska-Zajac A, Rogala B. Platelet activation during allergic inflammation. *Inflammation*. 2007;30(5):161-166.

[157] Katoh N. Platelets as versatile regulators of cutaneous inflammation. *J Dermatol Sci*. 2009;53(2):89-95.

[158] Tamagawa-Mineoka R, Katoh N, Ueda E, Masuda K, Kishimoto S. Elevated platelet activation in patients with atopic dermatitis and psoriasis: increased plasma levels of beta-thromboglobulin and platelet factor 4. *Allergol Int*. 2008;57(4):391-396.

[159] Tamagawa-Mineoka R, Katoh N, Ueda E, Masuda K, Kishimoto S. Platelet-derived microparticles and soluble P-selectin as platelet activation markers in patients with atopic dermatitis. *Clin Immunol*. 2009;131(3):495-500.

[160] Nastalek M, Potaczek DP, Wojas-Pelc A, Undas A. Plasma platelet activation markers in patients with atopic dermatitis and concomitant allergic diseases. *J Dermatol Sci*. 2011;64(1):79-82.

[161] Watanabe O, Natori K, Tamari M, Shiomoto Y, Kubo S, Nakamura Y. Significantly elevated expression of PF4 (platelet factor 4) and eotaxin in the NOA mouse, a model for atopic dermatitis. *J Hum Genet*. 1999;44(3):173-176.

[162] Yamamoto H, Nagata M, Tabe K, et al. The evidence of platelet activation in bronchial asthma. *J Allergy Clin Immunol*. 1993;91(1 Pt 1):79-87.

[163] Kasperska-Zajac A, Rogala B. Platelet activity measured by plasma levels of beta-thromboglobulin and platelet factor 4 in seasonal allergic rhinitis during natural pollen exposure. *Inflamm Res*. 2003;52(11):477-479.

[164] Benton AS, Kumar N, Lerner J, et al. Airway platelet activation is associated with airway eosinophilic inflammation in asthma. *J Investig Med*. 2010;58(8):987-990.

[165] Johansson MW, Han ST, Gunderson KA, Busse WW, Jarjour NN, Mosher DF. Platelet activation, P-selectin, and eosinophil beta1-integrin activation in asthma. *Am J Respir Crit Care Med*. 2012;185(5):498-507.

[166] Tuncel T, Uysal P, Hocaoglu AB, Erge DO, Karaman O, Uzuner N. Change of mean platelet volume values in asthmatic children as an inflammatory marker. *Allergol Immunopathol (Madr)*. 2012;40(2):104-107.

[167] Duarte D, Taveira-Gomes T, Sokhatska O, et al. Increased circulating platelet microparticles as a potential biomarker in asthma. *Allergy*. 2013;68(8):1073-1075.

[168] Pitchford SC, Yano H, Lever R, et al. Platelets are essential for leukocyte recruitment in allergic inflammation. *J Allergy Clin Immunol*. 2003;112(1):109-118.

[169] Pitchford SC, Riffo-Vasquez Y, Sousa A, et al. Platelets are necessary for airway wall remodeling in a murine model of chronic allergic inflammation. *Blood*. 2004;103(2): 639-647.

[170] Pitchford SC, Momi S, Giannini S, et al. Platelet P-selectin is required for pulmonary eosinophil and lymphocyte recruitment in a murine model of allergic inflammation. *Blood*. 2005;105(5):2074-2081.

[171] Pitchford SC, Momi S, Baglioni S, et al. Allergen induces the migration of platelets to lung tissue in allergic asthma. *Am J Respir Crit Care Med*. 2008;177(6):604-612.

[172] Tamagawa-Mineoka R, Katoh N, Ueda E, Takenaka H, Kita M, Kishimoto S. The role of platelets in leukocyte recruitment in chronic contact hypersensitivity induced by repeated elicitation. *Am J Pathol*. 2007;170(6):2019-2029.

[173] Joseph M, Capron A, Ameisen JC, et al. The receptor for IgE on blood platelets. *Eur J Immunol*. 1986;16(3):306-312.

[174] Joseph M, Gounni AS, Kusnierz JP, et al. Expression and functions of the high-affinity IgE receptor on human platelets and megakaryocyte precursors. *Eur J Immunol*. 1997;27(9):2212-2218.

[175] Hasegawa S, Pawankar R, Suzuki K, et al. Functional expression of the high affinity receptor for IgE (FcepsilonRI) in human platelets and its' intracellular expression in human megakaryocytes. *Blood*. 1999;93(8):2543-2551.

[176] Hasegawa S, Tashiro N, Matsubara T, Furukawa S, Ra C. A comparison of FcepsilonRI-mediated RANTES release from human platelets between allergic patients and healthy individuals. *Int Arch Allergy Immunol*. 2001;125 Suppl 1:42-47.

[177] Kameyoshi Y, Schroder JM, Christophers E, Yamamoto S. Identification of the cytokine RANTES released from platelets as an eosinophil chemotactic factor. *Int Arch Allergy Immunol*. 1994;104 Suppl 1(1):49-51.

[178] Klouche M, Klinger MH, Kuhnel W, Wilhelm D. Endocytosis, storage, and release of IgE by human platelets: differences in patients with type I allergy and nonatopic subjects. *J Allergy Clin Immunol*. 1997;100(2):235-241.

[179] Allen IC, Hartney JM, Coffman TM, Penn RB, Wess J, Koller BH. Thromboxane A2 induces airway constriction through an M3 muscarinic acetylcholine receptor-dependent mechanism. *Am J Physiol Lung Cell Mol Physiol*. 2006;290(3):L526-533.

[180] Yoshida A, Ohba M, Wu X, Sasano T, Nakamura M, Endo Y. Accumulation of platelets in the lung and liver and their degranulation following antigen-challenge in sensitized mice. *Br J Pharmacol*. 2002;137(2):146-152.

[181] Mannaioni PF, Di Bello MG, Masini E. Platelets and inflammation: role of platelet-derived growth factor, adhesion molecules and histamine. *Inflamm Res*. 1997;46(1): 4-18.

[182] Benveniste J, Henson PM, Cochrane CG. Leukocyte-dependent histamine release from rabbit platelets. The role of IgE, basophils, and a platelet-activating factor. *J Exp Med*. 1972;136(6):1356-1377.

[183] Kasperska-Zajac A, Brzoza Z, Rogala B. Platelet activating factor as a mediator and therapeutic approach in bronchial asthma. *Inflammation*. 2008;31(2):112-120.

[184] Durk T, Duerschmied D, Muller T, et al. Production of serotonin by tryptophan hydroxylase 1 and release via platelets contribute to allergic airway inflammation. *Am J Respir Crit Care Med*. 2013;187(5):476-485.

[185] Serhan CN, Hamberg M, Samuelsson B. Lipoxins: novel series of biologically active compounds formed from arachidonic acid in human leukocytes. *Proc Natl Acad Sci U S A*. 1984;81(17):5335-5339.

[186] Serhan CN, Sheppard KA. Lipoxin formation during human neutrophil-platelet interactions. Evidence for the transformation of leukotriene A4 by platelet 12-lipoxygenase in vitro. *J Clin Invest*. 1990;85(3):772-780.

[187] Edenius C, Stenke L, Lindgren JA. On the mechanism of transcellular lipoxin formation in human platelets and granulocytes. *Eur J Biochem*. 1991;199(2):401-409.

[188] Serhan CN. Pro-resolving lipid mediators are leads for resolution physiology. *Nature*. 2014;510(7503):92-101.

[189] de Boer JD, Majoor CJ, van 't Veer C, Bel EH, van der Poll T. Asthma and coagulation. *Bloo*d. 2012;119(14):3236-3244.

[190] Flad HD, Brandt E. Platelet-derived chemokines: pathophysiology and therapeutic aspects. Cell Mol Life Sci. 2010;67(14):2363-2386.

[191] Garbaraviciene J, Diehl S, Varwig D, et al. Platelet P-selectin reflects a state of cutaneous inflammation: possible application to monitor treatment efficacy in psoriasis. Exp Dermatol. 2010;19(8):736-741.

Chapter 4

# Platelet Interactions with Bacteria

Steven W. Kerrigan

Additional information is available at the end of the chapter

http://dx.doi.org/10.5772/60531

## 1. Introduction

It is well established that the primary function of platelets is their adhesion to endothelium or to matrix protein components at sites of the injured vessel wall in the initiation of haemostasis [1].Despite this critical role, platelets are poorly appreciated for their involvement in inflammatory or immune processes associated with host defence. The concept that platelets interact with bacteria is not new as there are many reports published throughout history describing this interaction. For example, the earliest report by Levaditi in 1901 demonstrated that platelets activated and 'clumped' when *Vibrio cholerae* were introduced into the circulation of rabbits [2]. In 1931 Dudgeon demonstrated platelet clumping occurred at 5 minutes of injecting S. aureus into rabbits [3]. More recently in the early 1970's Clawson and White demonstrated that bacteria were able to binding specifically to a platelet receptor, triggering a signal that resulted in aggregation and degranulation of intracellular contents [4-7]. These early studies provided observational evidence that platelets can respond to invading pathogens.

As our knowledge of basic platelet biology developed in more modern times it has become apparent that platelets are powerful multifunctional cells that are involved in processes outside their traditional role of thrombosis and haemostasis. For example, platelets share many similarities with professional leukocytes (white blood cells) well characterised for their role in immuno-protection following invasion by foreign invaders. Platelets can also recognise foreign invaders through specific receptors, release their granule contents and recruit immune cells.

Recently human platelets have been shown to express Toll Like Receptor (TLR) 1, 2, 4, 6, 8 and 9 [8-13]. These type I integral membrane receptors recognise common pathogen-associated molecular patterns found in foreign invaders. Platelets also express Intracellular Cell Adhesion Molecular (ICAM) 2 which binds to leukocyte β2 integrin, LFA-1 (α1β2, CD11a/CD18) and to dendritic cell specific ICAM grabbing nonintegrin (DC-SIGN). Trans interactions of platelet-derived Junctional Adhesion Molecules (A and C) have been found to support the luminal deposition of platelet chemokines and to enhance the recruitment of leukocytes. Upon activation CD40L is upregulated on the platelet surface which results in stimulation of endothelial cells through its cognate receptor CD40 and in increased expression of adhesion molecules, release of chemokines (eg. RANTES) enhancing recruitment of leukocytes [14].

As a result of such receptor mediated interactions platelets can secrete granular contents which have significant immuno-modulatory effects. Alpha granules contain proteins such as P-selectin which mediates adhesion of platelets to monocytes, neutrophils and lymphocytes, resulting in the formation of platelet leukocyte complexes [15-17]. Secretion also results in release of many chemotactic agents which lead to the recruitment of various inflammatory cells; platelet derived growth factor (PDGF) and 12-hydroxyeicosatetraenoic acid (12-HETE) which recruit neutrophils [18, 19]; platelet factor 4 and platelet derived histamine releasing factor (PDHRF) which recruit eosinophils in airway disease [20, 21]; PDGF and transforming growth factor β (TGF-β) which recruit monocytes and macrophages and TGF-β which recruits fibroblasts [22-24]. In addition the alpha granules also release many antimicrobial peptides such as beta-lysin, platelet microbial protein (PMP), neutrophil activating peptide (NAP-2), released upon activation normal T-cell expressed and secreted (RANTES) and fibrinopeptides A and B [25-29].

## 2. Common observations in platelet-bacterial interactions

Unlike typical platelet agonists that bind to specific platelet receptors and trigger a response, bacteria can interact with platelets using a number of different mechanisms.

*Direct interaction:* Bacteria express proteins that can directly interact with a surface receptor on the platelet. In this case they have ligand-mimetic domains that act as agonists on the platelet receptor. One such direct interaction is that with *Streptococcus sanguinis* which can directly to GPIbα, the vWf receptor on the platelet [30]. Other potential mediators of platelet activation are lipopolysaccharide (LPS) and lipoteichoic acid (LTA). LPS has been shown to activate platelets and LTA has been shown to inhibit platelet activation [11, 31].

*Indirect interaction (bridging protein):* Bacteria can also coat itself in a plasma protein and then use this mechanism as a bridge to its reciprocal platelet receptor. For example, Clumping factor A & B [32] and fibronectin binding protein [33] on *S. aureus* can both bind fibronectin and/or fibrinogen both of which are ligands for GPIIb/IIIa on the platelet. *Helicobacter pylori* can bind vWf which interacts with GPIbα on the platelet [34]. The most common bridging molecule for bacteria to use is IgG. IgG bound to the bacteria surface can interact with the platelet FcγRIIa receptor and while it appears that this alone cannot stimulate platelet activation it acts in conjunction with other bridging molecules [34-36]. In the absence of a second bridging molecule bound antibody can trigger complement formation which can mediate platelet activation via complement receptors in conjunction with the FcγRIIa receptor [36-38].

*Indirect interaction (secretion):* Bacteria also have the potential to secrete products that can in turn activate platelets. *Porphyromonas gingivalis* secretes gingipain, an enzyme that activates the thrombin receptor on platelets which leads to platelet activation [39] and *Escherichia coli* shiga toxin is associated with platelet activation [40] via a novel platelet glycosphingolipid [41]

Bacterial induced platelet aggregation is different in some respects to that seen with other platelet agonists. Bacterial-induced aggregation is an all-or-nothing response, in that no matter what concentration of bacteria are added to a platelet preparation the extent of aggregation will always be maximal (often less than that seen with other agonists) or else there is no aggregation. Unlike other agonists there is a lag time to aggregation. Adjusting the concentration of bacteria shortens the lag time to a minimum but never eliminates it. There are two categories of bacteria: those that have a short lag time of around 2-5 mins e.g. *S. aureus* and those with a long lag time of 15-20 mins e.g. *S. sanguinis* or *S. gordonii*. The short lag time usually indicates the presence of a direct interaction and is dependent on the levels of expression of the interacting protein on the bacterial surface [36]. The long lag time usually indicates a complement –dependent aggregation process.

Bacteria can finally support platelet adhesion, induce platelet spreading or trigger platelet aggregation and these interactions are often mediated by different platelet receptors and bacterial proteins. For example, *S. gordonii* supports platelet adhesion via a GPIbα – Hsa/GspB interaction, whereas platelet spreading is mediated by GPIIbIIIa –PadA interaction and finally platelet aggregation is mediated by GPIbα – Hsa/GspB/SspA/B interaction.

## 3. Platelet receptors recognised by bacteria

### 3.1. Glycoprotein Ibα

#### *3.1.1. Direct interaction with GPIbα*

*Streptococcus sanguinis* and *Streptococcus gordonii* are common commensals found in the oral cavity and have been found to bind directly to GPIbα. The interaction is mediated by a growing family of bacteria adhesins called Serine Rich Repeat (SRR) proteins. *Streptococcus sanguinis* expresses SrpA and *Streptococcus gordonii* expresses GspB and Hsa. [30, 42, 43]. The region on GspB and Hsa that bind to GPIbα has been localised to the non-repetitive region and interestingly does not contain any sequence similarity with vWf [44]. The non-repetitive ligand binding region of GspB has been worked out by crystallography studies as having a modular organization: helical domain; a Siglec domain (domain that binds sialic acids); and a unique domain [45]. A mammalian carbohydrate binding domain, identified as the Siglec domain, was found in Hsa and SrpA but not in the protein sequences of five other characterised SRR proteins on other bacteria suggesting that this domain is critical for the interaction with GPIbα [45]. Consistent with this finding is that at present Hsa and SrpA are the only streptococcal SRR proteins that have been found to bind to GPIbα. Interestingly, a point mutation in the Siglec domain at R484E showed a marked reduction in binding to purified GPIbα, in addition use of this mutated streptococcus reduced vegetative growth in a rat model of infective endocarditis [45]. *S. aureus* is also a common commensal of the human found predominately in the anterior nares of the nostrils and a opportunistic pathogen found in the blood stream. This bacteria also expresses a highly glycosylated SRR protein named SraP on its surface. A strain of *Staphylococcus aureus* deficient in expression of SraP led to the reduced virulence in a rabbit model of endocarditis [46]. Regardless of the fact that SraP shares significant similarities with a number of other SRR's found in the streptococci that have been found to bind to platelet GPIbα, it is currently unclear as to whether SraP binds to this platelet receptor.

*3.1.2. Indirect interaction with GPIbα*

Additional studies identified that bacterial interaction with platelets was abolished when plasma was removed, suggestive of the need for a plasma protein in the interaction. Subsequent studies identified that a number of bacteria bind vWf and bridge the bacteria to platelet GPIbα. For example, *S. aureus* expresses protein A (SpA) on its surface which binds to immobilised vWf under both static and shear based conditions which in turn bridges to platelet GPIbα. Site directed mutagenesis demonstrated that all five domains of SpA (A-E) can bind to the A1 domain of vWf with high affinity (low nM range) [47]. It is well established that GPIbα binding vWf can cross link to another platelet via GPIbα which represents agglutination rather than true platelet aggregation involving GPIIbIIIa and fibrinogen. Additional experiments are required to establish if the protein A-vWf interaction represents agglutination or true aggregation. *Helicobacter pylori* is the main causative organism of peptic ulcers and have been shown to induce platelet aggregation *in vitro* by binding to vWf which in turn bridges to platelet GPIbα triggering an activating response. Blocking vWf or GPIbα with inhibitory antibodies prevented the interaction. Patients lacking expression of GPIbα (Bernard Soulier Syndrome) fail to aggregate in response to *H. pylori* [34]. To date the *H. pylori* component that binds vWf has not yet been identified [48].

### 3.2. Glycoprotein IIbIIIa

*3.2.1. Direct interaction with GPIIbIIIa*

A number of different species of bacteria have been shown to bind directly to GPIIbIIIa. Physiological ligands mediate attachment to GPIIbIIIa via a short amino acid sequence, RGD. Consistent with this observation, several bacterial proteins have been identified to express an RGD-like sequence in their cell wall proteins. The serine/aspartate (SD) repeat family of proteins are among the most important cell wall components expressed on the surface of the skin commensal *Staphylococcus epidermidis*. SdrG, also referred to as Fbe, is expressed on up to 91% of clinical *S. epidermidis* strains [49]. Protein analysis identified a potential RGD-like sequence ($^{643}$RTD) in the B-domain of the SdrG protein. Platelet adhesion to a purified recombinant B-domain of SdrG was inhibited by using either a short synthetic peptide containing the RGD sequence or the GPIIbIIIa antagonist tirofiban (which spans the RGD site), suggesting that this sequence is responsible for directly interacting with GPIIbIIIa [50].

Under iron limited conditions *S. aureus* expresses a surface determinant called IsdB which also contains an RGD-like sequence ($^{248}$KYD) [51]. Surface plasmon resonance demonstrated that recombinant IsdB interacts directly with purified GPIIb/IIIa with high affinity with a dissociation constant ($K_D$) of 405±73.7nM. Platelet adhesion and aggregation was significantly reduced following preincubation of platelets with the GPIIbIIIa antagonist tirofiban or an inhibitory RGDS peptide mimetic. Furthermore, a strain defective in expression of IsdB also failed to bind to GPIIbIIIa [51].

*Streptococcus gordonii* expresses a large molecular weight protein on its surface (397kDa) designated platelet adherence protein A (PadA). Platelet adhesion to *S. gordonii* was inhibited by the GPIIbIIIa antagonist abciximab or an inhibitory peptide mimetic, RGDS [52]. Platelets adhering to immobilised *S. gordonii* or specific fragments of PadA underwent dramatic changes in morphology as observed by fluorescent confocal microscopy. Rearrangement of the platelet actin cytoskeleton led to filopodia and llamelipodia formation resulting in full platelet spreading [53]. Proteomic analysis identified that PadA contains integrin recognition motifs ($^{383}$RGT and $^{484}$AGD) that may act as binding sites for GPIIbIIIa. Using site directed mutagenesis the AGD or RGT sequence was replaced with a AAA. Platelet interaction with these mutants demonstrated that platelet adhesion was unaffected however platelet spreading was significantly reduced. In addition, replacement of the RGT sequence to AAA (but not the AGD sequence) significantly reduced granule secretion [54]. These results suggesting that there are potentially multiple sequences on PadA responsible for specific platelet functions. The sequence that is directly responsible for supporting platelet adhesion has currently not yet been identified.

### *3.2.2. Indirect interaction with GPIIbIIIa*

Both staphylococci and streptococci express a number of plasma protein binding proteins on their surface. Probably the most common are fibrinogen binding proteins, often expressed at different phase of bacterial growth. For example, *S. aureus* expresses clumping factor B (ClfB), fibronectin binding protein A (FnBPA), fibronectin binding protein B (FnBPB) in the early stage of growth (exponential phase) and clumping factor A (ClfA) in the late stage of growth (stationary phase). *S. epidermidis* expresses a fibrinogen binding protein, SdrG, at the exponential phase of growth. Group A (*Streptococcus pyogenes*) and Group B (*Streptococcus agalactiae*) streptococcus also express fibrinogen binding proteins called M protein and FbsA, respectively, in the exponential phase of growth.

The ligand binding sites of ClfA and ClfB have been mapped to residues 220 to 559 [55]. Interestingly the ligand binding sites of the two homologs are only 27% identical. In contrast to ClfA which recognises the extreme C-terminus of the $\gamma$-chain of fibrinogen, ClfB recognises the $\alpha$-chain of fibrinogen [56, 57]. The FnBPA or FnBPB can bind either fibronectin or fibrinogen. The N-terminal region of the fibronectin binding proteins (N1, N2 and N3) is structurally and functionally similar to the clumping factors, however in place of the serine-aspartate repeat region are tandemly repeated fibronectin-binding repeat domains. The FnBP's bind fibrinogen via the N1, N2 and N3 domains and fibronectin via the repeat domains (11 in FnBPA and 10 in FnBPB) [58]. SdrG (*S. epidermidis*) has the same structural organisation as the clumping factors and bind directly to the beta-chain of the fibrinogen molecule with a Kd in the range of 90-300nm [59, 60].

Group A streptococci (*Streptococcus pyogens*) express more than 80 types of the highly virulent factor, M-protein [61]. The fibrinogen binding motif differs between homologs of M-proteins, suggesting that this domain might have evolved independently in different M-protein lineages [62]. The exact binding site on fibrinogen that interacts with M-protein has not yet been defined, however in inhibitory peptide mimetic RGDS, abolishes platelet aggregation, suggesting the RGD site is involved [63]. Group B streptococcus (GBS) express three homologous proteins termed FbsA, FbsB and FbsC (BsaB). While all of these proteins have all been shown to bind fibrinogen to date only fsbA has been shown to be capable of binding fibrinogen and cross-linking to GPIIbIIIa [64]. Different GBS strains possess different numbers of repeat domains in the FbsA protein thus accounting for the size heterogeneity of the protein. Studies have demonstrated that a single repeat unit was capable of binding fibrinogen [65]. Although the site on the fibrinogen molecule that binds to FsbA was not identified, an RGDS peptide abolished the interaction suggesting that this motif on fibrinogen is critical [64].

A common observation is beginning to unfold in the light of all the fibrinogen binding proteins expressed on bacteria. Results demonstrate that where a bacterial protein binds fibrinogen and crosslinks to platelet GPIIbIIIa it is usually not enough to trigger an activating signal in the platelet and usually requires a co-stimulus In all cases outlined above the key co-stimulus is provided by the bacteria binding IgG and cross linking to its reciprocal receptor on platelets, FcγRIIa.

### 3.3. FcγRIIA

#### *3.3.1. Direct interaction with FcγRIIA*

Currently there are no reports of a bacterial protein binding directly to FcγRIIa on platelets, however there are a number of reports of an indirect interaction where bacterial proteins use IgG to cross link to platelet FcγRIIA.

#### *3.3.2. Indirect interaction with FcγRIIA*

FcγRIIA is fast becoming the most important receptor in platelet bacterial interactions as it has been shown to inhibit all bacterial induced platelet activation including those triggered by *S. aureus, S. epidermidis, S. sanguinis, S. gordonii, Streptococcus pneumonia, Streptococcus oralis, H. pylori* and *S. pyogenes* [30, 33, 34, 36, 50, 53, 66-70]. A key observation is that IgG is required for all of these bacteria to induce platelet aggregation, however antibody alone was not enough to trigger aggregation / activation of platelets. In all cases engagement of another platelet receptor was required such as GPIIbIIIa, GPIbα, or Toll Like Receptors (TLR's). These observations suggest that FcγRIIa requires receptor clustering in order to trigger platelet activation [69]. Indeed FcγRIIa has been shown to be physically associated with GPIIbIIIa and GPIbα and therefore plays an important role in their respective signalling in an IgG-independent manner [71].

http://dx.doi.org/10.5772/60531

| Platelet receptor | Bacteria & protein | Bridging protein | Reference |
|---|---|---|---|
| GPIbα | *S. gordonii* GspB/Hsa | Direct | 42,43,44 |
| | *S. sanguinis* SrpA | Direct | 30,94 |
| | *S. aureus* SraP | ? | 46 |
| | *S. aureus* SpA | vWf | 47 |
| | *H. pylori [unidenified]* | vWf | 48 |
| GPIIbIIIa | *S. epidermidis* SdrG | Direct | 49,50 |
| | *S. aureus* IsdB | Direct | 51 |
| | *S. gordonii* PadA | Direct | 52,53,54 |
| | *S. aureus* ClfA | Fibrinogen | 55,56 |
| | *S. aureus* ClfB | Fibrinogen | 57 |
| | *S. aureus* FnbpA/B | Fibronectin | 58 |
| | *S. epidermidis* SdrG | Fibrinogen | 59,60 |
| | *S. pyogenes* M1 | Fibrinogen | 62,63 |
| | *S. agalactiae* Fbs | Fibrinogen | 64,65 |
| FcγRIIa | *S. aureus* FnbpA/B | IgG | 33 |
| | *S. aurues* ClfA | IgG | 36 |
| | *S. aureus* ClfB | IgG | 72 |
| | *S. epidermidis* SdrG | IgG | 50 |
| | *H. pylori [unidentified]* | IgG | 34 |
| | *P. gingivalis [unidentified]* | IgG | 73 |
| gC1q-R/P32 | *S. aureus* SpA | direct | 74,75 |
| | *S. aureus* ClfA | ? | 32, 36 |
| | *S. aureus* ClfB | ? | 32,72 |
| | *S. sanguinis [unidentified]* | ? | 38,77 |
| TLR2 | *S. pneumoniae [unidentified]* | direct | 67 |
| | *P. gingivalis [unidentified]* | direct | 79 |

**Table 1.** Summary of interactions between bacteria and platelets. Bacteria can either interact with platelets directly or indirectly using a bridging protein, thus triggering activation. ClfA; clumping factor A, FnbpA; fibronectin binding protein A, SpA; protein A, PadA; platelet adhesion protein A, IsdB; iron-regulated surface determinant B, SdrG; Serine aspartate repeat G, Hsa; haemaglutinin salivary antigen, GspB; glycosylated spretococcal protein B, SrpA; serine rich protein A, IgG; immunoglobulin G, vWf; vonWillebrand Factor, C1q; complement 1q, GP; glycoprotein, TLR; Toll like receptor

| Platelet receptor | Bacteria | Bacterial toxin | Reference |
|---|---|---|---|
| TLR4 | *E. coli* | LPS | 81,82,83,84 |
| ? | *S. epidermidis* | LTA | 85,86,87,88 |
| ? | *P. gingivalis* | Gingipains | 39,89 |
| Glycospingolipids | *E.coli* | Verotoxin | 41,90 |
| ? | *S. aureus* | α-toxin | 91,92 |

**Table 2.** Summary of interactions between platelets and bacterial toxins. LPS; Lipopolysaccharide, LTA; Lipoteichoic acid

*S. aureus* and *S. epidermidis* induce platelet aggregation in an FcγRIIa dependent manner. *S. aureus* fails to induce platelet aggregation in the absence of plasma proteins. Addition of IgG alone is not enough to trigger aggregation induced by *S. aureus,* however addition of fibrinogen/fibronectin and IgG combined induces full aggregation [33, 36, 72]. Similarly S. epidermidis SdrG also induces platelet aggregation however requires concomitant binding of fibrinogen and IgG to the A-domain of SdrG and an unidentified cell wall component of *H. pylori* requires concomitant binding of vWf and IgG which crosslinks to GPIbα and FcγRIIa [34, 50].

All published reports of streptococcal induced platelet aggregation demonstrate their ability to induce platelet aggregation in an FcγRIIa dependent manner. Early reports suggested that streptococci could induce platelet aggregation in the absence of plasma proteins. However regardless of this, blocking FcγRIIa with a monoclonal antibody still abolished aggregation [30], suggesting that FcγRIIa may be playing a role in signal amplification. This observation is analogous to the role of FcγRIIa in promoting cell signalling/amplification through various platelets receptors such as GPIIbIIIa and GPIbα. Another oral bacteria, *S. oralis* on the other hand failed to induce platelet aggregation in gel filtered platelets [68]. The addition of plasma concentrations of fibrinogen to the gel filtered platelets failed to restore aggregation however addition of plasma concentrations of purified IgG fully restored platelet aggregation. More recently, Arman et al, demonstrated that *S. sanguinis, S. gordonii* but not *S. pneumoniae* require IgG's to induce platelet aggregation [69]. The site that IgG binds to was not identified in this study.

Oral bacteria, *Porphomonas gingivalis* expresses a surface protein called hgp44 which induces platelet aggregation in an FcγRIIA dependent manner [73]. The authors demonstrated that IgG was critical for the interaction. Preincubation of platelets with an anti-FcγRIIa antibody abolished *P. gingivalis* induced platelet aggregation. Furthermore, depletion of IgG from plasma also completely prevented aggregation. Interestingly recombinant hgp44 failed to induce platelet aggregation suggesting that hgp44 may be dependent on another *P. gingivalis* protein binding to platelets in order to crosslink receptors to trigger a signal that results in platelet aggregation.

### 3.4. gC1q-R/P33

#### *3.4.1. Direct interaction with gC1q-R/P33*

*S. aureus* SpA has been shown to be capable of binding directly to full length recombinant gC1qR (amino acids 1-282). Under resting conditions there is a low level of gC1qR expression on platelets, however upon activation expression levels significantly rises [74]. The latter suggests that another interaction between *S. aureus* and the platelet is required in order to express high levels of the receptor on the platelet surface. Binding was inhibited by both recombinant gC1qR and soluble purified protein A, however complement proteins did not appear to be required as the binding interaction occurs in the absence of complement proteins. Deletion of the C1q binding domain (amino acids 74-95) on the recombinant gC1qR resulted in loss of C1q binding but not *S. aureus* SpA suggesting that the SpA binding site is likely to reside outside of this domain [75].

#### *3.4.2. Indirect interaction*

Complement is part of the immune system that augments the opsonisation of bacteria by antibodies which in turn facilitates phagocytosis. There are three main pathways that lead to complement activation; the classical pathway can be triggered by antigen-antibody complexes; the alternative pathway can be triggered by binding specific complement proteins binding to the bacterial surface and finally the lectin pathway can be triggered by mannose binding protein binding the bacterial surface [76]. The lag time to platelet aggregation in response to *S. aureus* (mediated by ClfA or ClfB) is 2-4 mins and required the binding of fibrinogen and IgG to their respective receptors on platelets in order to trigger full activation and aggregation [32]. Subsequent studies on these interactions discovered that by deleting the fibrinogen binding domain on *S. aureus* ClfA (ClfA-PY) or ClfB (Q235A) it significantly extended the lag time to aggregation (12-15 mins) suggestive of a second much slower interaction [36, 72]. Heating plasma to destroy proteins abolished platelet activation and aggregation by both ClfA-PY and ClfB-Q235A. Further studies using zymosan, which removes complement proteins from plasma, also inhibited platelet activation and aggregation by both ClfA-PY and ClfB-Q235A. These studies suggested that complement played a key role in the second much slower interaction that resulted in platelet activation/aggregation. The receptor on platelets that binds bacteria coated complement proteins has not been identified yet.

The lag time to platelet aggregation varies with different strains of *S. sanguinis* [77], for example *S. sanguinis* can induce platelet aggregation with a lag time of 2-4 minutes or 12-15 minutes. The long lag time is indicative of the time taken for complement assembly [38]. Inactivation of complement by cobra venom or heat treatment abolished aggregation [38]. It is not known precisely how complement activation triggers platelet activation but it is possible that there is a threshold of bacterial-platelet interactions (capable of inducing strong or weak signals) which must be surpassed before triggering platelet aggregation however this remains to be investigated.

### 3.5. Toll like receptor 2

#### *3.5.1. Direct interaction with TLR2*

*Streptococcus pneumoniae* is a major pathogen usually found colonising the upper respiratory tract and nasopharynx. Following intense inflammatory response of the lungs the bacteria can gain entry to the bloodstream. *S. pneumonia* has been shown to bind induce platelet aggregation and dense granule secretion [67]. Preincubation of platelets with an inhibitory TLR2 antibody abolished platelet aggregation and dense granule secretion induced by *S. pneumoniae*. Both aggregation and dense granule secretion was dependent on FcγRIIa however antibody was not required for either to take place, further suggesting that this receptor plays a role in signal amplification possibly through recruitment of adapter proteins to initiate signaling. Interestingly stimulation of TLR2 by *S. pneumoniae* resulted in the activation of the PI3 kinase pathway [67]. PI3-kinase is typically a negative regulator of TLR2-dependent responses in several immune cells. However, in platelets many studies demonstrate that PI3-kinase acts as a positive regulator in various platelet functions such as adhesion, aggregation and spreading [78]. Therefore it appears that PI3 kinase is a positive regulator of *S. pneumoniae*-induced platelet aggregation. Oral bacteria, *Porphyromonas gingivalis* induced platelet-neutrophil aggregates in a TLR2 dependent manner. This response was significantly reduced in TLR2 deficient mice, highlighting the importance of this receptor in the platelet recognition of *P. gingivalis* [79]. Consistent with previous observations the authors also demonstrated that PI3 kinase was critically important in the signalling response mediated downstream of TLR2.

## 4. Secreted products

Lipopolysaccharide (LPS) is shed from the cell wall of gram negative bacteria into the local milieu and interacts with Toll-like receptors (TLR) on immune cells [80]. *Escherichia coli* LPS was shown to bind to and mediate activation of platelets in a TLR4-dependent manner [81] and to enhance platelet secretion of cytokines [82]. Chicken thymocytes were also shown to express TLR4 receptor and to become activated by LPS [83]. There seems to be variation in the ability of different types of LPS to bind to platelets and LPS from *E. coli* O157 appears to be the most potent [81]. Although LPS was found to bind to TLR4 on platelets, there is little evidence to suggest that binding leads to platelet activation. LPS bound platelets had increased affinity for neutrophils and only LPS-treated platelets were capable of inducing neutrophil activation [84]. LPS injected into wildtype mice induced thrombocytopenia that was neutrophil-dependent [13]. Thus, current understanding is that LPS binds to platelet TLR4 but does not generate an activation signal, at least not one than leads to platelet aggregation. However, LPS appears to prime the platelets allowing them to bind to and activate neutrophils.

In contrast Lipoteichoic acid (LTA) is secreted by Gram-positive bacteria. LTA binds to platelets and inhibits platelet aggregation by collagen [85]. LTA also supports platelet adhesion to *S. epidermidis* [86]. Some studies suggested that the anti-platelet effect of LTA was due to conformational changes in the membrane [87] and an increase in cAMP levels [88].

In a manner similar to thrombin activation of the Protease Activated Receptors on the platelet surface, *Porphyromonas gingivalis* secretes gingipains which are proteases that can directly activate platelets [39, 89]. Shiga-like toxin (verotoxin) is secreted by *E. coli* and triggers platelet aggregation [90] by binding to glycosphingolipid receptors on the platelet surface [41]. $\alpha$-toxin is a pore forming toxin produced by *S. aureus* which is responsible for haemolysis. It also leads to platelet activation [91] leading to the assembly of the pro-thrombinase complex on the platelet surface [92].

## 5. Animal studies versus clinically relevant models of infection

There are many reports in the literature investigating the interaction between bacteria and platelets *in vivo*. Translating animal studies to human disease is becoming increasingly difficult, especially with the identification that Fc$\gamma$RIIA is a key receptor involved in signal amplification in human platelets [69]. Fc$\gamma$RIIa is unique to higher primates and therefore calls into question the validity of using mouse, rat or rabbit animal models for studying platelet-bacterial interactions [93], as they do not express Fc$\gamma$RIIa. Although mouse, rat and rabbit platelets do aggregate in response to bacteria in vivo, the mechanism through which they signal must be different. Transgenic mice expressing human Fc$\gamma$RIIa are available commercially which can overcome this problem.

One potential possibility to overcome this problem is to develop a more clinically relevant model of infection using physiological conditions with human platelets. Using a parallel flow chamber with human platelets and shear conditions experienced under human physiological conditions a number of key interactions were observed. Under fluid shear conditions, human platelets rolled on immobilised *S. sanguinis* and *S. gordonii* at low shear rates (50s-1) followed by firm adhesion [42, 94]. This rolling behaviour was similar to the interaction between platelet GPIb$\alpha$ and vWf. Of key interest is that platelet rolling on vWf occurs under high shear conditions (>1000s-1) where the platelet rolling on bacteria occurs under low shear conditions (50s-1). Deletion of cell wall proteins *S. sanguinis* SrpA or *S. gordonii* Hsa abolished the rolling behaviour suggesting that these proteins must be in a conformation for direct interaction with platelet GPIb$\alpha$ under low shear conditions [42, 94]. Platelets rolled, adhered and formed micro thrombi on immobilised *S. oralis* at shear rates of 50s-1 to 800s-1. This interaction was also dependent on GPIb$\alpha$ as determined by anti-GPIb$\alpha$ antibodies and blood from a Bernard Soulier patient. Aggregate formation was dependent on *S. oralis* binding IgG, which cross-links to platelet Fc$\gamma$RIIa. This interaction also led to phosphorylation of the ITAM domain on Fc$\gamma$RIIa, resulting in dense granule secretion and amplification through the ADP receptor [68].

*S. pyogenes* interacts with platelets under high shear conditions. The major cell wall component M-protein was found to bind IgG and fibrinogen which cross link to Fc$\gamma$RIIa and GPIIbIIIa respectively to trigger thrombus formation [95]. *S. aureus* also triggered thrombus formation in the presence of human whole blood under high shear conditions (800s-1). These studies identified that deletion of major cell wall protein ClfA but not other cell wall proteins (FnBP's, SpA or SdrC) completely abolished thrombus formation. Thrombus formation was dependent on fibrinogen and IgG binding to platelets in order to trigger thrombus formation. Subsequent studies demonstrated that *S. aureus* ClfA bound IgG and fibrinogen crosslinked to FcγRIIa and GPIIbIIIa respectively thus triggering thrombus formation. Of particular interest is that *S. aureus* failed to interact with platelets under low shear [66].

## 6. Conclusion

Although the field of platelet bacterial interactions is in its infancy, significant advances have been made in identifying some of the molecular mechanisms. Through learning about these interactions it has provided strong evidence that platelets may indeed be acting as primitive immune cells. However a lot more research is required to gain a better understanding of the exact role platelets play in in the process. For example, by adhering, aggregating, spreading or forming a thrombus on the bacteria are the platelets trying to restrict spread of infection and then by releasing their granular contents orchestrate or control the immune response to the infection by recruiting defined numbers of leukocytes. Alternatively is it a clever move by the bacteria who coat themselves in non-professional immune cells (platelets) and therefore rendering themselves safe from attack from professional immune cells (leukocytes) and antibiotics, which cannot penetrate the platelet encapsulation to kill the bacteria thus allowing them to grow and divide in a safe environment.

## Author details

Steven W. Kerrigan

School of Pharmacy & Molecular and Cellular Therapeutics, Royal College of Surgeons in Ireland, Dublin, Ireland

## References

[1] Ruggeri, Z. M. (2009) Platelet adhesion under flow, *Microcirculation 16*, 58-83.

[2] Levaditi, C. (1901) Et des organism vaccines contre le vibron cholerique, *Ann Inst Pasteur 15*, 894-924.

[3] Dudgeon LS, G. H. (1931) The examination of the tissues and some observations on the blood platelets of rabbits at intervals of five minutes and later after intraveneous inoculations of Staphylococcus aureus and India ink, *J. Hyg (camb) 31*.

[4] Clawson, C. C., and White, J. G. (1971) Platelet interaction with bacteria. I. Reaction phases and effects of inhibitors, *The American journal of pathology 65*, 367-380.

[5] Clawson, C. C., and White, J. G. (1971) Platelet interaction with bacteria. II. Fate of the bacteria, *The American journal of pathology 65*, 381-397.

[6] Clawson, C. C. (1973) Platelet interaction with bacteria. 3. Ultrastructure, *The American journal of pathology 70*, 449-471.

[7] Clawson, C. C., Rao, G. H., and White, J. G. (1975) Platelet interaction with bacteria. IV. Stimulation of the release reaction, *The American journal of pathology 81*, 411-420.

[8] Cognasse, F., Hamzeh, H., Chavarin, P., Acquart, S., Genin, C., and Garraud, O. (2005) Evidence of Toll-like receptor molecules on human platelets, *Immunology and cell biology 83*, 196-198.

[9] Shiraki, R., Inoue, N., Kawasaki, S., Takei, A., Kadotani, M., Ohnishi, Y., Ejiri, J., Kobayashi, S., Hirata, K., Kawashima, S., and Yokoyama, M. (2004) Expression of Toll-like receptors on human platelets, *Thrombosis research 113*, 379-385.

[10] Aslam, R., Speck, E. R., Kim, M., Crow, A. R., Bang, K. W., Nestel, F. P., Ni, H., Lazarus, A. H., Freedman, J., and Semple, J. W. (2006) Platelet Toll-like receptor expression modulates lipopolysaccharide-induced thrombocytopenia and tumor necrosis factor-alpha production in vivo, *Blood 107*, 637-641.

[11] Zhang, G., Han, J., Welch, E. J., Ye, R. D., Voyno-Yasenetskaya, T. A., Malik, A. B., Du, X., and Li, Z. (2009) Lipopolysaccharide stimulates platelet secretion and potentiates platelet aggregation via TLR4/MyD88 and the cGMP-dependent protein kinase pathway, *Journal of immunology 182*, 7997-8004.

[12] Garraud, O., and Cognasse, F. (2010) Platelet Toll-like receptor expression: the link between "danger" ligands and inflammation, *Inflammation & allergy drug targets 9*, 322-333.

[13] Andonegui, G., Kerfoot, S. M., McNagny, K., Ebbert, K. V., Patel, K. D., and Kubes, P. (2005) Platelets express functional Toll-like receptor-4, *Blood 106*, 2417-2423.

[14] von Hundelshausen, P., and Weber, C. (2007) Platelets as immune cells: bridging inflammation and cardiovascular disease, *Circulation research 100*, 27-40.

[15] Diacovo, T. G., Puri, K. D., Warnock, R. A., Springer, T. A., and von Andrian, U. H. (1996) Platelet-mediated lymphocyte delivery to high endothelial venules, *Science 273*, 252-255.

[16] Diacovo, T. G., Roth, S. J., Buccola, J. M., Bainton, D. F., and Springer, T. A. (1996) Neutrophil rolling, arrest, and transmigration across activated, surface-adherent platelets via sequential action of P-selectin and the beta 2-integrin CD11b/CD18, *Blood 88*, 146-157.

[17] Larsen, E., Celi, A., Gilbert, G. E., Furie, B. C., Erban, J. K., Bonfanti, R., Wagner, D. D., and Furie, B. (1989) PADGEM protein: a receptor that mediates the interaction of activated platelets with neutrophils and monocytes, *Cell 59*, 305-312.

[18] Herd, C. M., and Page, C. P. (1994) Pulmonary immune cells in health and disease: platelets, *Eur Respir J 7*, 1145-1160.

[19] Mannaioni, P. F., Di Bello, M. G., and Masini, E. (1997) Platelets and inflammation: role of platelet-derived growth factor, adhesion molecules and histamine, *Inflamm Res 46*, 4-18.

[20] Brindley, L. L., Sweet, J. M., and Goetzl, E. J. (1983) Stimulation of histamine release from human basophils by human platelet factor 4, *J Clin Invest 72*, 1218-1223.

[21] Frigas, E., and Gleich, G. J. (1986) The eosinophil and the pathophysiology of asthma, *J Allergy Clin Immunol 77*, 527-537.

[22] Deuel, T. F., Senior, R. M., Huang, J. S., and Griffin, G. L. (1982) Chemotaxis of monocytes and neutrophils to platelet-derived growth factor, *J Clin Invest 69*, 1046-1049.

[23] Tzeng, D. Y., Deuel, T. F., Huang, J. S., and Baehner, R. L. (1985) Platelet-derived growth factor promotes human peripheral monocyte activation, *Blood 66*, 179-183.

[24] Wahl, S. M., Hunt, D. A., Wakefield, L. M., McCartney-Francis, N., Wahl, L. M., Roberts, A. B., and Sporn, M. B. (1987) Transforming growth factor type beta induces monocyte chemotaxis and growth factor production, *Proc Natl Acad Sci U S A 84*, 5788-5792.

[25] Johnson, F. B., and Donaldson, D. M. (1968) Purification of staphylocidal beta-lysin from rabbit serum, *J Bacteriol 96*, 589-595.

[26] Donaldson, D. M., and Tew, J. G. (1977) beta-Lysin of platelet origin, *Bacteriol Rev 41*, 501-513.

[27] Kameyoshi, Y., Dorschner, A., Mallet, A. I., Christophers, E., and Schroder, J. M. (1992) Cytokine RANTES released by thrombin-stimulated platelets is a potent attractant for human eosinophils, *J Exp Med 176*, 587-592.

[28] Yeaman, M. R., Tang, Y. Q., Shen, A. J., Bayer, A. S., and Selsted, M. E. (1997) Purification and in vitro activities of rabbit platelet microbicidal proteins, *Infect Immun 65*, 1023-1031.

[29] Krijgsveld, J., Zaat, S. A., Meeldijk, J., van Veelen, P. A., Fang, G., Poolman, B., Brandt, E., Ehlert, J. E., Kuijpers, A. J., Engbers, G. H., Feijen, J., and Dankert, J. (2000) Thrombocidins, microbicidal proteins from human blood platelets, are C-terminal deletion products of CXC chemokines, *J Biol Chem 275*, 20374-20381.

[30] Kerrigan, S. W., Douglas, I., Wray, A., Heath, J., Byrne, M. F., Fitzgerald, D., and Cox, D. (2002) A role for glycoprotein Ib in Streptococcus sanguis-induced platelet aggregation, *Blood 100*, 509-516.

[31] Waller, A. K., Sage, T., Kumar, C., Carr, T., Gibbins, J. M., and Clarke, S. R. (2013) Staphylococcus aureus lipoteichoic acid inhibits platelet activation and thrombus formation via the Paf receptor, *The Journal of infectious diseases 208*, 2046-2057.

[32] O'Brien, L., Kerrigan, S. W., Kaw, G., Hogan, M., Penades, J., Litt, D., Fitzgerald, D. J., Foster, T. J., and Cox, D. (2002) Multiple mechanisms for the activation of human platelet aggregation by Staphylococcus aureus: roles for the clumping factors ClfA and ClfB, the serine-aspartate repeat protein SdrE and protein A, *Molecular microbiology 44*, 1033-1044.

[33] Fitzgerald, J. R., Loughman, A., Keane, F., Brennan, M., Knobel, M., Higgins, J., Visai, L., Speziale, P., Cox, D., and Foster, T. J. (2006) Fibronectin-binding proteins of Staphylococcus aureus mediate activation of human platelets via fibrinogen and fibronectin bridges to integrin GPIIb/IIIa and IgG binding to the FcgammaRIIa receptor, *Molecular microbiology 59*, 212-230.

[34] Byrne, M. F., Kerrigan, S. W., Corcoran, P. A., Atherton, J. C., Murray, F. E., Fitzgerald, D. J., and Cox, D. M. (2003) Helicobacter pylori binds von Willebrand factor and interacts with GPIb to induce platelet aggregation, *Gastroenterology 124*, 1846-1854.

[35] Fitzgerald, J. R., Foster, T. J., and Cox, D. (2006) The interaction of bacterial pathogens with platelets, *Nat Rev Microbiol 4*, 445-457.

[36] Loughman, A., Fitzgerald, J. R., Brennan, M. P., Higgins, J., Downer, R., Cox, D., and Foster, T. J. (2005) Roles for fibrinogen, immunoglobulin and complement in platelet activation promoted by Staphylococcus aureus clumping factor A, *Molecular microbiology 57*, 804-818.

[37] Ford, I., Douglas, C. W., Cox, D., Rees, D. G., Heath, J., and Preston, F. E. (1997) The role of immunoglobulin G and fibrinogen in platelet aggregation by Streptococcus sanguis, *Br J Haematol 97*, 737-746.

[38] Ford, I., Douglas, C. W., Heath, J., Rees, C., and Preston, F. E. (1996) Evidence for the involvement of complement proteins in platelet aggregation by Streptococcus sanguis NCTC 7863, *British journal of haematology 94*, 729-739.

[39] Lourbakos, A., Yuan, Y. P., Jenkins, A. L., Travis, J., Andrade-Gordon, P., Santulli, R., Potempa, J., and Pike, R. N. (2001) Activation of protease-activated receptors by gingipains from Porphyromonas gingivalis leads to platelet aggregation: a new trait in microbial pathogenicity, *Blood 97*, 3790-3797.

[40] Proulx, F., Seidman, E. G., and Karpman, D. (2001) Pathogenesis of Shiga toxin-associated hemolytic uremic syndrome, *Pediatr Res 50*, 163-171.

[41] Cooling, L. L., Walker, K. E., Gille, T., and Koerner, T. A. (1998) Shiga toxin binds human platelets via globotriaosylceramide (Pk antigen) and a novel platelet glycosphingolipid, *Infect Immun 66*, 4355-4366.

[42] Kerrigan, S. W., Jakubovics, N. S., Keane, C., Maguire, P., Wynne, K., Jenkinson, H. F., and Cox, D. (2007) Role of Streptococcus gordonii surface proteins SspA/SspB and Hsa in platelet function, *Infection and immunity 75*, 5740-5747.

[43] Bensing, B. A., Lopez, J. A., and Sullam, P. M. (2004) The Streptococcus gordonii surface proteins GspB and Hsa mediate binding to sialylated carbohydrate epitopes on the platelet membrane glycoprotein Ibalpha, *Infection and immunity 72*, 6528-6537.

[44] Takamatsu, D., Bensing, B. A., Cheng, H., Jarvis, G. A., Siboo, I. R., Lopez, J. A., Griffiss, J. M., and Sullam, P. M. (2005) Binding of the Streptococcus gordonii surface glycoproteins GspB and Hsa to specific carbohydrate structures on platelet membrane glycoprotein Ibalpha, *Molecular microbiology 58*, 380-392.

[45] Pyburn, T. M., Bensing, B. A., Xiong, Y. Q., Melancon, B. J., Tomasiak, T. M., Ward, N. J., Yankovskaya, V., Oliver, K. M., Cecchini, G., Sulikowski, G. A., Tyska, M. J., Sullam, P. M., and Iverson, T. M. (2011) A structural model for binding of the serine-rich repeat adhesin GspB to host carbohydrate receptors, *PLoS pathogens 7*, e1002112.

[46] Siboo, I. R., Chambers, H. F., and Sullam, P. M. (2005) Role of SraP, a Serine-Rich Surface Protein of Staphylococcus aureus, in binding to human platelets, *Infection and immunity 73*, 2273-2280.

[47] O'Seaghdha, M., van Schooten, C. J., Kerrigan, S. W., Emsley, J., Silverman, G. J., Cox, D., Lenting, P. J., and Foster, T. J. (2006) Staphylococcus aureus protein A binding to von Willebrand factor A1 domain is mediated by conserved IgG binding regions, *The FEBS journal 273*, 4831-4841.

[48] Corcoran, P. A., Atherton, J. C., Kerrigan, S. W., Wadstrom, T., Murray, F. E., Peek, R. M., Fitzgerald, D. J., Cox, D. M., and Byrne, M. F. (2007) The effect of different strains of Helicobacter pylori on platelet aggregation, *Canadian journal of gastroenterology = Journal canadien de gastroenterologie 21*, 367-370.

[49] Arciola, C. R., Campoccia, D., Gamberini, S., Donati, M. E., and Montanaro, L. (2004) Presence of fibrinogen-binding adhesin gene in Staphylococcus epidermidis isolates from central venous catheters-associated and orthopaedic implant-associated infections, *Biomaterials 25*, 4825-4829.

[50] Brennan, M. P., Loughman, A., Devocelle, M., Arasu, S., Chubb, A. J., Foster, T. J., and Cox, D. (2009) Elucidating the role of Staphylococcus epidermidis serine-aspartate repeat protein G in platelet activation, *Journal of thrombosis and haemostasis : JTH 7*, 1364-1372.

[51] Miajlovic, H., Zapotoczna, M., Geoghegan, J. A., Kerrigan, S. W., Speziale, P., and Foster, T. J. (2010) Direct interaction of iron-regulated surface determinant IsdB of Staphylococcus aureus with the GPIIb/IIIa receptor on platelets, *Microbiology 156*, 920-928.

[52] Petersen, H. J., Keane, C., Jenkinson, H. F., Vickerman, M. M., Jesionowski, A., Waterhouse, J. C., Cox, D., and Kerrigan, S. W. (2010) Human platelets recognize a novel surface protein, PadA, on Streptococcus gordonii through a unique interaction involving fibrinogen receptor GPIIbIIIa, *Infection and immunity 78*, 413-422.

[53] Keane, C., Petersen, H., Reynolds, K., Newman, D. K., Cox, D., Jenkinson, H. F., Newman, P. J., and Kerrigan, S. W. (2010) Mechanism of outside-in {alpha}IIb{beta}3-mediated activation of human platelets by the colonizing Bacterium, Streptococcus gordonii, *Arteriosclerosis, thrombosis, and vascular biology 30*, 2408-2415.

[54] Keane, C., Petersen, H. J., Tilley, D. O., Haworth, J., Cox, D., Jenkinson, H. F., and Kerrigan, S. W. (2013) Multiple sites on Streptococcus gordonii surface protein PadA bind to platelet GPIIbIIIa, *Thrombosis and haemostasis 110*, 1278-1287.

[55] McDevitt, D., Francois, P., Vaudaux, P., and Foster, T. J. (1995) Identification of the ligand-binding domain of the surface-located fibrinogen receptor (clumping factor) of Staphylococcus aureus, *Molecular microbiology 16*, 895-907.

[56] McDevitt, D., Nanavaty, T., House-Pompeo, K., Bell, E., Turner, N., McIntire, L., Foster, T., and Hook, M. (1997) Characterization of the interaction between the Staphylococcus aureus clumping factor (ClfA) and fibrinogen, *European journal of biochemistry / FEBS 247*, 416-424.

[57] Walsh, E. J., Miajlovic, H., Gorkun, O. V., and Foster, T. J. (2008) Identification of the Staphylococcus aureus MSCRAMM clumping factor B (ClfB) binding site in the alphaC-domain of human fibrinogen, *Microbiology 154*, 550-558.

[58] Wann, E. R., Gurusiddappa, S., and Hook, M. (2000) The fibronectin-binding MSCRAMM FnbpA of Staphylococcus aureus is a bifunctional protein that also binds to fibrinogen, *The Journal of biological chemistry 275*, 13863-13871.

[59] Davis, S. L., Gurusiddappa, S., McCrea, K. W., Perkins, S., and Hook, M. (2001) SdrG, a fibrinogen-binding bacterial adhesin of the microbial surface components recognizing adhesive matrix molecules subfamily from Staphylococcus epidermidis, targets the thrombin cleavage site in the Bbeta chain, *The Journal of biological chemistry 276*, 27799-27805.

[60] Hartford, O., O'Brien, L., Schofield, K., Wells, J., and Foster, T. J. (2001) The Fbe (SdrG) protein of Staphylococcus epidermidis HB promotes bacterial adherence to fibrinogen, *Microbiology 147*, 2545-2552.

[61] Cunningham, M. W. (2000) Pathogenesis of group A streptococcal infections, *Clinical microbiology reviews 13*, 470-511.

[62] Carlsson, F., Sandin, C., and Lindahl, G. (2005) Human fibrinogen bound to Streptococcus pyogenes M protein inhibits complement deposition via the classical pathway, *Molecular microbiology 56*, 28-39.

[63] Shannon, O., Hertzen, E., Norrby-Teglund, A., Morgelin, M., Sjobring, U., and Bjorck, L. (2007) Severe streptococcal infection is associated with M protein-induced platelet activation and thrombus formation, *Molecular microbiology 65*, 1147-1157.

[64] Pietrocola, G., Schubert, A., Visai, L., Torti, M., Fitzgerald, J. R., Foster, T. J., Reinscheid, D. J., and Speziale, P. (2005) FbsA, a fibrinogen-binding protein from Streptococcus agalactiae, mediates platelet aggregation, *Blood 105*, 1052-1059.

[65] Schubert, A., Zakikhany, K., Schreiner, M., Frank, R., Spellerberg, B., Eikmanns, B. J., and Reinscheid, D. J. (2002) A fibrinogen receptor from group B Streptococcus interacts with fibrinogen by repetitive units with novel ligand binding sites, *Molecular microbiology 46*, 557-569.

[66] Kerrigan, S. W., Clarke, N., Loughman, A., Meade, G., Foster, T. J., and Cox, D. (2008) Molecular basis for Staphylococcus aureus-mediated platelet aggregate formation under arterial shear in vitro, *Arteriosclerosis, thrombosis, and vascular biology 28*, 335-340.

[67] Keane, C., Tilley, D., Cunningham, A., Smolenski, A., Kadioglu, A., Cox, D., Jenkinson, H. F., and Kerrigan, S. W. (2010) Invasive Streptococcus pneumoniae trigger platelet activation via Toll-like receptor 2, *Journal of thrombosis and haemostasis : JTH 8*, 2757-2765.

[68] Tilley, D. O., Arman, M., Smolenski, A., Cox, D., O'Donnell, J. S., Douglas, C. W., Watson, S. P., and Kerrigan, S. W. (2013) Glycoprotein Ibalpha and FcgammaRIIa play key roles in platelet activation by the colonizing bacterium, Streptococcus oralis, *Journal of thrombosis and haemostasis : JTH 11*, 941-950.

[69] Arman, M., Krauel, K., Tilley, D. O., Weber, C., Cox, D., Greinacher, A., Kerrigan, S. W., and Watson, S. P. (2014) Amplification of bacteria-induced platelet activation is triggered by FcgammaRIIA, integrin alphaIIbbeta3, and platelet factor 4, *Blood 123*, 3166-3174.

[70] Svensson, L., Baumgarten, M., Morgelin, M., and Shannon, O. (2014) Platelet Activation by Streptococcus pyogenes Leads to Entrapment in Platelet Aggregates, from Which Bacteria Subsequently Escape, *Infection and immunity 82*, 4307-4314.

[71] Sullam, P. M., Hyun, W. C., Szollosi, J., Dong, J., Foss, W. M., and Lopez, J. A. (1998) Physical proximity and functional interplay of the glycoprotein Ib-IX-V complex and the Fc receptor FcgammaRIIA on the platelet plasma membrane, *The Journal of biological chemistry 273*, 5331-5336.

[72] Miajlovic, H., Loughman, A., Brennan, M., Cox, D., and Foster, T. J. (2007) Both complement- and fibrinogen-dependent mechanisms contribute to platelet aggregation mediated by Staphylococcus aureus clumping factor B, *Infection and immunity 75*, 3335-3343.

[73] Naito, M., Sakai, E., Shi, Y., Ideguchi, H., Shoji, M., Ohara, N., Yamamoto, K., and Nakayama, K. (2006) Porphyromonas gingivalis-induced platelet aggregation in plasma depends on Hgp44 adhesin but not Rgp proteinase, *Molecular microbiology 59*, 152-167.

[74] Peerschke, E. I., Murphy, T. K., and Ghebrehiwet, B. (2003) Activation-dependent surface expression of gC1qR/p33 on human blood platelets, *Thrombosis and haemostasis 89*, 331-339.

[75] Nguyen, T., Ghebrehiwet, B., and Peerschke, E. I. (2000) Staphylococcus aureus protein A recognizes platelet gC1qR/p33: a novel mechanism for staphylococcal interactions with platelets, *Infection and immunity 68*, 2061-2068.

[76] Sarma, J. V., and Ward, P. A. (2011) The complement system, *Cell and tissue research 343*, 227-235.

[77] Ford, I., Douglas, C. W., Preston, F. E., Lawless, A., and Hampton, K. K. (1993) Mechanisms of platelet aggregation by Streptococcus sanguis, a causative organism in infective endocarditis, *British journal of haematology 84*, 95-100.

[78] Jackson, S. P., Yap, C. L., and Anderson, K. E. (2004) Phosphoinositide 3-kinases and the regulation of platelet function, *Biochemical Society transactions 32*, 387-392.

[79] Blair, P., Rex, S., Vitseva, O., Beaulieu, L., Tanriverdi, K., Chakrabarti, S., Hayashi, C., Genco, C. A., Iafrati, M., and Freedman, J. E. (2009) Stimulation of Toll-like receptor 2 in human platelets induces a thromboinflammatory response through activation of phosphoinositide 3-kinase, *Circulation research 104*, 346-354.

[80] Beutler, B., Hoebe, K., Du, X., and Ulevitch, R. J. (2003) How we detect microbes and respond to them: the Toll-like receptors and their transducers, *J Leukoc Biol 74*, 479-485.

[81] Stahl, A. L., Svensson, M., Morgelin, M., Svanborg, C., Tarr, P. I., Mooney, J. C., Watkins, S. L., Johnson, R., and Karpman, D. (2006) Lipopolysaccharide from enterohemorrhagic Escherichia coli binds to platelets through TLR4 and CD62 and is detected on circulating platelets in patients with hemolytic uremic syndrome, *Blood 108*, 167-176.

[82] Cognasse, F., Hamzeh-Cognasse, H., Lafarge, S., Delezay, O., Pozzetto, B., McNicol, A., and Garraud, O. (2008) Toll-like receptor 4 ligand can differentially modulate the release of cytokines by human platelets, *Br J Haematol 141*, 84-91.

[83] Scott, T., and Owens, M. D. (2008) Thrombocytes respond to lipopolysaccharide through Toll-like receptor-4, and MAP kinase and NF-kappaB pathways leading to expression of interleukin-6 and cyclooxygenase-2 with production of prostaglandin E2, *Mol Immunol 45*, 1001-1008.

[84] Clark, S. R., Ma, A. C., Tavener, S. A., McDonald, B., Goodarzi, Z., Kelly, M. M., Patel, K. D., Chakrabarti, S., McAvoy, E., Sinclair, G. D., Keys, E. M., Allen-Vercoe, E., Devinney, R., Doig, C. J., Green, F. H., and Kubes, P. (2007) Platelet TLR4 activates neutrophil extracellular traps to ensnare bacteria in septic blood, *Nat Med 13*, 463-469.

[85] Beachey, E. H., Chiang, T. M., Ofek, I., and Kang, A. H. (1977) Interaction of lipoteichoic acid of group A streptococci with human platelets, *Infect Immun 16*, 649-654.

[86] Chugh, T. D., Burns, G. J., Shuhaiber, H. J., and Bahr, G. M. (1990) Adherence of Staphylococcus epidermidis to fibrin-platelet clots in vitro mediated by lipoteichoic acid, *Infect Immun 58*, 315-319.

[87] Sheu, J. R., Lee, C. R., Lin, C. H., Hsiao, G., Ko, W. C., Chen, Y. C., and Yen, M. H. (2000) Mechanisms involved in the antiplatelet activity of Staphylococcus aureus lipoteichoic acid in human platelets, *Thromb Haemost 83*, 777-784.

[88] Sheu, J. R., Hsiao, G., Lee, C., Chang, W., Lee, L. W., Su, C. H., and Lin, C. H. (2000) Antiplatelet activity of Staphylococcus aureus lipoteichoic acid is mediated through a cyclic AMP pathway, *Thromb Res 99*, 249-258.

[89] Lourbakos, A., Potempa, J., Travis, J., D'Andrea, M. R., Andrade-Gordon, P., Santulli, R., Mackie, E. J., and Pike, R. N. (2001) Arginine-specific protease from Porphyromonas gingivalis activates protease-activated receptors on human oral epithelial cells and induces interleukin-6 secretion, *Infect Immun 69*, 5121-5130.

[90] Rose, P. E., Armour, J. A., Williams, C. E., and Hill, F. G. (1985) Verotoxin and neuraminidase induced platelet aggregating activity in plasma: their possible role in the pathogenesis of the haemolytic uraemic syndrome, *J Clin Pathol 38*, 438-441.

[91] Bhakdi, S., Muhly, M., Mannhardt, U., Hugo, F., Klapettek, K., Mueller-Eckhardt, C., and Roka, L. (1988) Staphylococcal alpha toxin promotes blood coagulation via attack on human platelets, *J Exp Med 168*, 527-542.

[92] Arvand, M., Bhakdi, S., Dahlback, B., and Preissner, K. T. (1990) Staphylococcus aureus alpha-toxin attack on human platelets promotes assembly of the prothrombinase complex, *J Biol Chem 265*, 14377-14381.

[93] Ramsland, P. A., Farrugia, W., Bradford, T. M., Sardjono, C. T., Esparon, S., Trist, H. M., Powell, M. S., Tan, P. S., Cendron, A. C., Wines, B. D., Scott, A. M., and Hogarth, P. M. (2011) Structural basis for Fc gammaRIIa recognition of human IgG and formation of inflammatory signaling complexes, *Journal of immunology 187*, 3208-3217.

[94] Plummer, C., Wu, H., Kerrigan, S. W., Meade, G., Cox, D., and Ian Douglas, C. W. (2005) A serine-rich glycoprotein of Streptococcus sanguis mediates adhesion to platelets via GPIb, British journal of haematology 129, 101-109.

[95] Sjobring, U., Ringdahl, U., and Ruggeri, Z. M. (2002) Induction of platelet thrombi by bacteria and antibodies, Blood 100, 4470-4477.

Chapter 5

# Platelet Interactions with Viruses and Parasites

Ana Lopez Alonso and Dermot Cox

Additional information is available at the end of the chapter

http://dx.doi.org/10.5772/60747

## 1. Introduction

Over the last few years our understanding of the role of platelets has evolved. While originally considered to be solely involved in thrombus formation recent studies suggest that they play an important role in the innate immune system. As the most numerous particles in the blood platelets are the first responders to any breaches in the vasculature where they bind to the damaged vessel and aggregate to seal the leak. They also become activated and secrete the contents of their granules, which contain anti-microbial peptides, which acts to sterilise the wound and to recruit other immune cells. As a result thrombocytopenia is a common response to infection by many different organisms [1, 2].

As part of the innate immune system platelets express many different pathogen recognition molecules that are involved in immune function rather than thrombosis. Thus platelets express Toll-Like Receptors (TLRs), which are pathogen recognition receptors [3] and in particular platelet TLR2 [4], TLR4 [5] and TLR7 [6] have been shown to be functional. Another important immune receptor is FcγRIIa, a receptor for the Fc-portion of IgG, which is typically expressed on phagocytic cells [7]. While platelets express functional FcγRIIa there is evidence of limited phagocytic ability for platelets [8-11]. DC-SIGN is another important pattern recognition molecule [12] that has been identified on platelets and found to be functional [13]. While both immune-mediated and haemostasis-mediated platelet activation result in activated platelets the platelet response is quite different in both cases [14].

The best-studied example of a role of platelets in infection is that with bacterial infection. While most effort has focused on Gram-positive bacteria many bacteria have been shown to activate platelets and these studies show a number of common features. The interaction of bacteria with platelets typically occurs due to direct binding to platelets, binding of a platelet-binding plasma protein to the bacteria or the secretion of a substance that activates platelets [1, 15, 16]. Typically streptococcal species such as *S. sanguinis* and *S. gordonii* bind directly to platelet GPIb.

In contrast *Staphylococcus aureus* binds fibrinogen, which in turn binds to GPIIb/IIIa on the platelet surface. *S. aureus* also produces toxins that activate platelets [17]. For the majority of bacteria that activate platelets, binding of IgG is required. This binds to FcγRIIa on the platelet surface triggering platelet activation [18]

## 2. Platelets in viral infection

While thrombocytopenia and in severe cases disseminated intravascular coagulation (DIC) are associated with bacterial infection this is also true for viral infection. Viral Haemorrhagic Fever (VHF) is similar to sepsis and both can be considered as forms of Systemic Inflammatory Response Syndrome (SIRS) [19, 20]. Equally thrombocytopenia is a common response to viral infections. However, it is worth noting that in some case the use of anti-viral agents may mediate the thrombocytopenia such as where neuraminidase inhibitors are associated with an immune thrombocytopenia [21] and abacavir enhances platelet activity by inhibiting guanylate cyclase [22].

### 2.1. Viral Haemorrhagic fever

Unlike with bacteria where virtually any species can lead to sepsis the viral equivalent (VHF) only occurs with members of 4 families of viruses known collectively as VHF viruses [20, 23].

**Flaviviruses.** These include Dengue virus (DENV) [24] and Yellow fever virus, which are transmitted by mosquitos and Omsk hemorrhagic fever virus [25] and Kyanasur Forest virus [26], which are transmitted by ticks. DENV is the most studied flavivirus due primarily to the 100 million infections per year with case fatality rates between 1-15% [27, 28]. Of these around 500,000 will progress to develop Dengue haemorrhagic fever (DHF) [27-30].

Dengue haemorrhagic fever is unusual as it typically occurs in response to a secondary infection with the primary infection producing relatively minor 'flu-like symptoms. In fact there are 4 serotypes of DENV and it is infection with a second serotype that leads to dengue haemorrhagic fever. This suggests that the presence of anti-DENV antibodies is necessary for DHF to occur and this process is known as antibody-dependent enhancement (ADE) [31, 32]. These antibodies have been shown to enhance virus uptake and replication through an interaction with Fc receptors [32-35]. However, just as antibody binding to bacteria can trigger platelet activation it is likely that antibody binding to DENV will also activate platelets in an FcγRIIa-dependent manner. This platelet activation has been shown to lead to enhanced permeability [36]. Bone marrow infection occurs in animal models of Dengue [37], which could lead to thrombocytopenia due to impaired platelet production.

**Filoviruses.** Filoviruses are primarily represented by Ebola and Marburg viruses both of which cause a very severe VHF. The Ebola virus is transmitted by fruit bats. Very little is known about the pathogenesis of filovirus-induced VHF although, not surprisingly there is evidence of platelet activation [38, 39]. Sudan virus (SUDV) has been shown to be associated with an increase in von Willebrand factor (vWf) levels, which is associated with poor outcome as well as haemorrhagic presentation [40].

http://dx.doi.org/10.5772/60747

**Bunyaviruses.** This family includes the Phleboviruses (Rift Valley fever virus), Nairoviruses (Crimean-Congo Haemorrhagic fever, CCHF) and Hantaviruses (Hantaan virus). Thrombocytopenia and an increase in mean platelet volume are associated with CCHF [41]. Thrombocytopenia is a common feature of Severe fever with thrombocytopenia syndrome (a Phlebovirus infection) and is a predictor of fatal outcome [42] and direct binding to platelets was demonstrated [43]. Thrombocytopenia in Hantaan virus infection is also associated with poor outcome [44]. The use of steroids and IVIg was found to be successful in the treatment of CCHF in twelve patients [45] and as IVIg has been shown to act as an inhibitor of FcγRIIa [46] it suggests a potential role for FcγRIIa in CCHF.

**Arenaviruses.** These include the Old World Lassa fever virus and lymphocytic choriomeningitis virus (LCMV) and the New World Junin, Guanarito, Machupo and Sabia viruses [47]. Little is known about the pathogenesis on Arenavirus VHF although there is evidence that partial platelet depletion increases disease severity in LCMV infection [48-50].

### 2.2. Other viral infections

Although there is a paucity of data on the mechanisms involved thrombocytopenia is a common response to many viral infection and not just VHF. However, in general, viral-induced thrombocytopenia is either due to platelet activation leading to consumption or infection of the megakaryocytes leading to impaired platelet production.

**Viral-induced platelet activation.** Coxsackieviruses B infection is associated with thrombocytopenia and has been shown to directly infect platelets. This appears to be beneficial as thrombocytopenic mice had higher mortality rates than normal mice. Thus, platelets appear to act as a sponge mopping up virus particles [51]. Platelets have been shown to express Toll-like receptors that play a role in the response to infection. Recently TLR-7 has been shown to be functional in platelets and to trigger platelet activation in response to encephalomyocarditis virus in a mouse model [6]. Cytomegalovirus binds to platelet TLR-2 leading to platelet activation [52]. On the other hand platelet activation leads to secretion of CXCL4, which prevents HIV-1 infection of neighbouring T-cells [53] as well as secretion of other pro-inflammatory factors such as CD40L [54]. FcγRIIa also plays an important role in platelet activation by viruses just as happens with bacteria. Influenza A $H_1N_1$ forms immune complexes that can trigger platelet activation in a FcγRIIa-dependent manner [55]. DC-SIGN is present on the platelet surface and is implicated in the binding of HIV-1 [56] and Dengue virus [13]. In the case of HIV-1 it acts in conjunction with CLEC-2 [57]. Adenovirus Type 3 enhanced ADP-induced platelet activation [58]. Enhanced platelet activation and sequestration was found with Hepatitis B infection [59]. Co-infection of influenza H1N1 and *Staphylococcus aureus* greatly increased the chances of developing DIC [60]. SIV infection in macaques leads to thrombocytopenia [61]. The occurrence of thrombocytopenia in influenza H1N1 infection is associated with mortality [62].

**Platelet interaction with other cells.** HIV-1 infection increases platelet-monocyte interactions, which is associated with neuroinflammation [63]. Influenza infection of endothelial cells leads to activation and recruitment of platelets, which can further increase permeability and reduce platelet count [64]. HIV-1 infection leads to increased levels of platelet-derived CD40L and platelet-monocyte aggregates. This results in monocyte activation and enhanced levels of extravasation especially in the brain microvasculature. It is proposed that this may play a role in the cognitive decline seen in AIDS [63-66]. The enhanced platelet activity seen in HIV patients can be reduced by treatment with aspirin [67]. The enhanced inflammation and endothelial cell activation seen in HIV [68] has been shown to persist even being present 12-years after anti-retroviral therapy [69]. Anti-retroviral therapy was found to reduce the thrombocytopenia that was found to re-occur if treatment was stopped. Re-starting treatment resolved the thrombocytopenia [70]. HIV-1-derived Tat has been shown to directly bind to platelets and activate them in a process dependent on CCR3 and $\beta_3$-integrins [71]. SIV infection in macaques leads to increased platelet-monocyte interactions [61]. Platelets interact with neutrophil extracellular traps (NETs) and facilitate their ability to neutralise poxvirus [72]. In hepatitis there is evidence that platelet are being sequestered to the liver which may play a significant role in hepatitis-associated thrombocytopenia [73].

**Effect of viruses on platelet production.** In SIV, TGFβ-mediated down-regulation of thrombopoietin leads to reduced production of platelets [74]. Reduced platelet production has also been seen in Dengue-infected mice [75] and megakaryocytes have been shown to be infected by Dengue virus [76]. Platelets are involved in hepatocellular carcinoma in mice infected with hepatitis B [77] and aspirin and clopidogrel therapy reduced the incidence in infected patients [78]. Respiratory syncytial virus (RSV) is associated with a decrease in mean platelet volume (MPV) [79] as is rotavirus [80] while HIV infection is associated with an increase in MPV [81]. Infection of mice with γ-herpes virus has also been shown to induce the formation of anti-platelet antibodies, which leads to an immune thrombocytopenia [82].

**Pathogen inactivation.** A major problem with blood transfusions is the potential for passing on both bacterial and viral infections. This was a major cause of transmission with both HIV and Hepatitis C. As a result strategies for pathogen inactivation have been developed. One of the challenges in this area is that it is necessary to develop strategies that will be effective against known pathogens such as HIV and hepatitis C as well as pathogens that we are not aware of yet. There are two specific products that need to be treated requiring different strategies. In the case of plasma solvent-detergent treatment can be effective however, this cannot be used for cell-based products such as red blood cells or platelets [83-86].

**Conclusion.** The platelet response to viral infection has many of the similarities of the response to bacterial infection. The primary purpose of this is host-defence and in this context there is evidence that platelets act as sponges to absorb the viruses and subsequently being cleared from the circulation. However, thrombocytopenia can also arise from infection of the endothelium, which binds platelets and removes them from the circulation. The other cause of viral-induced thrombocytopenia is impaired platelet production in response to megakaryocyte infection. There is evidence to support all of these mechanisms with different viruses having different effects. In fact even with a single virus multiple effects on platelets can be seen just as different bacteria have different mechanisms for activating platelet [1, 16] and even individual bacteria have multiple mechanism that depend on the shear stress of the local environment [87].

While the strategy of an anti-viral sponge is effective it is not without its problems. Excessive platelet activation can lead to disseminated intravascular coagulation such as occurs in an

http://dx.doi.org/10.5772/60747

extreme form in VHF. Correcting this DIC is critical for survival of the patient. Equally the prolonged hyper-activity of platelets in HIV-positive patients is a risk factor for cardiovascular disease in these patients. There is some evidence that anti-platelet agents can play a role here but as they inhibit platelet activity they may not be the ideal solution especially in DIC. A better strategy is to identify the mechanisms involved in the thrombocytopenia and to develop an inhibitor of the virus-platelet interaction without compromising platelet function (Figure 1). Interestingly FcγRIIa has been found to be an important drug target in bacteria-platelet interactions [1, 16] and there is evidence that with some viruses it may also be an important drug target as well [55].

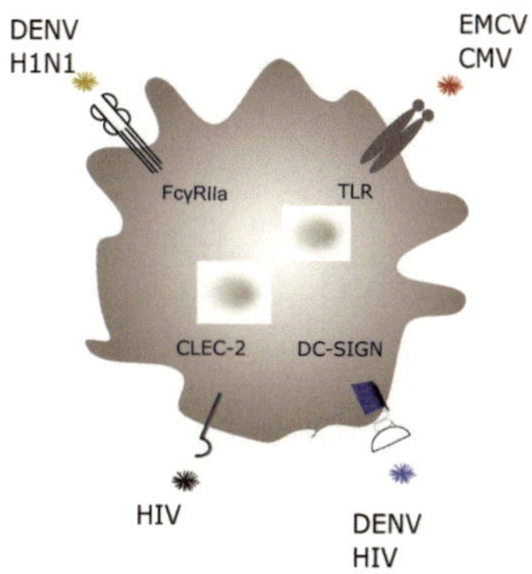


**Figure 1.** Virus can interact with platelets through multiple different receptors. Dengue (DENV) and Influenza H1N1 bind to FcγRIIa; HIV binds to CLEC-2; DENV and HIV can bind to DC-SIGN and Cytomegalovirus virus (CMV) and encephalomyocarditis (EMCV) bind to Toll-like receptors (TLR).

## 3. Parasites

As platelets are part of the innate immune system and interact with bacteria and viruses they also interact with parasites. In this context they bind to parasites and in some cases will kill them. As a result there can be a thrombocytopenia as well as evidence of micro-thrombi formation. The most studied parasites that interacts with platelets are the malaria parasites [88] although there has been some work on other parasites as well.

### 3.1. Malaria

Malaria is a mosquito borne parasite infection (*Plasmodium*), which is transmitted to humans through the *Anopheles* mosquito. Malaria is a major cause of morbidity and mortality in the developing world with 207 million cases of malaria in 2012 and an estimated 627 000 deaths, mostly children under five and pregnant women who live in Sub-Saharan Africa (WHO 2013). Malaria is caused by infection with *Plasmodium falciparum*, *P. vivax*, *P. ovale*, *P. malariae* or *P. knowlesi*. Most of the deaths are due to infection by *P. falciparum* as it is the most severe infection as well as the dominant infection. *P. bergei* and *P. chabaudi* infect mice and are frequently used for animal studies. Most cases of malaria present as uncomplicated malaria with characteristic symptoms of fever, nausea and aches, however, some can present with severe malaria that involves impaired function of various organs. The most serious form of severe malaria is cerebral malaria, which is estimated to occur in 10% of hospitalised cases and is associated with 80% of deaths. Cerebral malaria occurs when infected red blood cells (RBCs) occlude cerebral blood vessels [89].

**Thrombocytopenia in malaria.** Thrombocytopenia is a common feature in malaria [90, 91]. In fact it is considered to be diagnostic in suspect febrile patients [92, 93]. The extent of the thrombocytopenia is also a predictor of outcome [94-96]. There are a few studies suggesting that malarial thrombocytopenia is driven by platelet activation in patients with malaria [97, 98], and infected mice [99, 100]. A possible explanation for platelet activation in malaria is complement formation. The formation of C3d, indicating complement activation, was associated with thrombocytopenia in malaria-infected patients [101]. Nevertheless activation of platelets in malaria could also be related to direct interaction with the parasites [102, 103]. There is also evidence of immune-mediated clearance with two studies identifying an increased level of platelet-associated antibodies in thrombocytopenic malaria patients [104, 105]. This was further supported by a study that showed an association between polymorphisms in FcγRIIa, the platelet IgG receptor and disease severity [106]. IgE levels have also been associated with severity of malaria [107].

Platelets have been shown to be involved in clumping of parasitized red cells [108] and they have been found to accumulate in the brains of patients with cerebral malaria [108, 109].

**Plasmodium and platelet interaction.** GPIV (CD36) is a glycosylated protein [110] present in platelets - other cells such as macrophages, dendritic cells, adipocytes, muscle and some types of endothelial cells. While CD36 is a cell receptor for *P. falciparum*-infected erythrocytes [111, 112] there is evidence for other interactions, as antibodies to CD36 did not inhibit interactions with all isolates [95, 113]. The complement receptor gC1qR/HABP1/p32 on both endothelial cells and platelets has been shown to support an interaction with infected RBC's and supports platelet mediated clumping of infected RBC's although the parasite ligand is not known [113]. PECAM-1 was also shown to be an endothelial receptor for infected RBC's [114] and as this is also expressed on the platelet surface it is likely to mediate an interaction with platelets as well.

***Plasmodium falciparum*** **erythrocyte membrane protein 1 (PfEMP1).** Some strains of falciparum malaria parasites induce the formation of small membrane protrusions known as knobs on erythrocytes. These knobs have been identified as the site of contact with endothelial cells and high molecular weight malarial proteins expressed on these knobs mediate this interaction [115-117]. PfEMP1 was subsequently identified as the knob protein that binds to CD36 [118] but also to ICAM-1 and VCAM-1and it contains a number of different binding domains. PfEMP1 contains two different modules, the Duffy binding-like domain (DBL) of which there are six and the cysteine-rich inter-domain regions (CIDR) of which there are three [119]. The CD36 binding domain has been localized to one of the CIDR's, CIDR$\alpha$. A C-terminal 166 amino acid sequence appears to be responsible for the interaction with CD36 and that amino acids 106-166 appear to be especially important [120]. The region of CD36 that binds to PfEMP1 has been located to the region between amino acids 139-184 [121]. While PfEMP1 can directly bind to CD36 and a number of CD36 ligands can induce platelet aggregation there is no evidence that PfEMP1 triggers platelet activation. However, *P. falciparum* does trigger clumping of infected erythrocytes that is mediated by platelets in a CD36-dependent manner [95] and thus it is possible that this may be due to PfEMP1-CD36 mediated platelet activation.

### 3.2. Role of the endothelium

The endothelium plays an important role in the pathogenesis of malaria. The clumped RBC's bind to the endothelium and can ultimately occlude smaller blood vessels, especially in the brain. Activated endothelium is a key component of cerebral malaria and has been shown to occur in children [122]. Overproduction of cytokines plays a major role in the activation of the endothelium [123, 124]. One of the key cytokines involved is TNF, which is produced by macrophages in response to malaria antigens [125], possibly acting on TNFR2 [126]. Platelets play a significant role in the destruction of TNF-activated endothelial cells [127-129] while $TGF\beta_1$ released from activated platelets can kill TNF-activated endothelial cells [130].

A recent model has been proposed that draws together many of these observations in malaria (Figure 2). Activated endothelial cells secrete high molecular weight vWf, which form strings under high shear. Platelets bind to these strings, which also bind to the activated endothelial cells. Infected RBCs can then in turn bind to the immobilised platelets ultimately occluding the blood vessel which if in the cerebral micro-circulation leads to cerebral malaria [131].

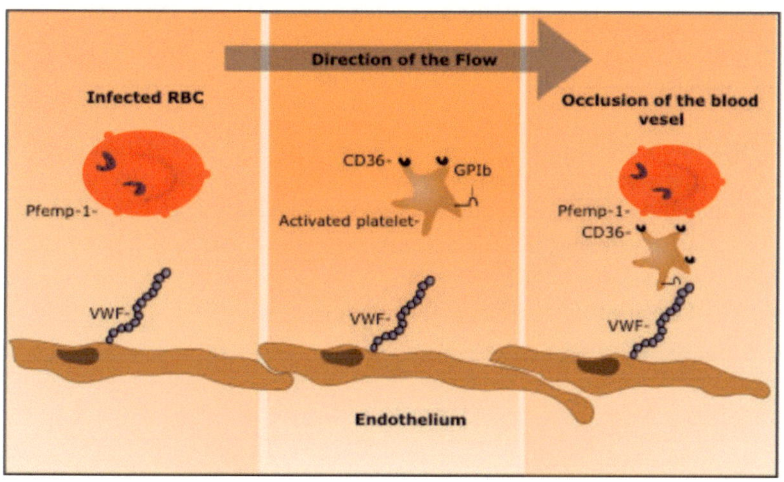


**Figure 2.** Platelets mediate plasmodium-infected red blood cells binding to the endothelium by GPIb binding to von Willebrand factor (vWf) strings on the endothelium and CD36 binding to *Plasmodium falciparum* erythrocyte membrane protein 1 (PfEMP1) on the red blood cell.

**Platelets as a double-edged sword.** The role of platelets in malaria is complex. On one hand platelet activation is critical in mediating the binding of infected RBCs to the endothelium and subsequent aggregate formation that is cause of cerebral malaria and animal studies suggest that blocking platelet function in mice is beneficial [124, 132, 133]. On the other hand platelets as part of the innate immune system play an important role in mediating the initial immune response to infection. Studies suggest that platelets play a beneficial role in malaria [134, 135] and mice rendered thrombocytopenic prior to infection had a much higher mortality rate compared with normal mice and thrombocytopenia only occurred in normal rats and not in splenectomised although mortality was much higher in splenectomised rats [134, 136]. Platelets also have been shown to be cytotoxic to plasmodium [137] and that platelet factor 4 (CXCL4) plays a key role in mediating this cytotoxicity [138, 139].

### 3.3. Other parasites

Schistosomes are trematodes and a major pathogen that causes over 200 million cases of schistosomiasis per year. Thrombocytopenia is a common symptom of infection with *Schistosoma mansoni* primarily due to platelets gathering in the spleen. There is also an increase in vWf and an increase in MPV [140]. Induction of thrombocytopenia prior to infection has been shown to significantly increase *S. mansoni* growth and platelets have been shown to bind to and kill the schistosomes [141, 142]. It appears that the cytotoxicity of platelets is enhanced significantly by factors secreted from immune cells such as interferon, tumour necrosis factor and IL-6 [143].

Trypanosomatids are unicellular parasites with a single flagellum and there are two clinically relevant genera. Genus *Trypanosma* has two major pathogenic species: *T. brucei* which is transmitted by the Tsetse fly and causes African sleeping sickness (a neurological disorder) [144] and *T. cruzi* which is transmitted by triatomine bugs and causes Chagas disease (a cardiac disease) [145]. Genus *Leshmania* contains a large number of species that cause leshmaniasis in humans and are transmitted by sandflies. *T. cruzi* infection of mice causes thrombocytopenia [146]. Chagas disease is associated with thromboembolism leading to stroke [145] and interestingly pentamidine which is often used to treat Chagas disease is also an anti-platelet agent (GPIIb/IIIa antagonist) [147] and *T. cruzi* binds fibronectin which could facilitate an interaction with platelets [148]. Trans-sialidase secreted from the trypanosome has been implicated in Chagas-associated thrombocytopenia as it cleaves sialic acid residues from platelets, which are then cleared from the circulation by Kupffer cells [149]. Kala Azar, a form of leshmaniasis is associated with thrombocytopenia and DIC [150]. In dogs with leshmaniasis there is evidence of an immune mediated thrombocytopenia [151].

## 4. Conclusions

It is clear that platelets are a key component of the innate immune system where they are the initial responders to infection. They appear to respond to the full range of pathogens including bacteria, parasites and viruses. Thus, thrombocytopenia is a characteristic symptom of infection by any organism. The response to bacteria infection is the best studied and a key role of the platelets is the secretion of anti-microbial peptides that as their name implies kill bacteria. While there is evidence that this also occurs with parasites it may not be true of viruses as they are not cells. There are what appear to be conflicting data on the role of platelets in infection. On one hand severe thrombocytopenia is associated with poor outcome suggesting that platelet activation is important in pathogenesis. On the other hand thrombocytopenic animals are more likely to have a poor outcome suggesting that platelets prevent the disease.

These conflicting data can be resolved in a model where platelets have a dual role. Upon initial exposure to a pathogen there is a decline in platelet number due to the initial immune response. Platelets are activated and bind the pathogen. This then results in pathogen killing or at least clearance of the platelet-pathogen complex from the circulation. If that works then it is the end of the story. The pathogen is ultimately cleared and the disease resolves. However, sometimes platelets fail to clear the pathogen or pathogen replication exceeds the clearance. As a result there is excessive platelet activation that can progress to disseminated intravascular coagulation. Thus, in the early stage of infection platelets are good as they help clear the pathogen, however, in the later stages of infection platelets are bad as they are contributing to the problem.

This then leads to the question of whether platelets are a good target for treating infection. It has been proposed that anti-platelet agents may not be wise in patients with malaria since they are protective [152]. However, it is important to appreciate the stage of the disease. During the early stages of an infection an anti-platelet agent would be undesirable, as it would inhibit the immune functions of the platelets. However, as the disease progresses towards DIC an anti-platelet agent would be desirable as at this point platelets are now part of the problem and their excessive activation must be contained. While conventional anti-platelet agents may be useful in a patient with VHF or DIC this may not be advisable. The result may be that platelet number is preserved but the price paid would be platelet function, which in VHF would exacerbate the bleeding problems. Thus, a better approach may be targeting the platelet receptors that mediate the interactions with the pathogen. This would prevent platelet activation while maintaining platelet function. While some of these targets are likely to be pathogen specific a good target may be FcγRIIa. It has been shown to be critical in bacteria-induced platelet activation but also appears to play a role in some viral infections.

## Author details

Ana Lopez Alonso and Dermot Cox*

*Address all correspondence to: dcox@rcsi.ie

Molecular & Cellular Therapeutics, Royal College of Surgeons in Ireland, Dublin, Ireland

## References

[1] Cox D, Kerrigan SW, Watson SP. Platelets and the innate immune system: mechanisms of bacterial-induced platelet activation. *Journal of Thrombosis and Haemostasis.* 2011; 9: 1097-107.

[2] Semple JW, Italiano JE, Freedman J. Platelets and the immune continuum. *Nat Rev Immunol.* 2011; 11: 264-74.

[3] Keogh B, Parker AE. Toll-like receptors as targets for immune disorders. *Trends in Pharmacological Sciences*. 2011; 32: 435-42.

[4] Keane C, Tilley D, Cunningham A, Smolenski A, Kadioglu A, Cox D, Jenkinson HF, Kerrigan SW. Invasive *Streptococcus pneumoniae* trigger platelet activation via Toll-like receptor 2. *J Thrombos Haemost*. 2010; 8: 2757-65.

[5] Clark SR, Ma AC, Tavener SA, McDonald B, Goodarzi Z, Kelly MM, Patel KD, Chakrabarti S, McAvoy E, Sinclair GD, Keys EM, Allen-Vercoe E, Devinney R, Doig CJ, Green FH, Kubes P. Platelet TLR4 activates neutrophil extracellular traps to ensnare bacteria in septic blood. *Nature medicine*. 2007; 13: 463-9.

[6] Koupenova M, Vitseva O, MacKay CR, Beaulieu LM, Benjamin EJ, Mick E, Kurt-Jones EA, Ravid K, Freedman JE. *Platelet-TLR7 mediates host survival and platelet count during viral infection in the absence of platelet-dependent thrombosis*. 2014.

[7] Hogarth PM, Pietersz GA. Fc receptor-targeted therapies for the treatment of inflammation, cancer and beyond. *Nat Rev Drug Discov*. 2012; 11: 311-31.

[8] Riaz AH, Tasma BE, Woodman ME, Wooten RM, Worth RG. Human platelets efficiently kill IgG-opsonized E. coli. *FEMS Immunology & Medical Microbiology*. 2012; 65: 78-83.

[9] Antczak AJ, Vieth JA, Singh N, Worth RG. Internalization of IgG-Coated Targets Results in Activation and Secretion of Soluble CD40 Ligand and RANTES by Human Platelets. *Clin Vaccine Immunol*. 2011; 18: 210-6.

[10] Fitzgerald JR, Loughman A, Keane F, Brennan M, Knobel M, Higgins J, Visai L, Speziale P, Cox D, Foster TJ. Fibronectin-binding proteins of *Staphylococcus aureus* mediate activation of human platelets via fibrinogen and fibronectin bridges to integrin GPIIb/IIIa and IgG binding to the FcgRIIa receptor. *Mol Microbiol*. 2006; 59: 212-30.

[11] Huang Z-Y, Chien P, Indik ZK, Schreiber AD. Human platelet Fc[gamma]RIIA and phagocytes in immune-complex clearance. *Molecular Immunology*. 2011; 48: 691-6.

[12] Garcia-Vallejo JJ, van Kooyk Y. The physiological role of DC-SIGN: A tale of mice and men. *Trends in Immunology*. 2013; 34: 482-6.

[13] Hottz ED, Oliveira MF, Nunes PC, Nogueira RM, Valls-de-Souza R, Da Poian AT, Weyrich AS, Zimmerman GA, Bozza PT, Bozza FA. Dengue induces platelet activation, mitochondrial dysfunction and cell death through mechanisms that involve DC-SIGN and caspases. *J Thromb Haemost*. 2013; 11: 951-62.

[14] Rex S, Beaulieu L, Perlman D, Vitseva O, Blair P, McComb M, Costello C, Freedman J. Immune versus thrombotic stimulation of platelets differentially regulates signalling pathways, intracellular protein-protein interactions, and alpha-granule release. *Thromb Haemost*. 2009; 102: 97-110.

[15] Cox D. Bacteria-platelet interactions. *Journal of Thrombosis and Haemostasis*. 2009; 7: 1865-6.

[16] Fitzgerald JR, Foster TJ, Cox D. The interaction of bacterial pathogens with platelets. *Nat Rev Microbiol*. 2006; 4: 445-57.

[17] Kerrigan S, Cox D. The Effect of Bacterial Toxins on Platelet Function. In: Kini RM, Clemetson KJ, Markland FS, McLane MA, Morita T, eds. *Toxins and Hemostasis From Bench to Bedside*. Heidelberg: Springer, 2010, 637-51.

[18] Arman M, Krauel K, Tilley DO, Weber C, Cox D, Greinacher A, Kerrigan SW, Watson SP. Amplification of bacteria-induced platelet activation is triggered by FcgammaRIIA, integrin alphaIIbbeta3, and platelet factor 4. *Blood*. 2014; 123: 3166-74.

[19] Bosmann M, Ward PA. The inflammatory response in sepsis. *Trends in Immunology*. 2013; 34: 129-36.

[20] Cox D, Salvato M, Zapata J. The Role of Platelets in Viral Hemorrhagic Fevers. *J Bioterr Biodef*. 2013: S12-003.

[21] Harada-Shirado K, Ikeda K, Furukawa M, Sukegawa M, Takahashi H, Shichishima-Nakamura A, Ohkawara H, Noji H, Kawabata K, Saito S-i, Ohto H, Ogawa K, Takeishi Y. Severe Immune Thrombocytopenia Possibly Elicited by the Anti-influenza Viral Agent Peramivir. *Internal Medicine*. 2014; 53: 2369-71.

[22] Baum PD, Sullam PM, Stoddart CA, McCune JM. Abacavir increases platelet reactivity via competitive inhibition of soluble guanylyl cyclase. *AIDS*. 2011; 25: 2243-8.

[23] Zapata JC, Cox D, Salvato MS. The Role of Platelets in the Pathogenesis of Viral Hemorrhagic Fevers. *PLoS Negl Trop Dis*. 2014; 8: e2858.

[24] Leyssen P, De Clercq E, Neyts J. Perspectives for the treatment of infections with Flaviviridae. *Clin Microbiol Rev*. 2000; 13: 67-82, table of contents.

[25] Ruzek D, Yakimenko VV, Karan LS, Tkachev SE. Omsk haemorrhagic fever. *Lancet*. 2010; 376: 2104-13.

[26] Kyasanur Forest Disease. CDC, 2012.

[27] Scientific working group report on dengue. WHO, 2006.

[28] Dengue - Guidelines for diagnosis, Treatment, prevention and control. Geneva, Switzerland: World Health Organization, 2009.

[29] Gibbons RV, Vaughn DW. Dengue: an escalating problem. *BMJ*. 2002; 324: 1563-6.

[30] Guzman MG, Kouri G. Dengue and dengue hemorrhagic fever in the Americas: lessons and challenges. *J Clin Virol*. 2003; 27: 1-13.

[31] Cummings DA, Schwartz IB, Billings L, Shaw LB, Burke DS. Dynamic effects of antibody-dependent enhancement on the fitness of viruses. *Proc Natl Acad Sci U S A*. 2005; 102: 15259-64.

[32] Schmidt AC. Response to Dengue Fever — The Good, the Bad, and the Ugly? *New England Journal of Medicine*. 2010; 363: 484-7.

[33] Goncalvez AP, Engle RE, St Claire M, Purcell RH, Lai CJ. Monoclonal antibody-mediated enhancement of dengue virus infection in vitro and in vivo and strategies for prevention. *Proc Natl Acad Sci U S A*. 2007; 104: 9422-7.

[34] Rodenhuis-Zybert IA, van der Schaar HM, da Silva Voorham JM, van der Ende-Metselaar H, Lei HY, Wilschut J, Smit JM. Immature dengue virus: a veiled pathogen? *PLoS pathogens*. 2010; 6: e1000718.

[35] Moi ML, Lim C-K, Takasaki T, Kurane I. Involvement of the Fc{gamma} receptor IIA cytoplasmic domain in antibody-dependent enhancement of dengue virus infection. *J Gen Virol*. 2010; 91: 103-11.

[36] Hottz ED, Lopes JF, Freitas C, Valls-de-Souza R, Oliveira MF, Bozza MT, Da Poian AT, Weyrich AS, Zimmerman GA, Bozza FA, Bozza PT. *Platelets mediate increased endothelium permeability in dengue through NLRP3-inflammasome activation*. 2013.

[37] Noisakran S, Onlamoon N, Hsiao H-M, Clark KB, Villinger F, Ansari AA, Perng GC. Infection of bone marrow cells by dengue virus in vivo. *Experimental hematology*. 2012; 40: 250-9.e4.

[38] Fisher-Hoch SP, Platt GS, Lloyd G, Simpson DI, Neild GH, Barrett AJ. Haematological and biochemical monitoring of Ebola infection in rhesus monkeys: implications for patient management. *Lancet*. 1983; 2: 1055-8.

[39] Fisher-Hoch SP, Platt GS, Neild GH, Southee T, Baskerville A, Raymond RT, Lloyd G, Simpson DI. Pathophysiology of shock and hemorrhage in a fulminating viral infection (Ebola). *J Infect Dis*. 1985; 152: 887-94.

[40] McElroy AK, Erickson BR, Flietstra TD, Rollin PE, Towner JS, Nichol ST, Spiropoulou CF. Von Willebrand Factor Is Elevated in Individuals Infected with Sudan Virus and Is Associated with Adverse Clinical Outcomes. *Viral Immunol*. 2014.

[41] Ekiz F, Gurbuz Y, Basar O, Aytekin G, Ekiz O, Senturk CS, Aktas B, Yilmaz B, Altinbas A, Coban S, Sencan I. Mean platelet volume in the diagnosis and prognosis of Crimean-Congo hemorrhagic fever. *Clin Appl Thromb Hemost*. 2013; 19: 441-4.

[42] Cui N, Bao X-L, Yang Z-D, Lu Q-B, Hu C-Y, Wang L-Y, Wang B-J, Wang H-Y, Liu K, Yuan C, Fan X-J, Wang Z, Zhang L, Zhang X-A, Hu L-P, Liu W, Cao W-C. Clinical progression and predictors of death in patients with severe fever with thrombocytopenia syndrome in China. *Journal of Clinical Virology*. 2014; 59: 12-7.

[43] Jin C, Liang M, Ning J, Gu W, Jiang H, Wu W, Zhang F, Li C, Zhang Q, Zhu H, Chen T, Han Y, Zhang W, Zhang S, Wang Q, Sun L, Liu Q, Li J, Wang T, Wei Q, Wang S,

Deng Y, Qin C, Li D. Pathogenesis of emerging severe fever with thrombocytopenia syndrome virus in C57/BL6 mouse model. *Proc Natl Acad Sci U S A*. 2012; 109: 10053-8.

[44] Wang M, Wang J, Wang T, Li J, Hui L, Ha X. Thrombocytopenia as a predictor of severe acute kidney injury in patients with Hantaan virus infections. *PLoS One*. 2013; 8: e53236.

[45] Erduran E, Bahadir A, Palanci N, Gedik Y. The treatment of crimean-congo hemorrhagic fever with high-dose methylprednisolone, intravenous immunoglobulin, and fresh frozen plasma. *J Pediatr Hematol Oncol*. 2013; 35: e19-24.

[46] van Mirre E, Teeling JL, van der Meer JWM, Bleeker WK, Hack CE. Monomeric IgG in Intravenous Ig Preparations Is a Functional Antagonist of Fc{gamma}RII and Fc{gamma}RIIIb. *J Immunol*. 2004; 173: 332-9.

[47] Cummins D. Arenaviral haemorrhagic fevers. *Blood Rev*. 1991; 5: 129-37.

[48] Loria GD, Romagnoli PA, Moseley NB, Rucavado A, Altman JD. Platelets support a protective immune response to LCMV by preventing splenic necrosis. *Blood*. 2013; 121: 940-50.

[49] Gómez RM, Schattner M. *Arenaviruses bite the "dust"*. 2013.

[50] Schattner M, Rivadeneyra L, Pozner R, Gómez R. Pathogenic Mechanisms Involved in the Hematological Alterations of Arenavirus-induced Hemorrhagic Fevers. *Viruses*. 2013; 5: 340-51.

[51] Negrotto S, Jaquenod de Giusti C, Rivadeneyra L, Ure AE, Mena HA, Schattner M, Gomez RM. Platelets interact with Coxsackieviruses B and have a critical role in the pathogenesis of virus-induced myocarditis. *J Thromb Haemost*. 2014.

[52] Assinger A, Kral JB, Yaiw KC, Schrottmaier WC, Kurzejamska E, Wang Y, Mohammad A-A, Religa P, Rahbar A, Schabbauer G, Butler LM, Söderberg-Naucler C. Human Cytomegalovirus–Platelet Interaction Triggers Toll-Like Receptor 2–Dependent Proinflammatory and Proangiogenic Responses. *Arteriosclerosis, Thrombosis, and Vascular Biology*. 2014; 34: 801-9.

[53] Solomon Tsegaye T, GnirSZ K, Rahe-Meyer N, Kiene M, Kramer-Kuhl A, Behrens G, Munch J, Pohlmann S. Platelet activation suppresses HIV-1 infection of T cells. *Retrovirology*. 2013; 10: 48.

[54] Damien P, Cognasse F, Lucht F, Suy F, Pozzetto B, Garraud O, Hamzeh-Cognasse H. Highly Active Antiretroviral Therapy Alters Inflammation Linked to Platelet Cytokines in HIV-1–Infected Patients. *Journal of Infectious Diseases*. 2013; 208: 868-70.

[55] Boilard E, Paré G, Rousseau M, Cloutier N, Dubuc I, Lévesque T, Borgeat P, Flamand L. *Influenza virus H1N1 activates platelets through FcγRIIA signaling and thrombin generation*. 2014.

[56] Beck Z, Jagodzinski LL, Eller MA, Thelian D, Matyas GR, Kunz AN, Alving CR. Platelets and Erythrocyte-Bound Platelets Bind Infectious HIV-1 in Plasma of Chronically Infected Patients. *PLoS ONE*. 2013; 8: e81002.

[57] Chaipan C, Soilleux EJ, Simpson P, Hofmann H, Gramberg T, Marzi A, Geier M, Stewart EA, Eisemann J, Steinkasserer A, Suzuki-Inoue K, Fuller GL, Pearce AC, Watson SP, Hoxie JA, Baribaud F, Pohlmann S. DC-SIGN and CLEC-2 mediate human immunodeficiency virus type 1 capture by platelets. *J Virol*. 2006; 80: 8951-60.

[58] Jin YY, Yu XN, Qu ZY, Zhang AA, Xing YL, Jiang LX, Shang L, Wang YC. Adenovirus type 3 induces platelet activation in vitro. *Mol Med Rep*. 2014; 9: 370-4.

[59] Dou J, Lou Y, Wu J, Lu Y, Jin Y. Thrombocytopenia in patients with hepatitis B virus-related chronic hepatitis: Evaluation of the immature platelet fraction. *Platelets*. 2014; 25: 399-404.

[60] Nguyen T, Kyle UG, Jaimon N, Tcharmtchi MH, Coss-Bu JA, Lam F, Teruya J, Loftis L. Coinfection with Staphylococcus aureus increases risk of severe coagulopathy in critically ill children with influenza A (H1N1) virus infection. *Crit Care Med*. 2012; 40: 3246-50.

[61] Metcalf Pate KA, Lyons CE, Dorsey JL, Shirk EN, Queen SE, Adams RJ, Gama L, Morrell CN, Mankowski JL. Platelet Activation and Platelet-Monocyte Aggregate Formation Contribute to Decreased Platelet Count During Acute Simian Immunodeficiency Virus Infection in Pig-tailed Macaques. *Journal of Infectious Diseases*. 2013; 208: 874-83.

[62] Lopez-Delgado JC, Rovira A, Esteve F, Rico N, Manez Mendiluce R, Ballus Noguera J, Berrade J. Thrombocytopenia as a mortality risk factor in acute respiratory failure in H1N1 influenza. *Swiss Med Wkly*. 2013; 143: w13788.

[63] Singh MV, Davidson DC, Jackson JW, Singh VB, Silva J, Ramirez SH, Maggirwar SB. Characterization of Platelet–Monocyte Complexes in HIV-1–Infected Individuals: Possible Role in HIV-Associated Neuroinflammation. *The Journal of Immunology*. 2014; 192: 4674-84.

[64] Armstrong SM, Darwish I, Lee WL. Endothelial activation and dysfunction in the pathogenesis of influenza A virus infection. *Virulence*. 2013; 4: 537-42.

[65] Davidson D, Jackson J, Maggirwar S. Targeting platelet-derived soluble CD40 ligand: a new treatment strategy for HIV-associated neuroinflammation? *Journal of Neuroinflammation*. 2013; 10: 144.

[66] Bethel-Brown C, Yao H, Hu G, Buch S. Platelet-derived growth factor (PDGF)-BB-mediated induction of monocyte chemoattractant protein 1 in human astrocytes: implications for HIV-associated neuroinflammation. *J Neuroinflammation*. 2012; 9: 262.

[67] O'Brien M, Montenont E, Hu L, Nardi MA, Valdes V, Merolla M, Gettenberg G, Cavanagh K, Aberg JA, Bhardwaj N, Berger JS. Aspirin attenuates platelet activation and

immune activation in HIV-1-infected subjects on antiretroviral therapy: a pilot study. *J Acquir Immune Defic Syndr*. 2013; 63: 280-8.

[68] Gresele P, Falcinelli E, Sebastiano M, Baldelli F. Endothelial and platelet function alterations in HIV-infected patients. *Thromb Res*. 2012; 129: 301-8.

[69] Ronsholt FF, Ullum H, Katzenstein TL, Gerstoft J, Ostrowski SR. Persistent inflammation and endothelial activation in HIV-1 infected patients after 12 years of antiretroviral therapy. *PLoS One*. 2013; 8: e65182.

[70] Zetterberg E, Neuhaus J, Baker JV, Somboonwit C, Llibre JM, Palfreeman A, Chini M, Lundgren JD, Group ISS. Platelet count kinetics following interruption of antiretroviral treatment. *AIDS*. 2013; 27: 59-68.

[71] Wang J, Zhang W, Nardi MA, Li Z. HIV-1 Tat-induced platelet activation and release of CD154 contribute to HIV-1-associated autoimmune thrombocytopenia. *Journal of Thrombosis and Haemostasis*. 2011; 9: 562-73.

[72] Jenne Craig N, Wong Connie HY, Zemp Franz J, McDonald B, Rahman Masmudur M, Forsyth Peter A, McFadden G, Kubes P. Neutrophils Recruited to Sites of Infection Protect from Virus Challenge by Releasing Neutrophil Extracellular Traps. *Cell Host & Microbe*. 2013; 13: 169-80.

[73] Kondo R, Yano H, Nakashima O, Tanikawa K, Nomura Y, Kage M. Accumulation of platelets in the liver may be an important contributory factor to thrombocytopenia and liver fibrosis in chronic hepatitis C. *J Gastroenterol*. 2013; 48: 526-34.

[74] Metcalf Pate KA, Lyons CE, Dorsey JL, Queen SE, Adams RJ, Morrell CN, Mankowski JL. TGFbeta-Mediated Downregulation of Thrombopoietin Is Associated With Platelet Decline in Asymptomatic SIV Infection. *J Acquir Immune Defic Syndr*. 2014; 65: 510-6.

[75] Sridharan A, Chen Q, Tang KF, Ooi EE, Hibberd ML, Chen J. Inhibition of Megakaryocyte Development in the Bone Marrow Underlies Dengue Virus-Induced Thrombocytopenia in Humanized Mice. *Journal of Virology*. 2013; 87: 11648-58.

[76] Clark KB, Noisakran S, Onlamoon N, Hsiao HM, Roback J, Villinger F, Ansari AA, Perng GC. Multiploid CD61+ Cells Are the Pre-Dominant Cell Lineage Infected during Acute Dengue Virus Infection in Bone Marrow. *PLoS One*. 2012; 7: e52902.

[77] Sitia G, Aiolfi R, Di Lucia P, Mainetti M, Fiocchi A, Mingozzi F, Esposito A, Ruggeri ZM, Chisari FV, Iannacone M, Guidotti LG. Antiplatelet therapy prevents hepatocellular carcinoma and improves survival in a mouse model of chronic hepatitis B. *Proceedings of the National Academy of Sciences*. 2012; 109: E2165–E72.

[78] Sitia G, Iannacone M, Guidotti LG. Anti-platelet therapy in the prevention of hepatitis B virus-associated hepatocellular carcinoma. *Journal of Hepatology*. 2013; 59: 1135-8.

[79] Renshaw AA, Drago B, Toraya N, Gould EW. Respiratory syncytial virus infection is strongly correlated with decreased mean platelet volume. *International Journal of Infectious Diseases*. 2013; 17: e678-e80.

[80] Mete E, Akelma AZ, Cizmeci MN, Bozkaya D, Kanburoglu MK. Decreased mean platelet volume in children with acute rotavirus gastroenteritis. *Platelets*. 2014; 25: 51-4.

[81] Mena A, Meijide H, Vazquez P, Castro A, Lopez S, Bello L, Serrano J, Balinas J, Pedreira JD. HIV increases mean platelet volume during asymptomatic HIV infection in treatment-naive patients. *J Acquir Immune Defic Syndr*. 2011; 57: e112-3.

[82] Freeman ML, Burkum CE, Lanzer KG, Roberts AD, Pinkevych M, Itakura A, Kummer LW, Szaba FM, Davenport MP, McCarty OJ, Woodland DL, Smiley ST, Blackman MA. Gammaherpesvirus latency induces antibody-associated thrombocytopenia in mice. *J Autoimmun*. 2013; 42: 71-9.

[83] Schlenke P. Pathogen Inactivation Technologies for Cellular Blood Components: an Update. *Transfusion Medicine and Hemotherapy*. 2014; 41: 309-25.

[84] Lozano M, Cid J. Pathogen inactivation: coming of age. *Curr Opin Hematol*. 2013; 20: 540-5.

[85] Seltsam A, Muller TH. Update on the use of pathogen-reduced human plasma and platelet concentrates. *Br J Haematol*. 2013; 162: 442-54.

[86] Prowse CV. Component pathogen inactivation: a critical review. *Vox Sang*. 2013; 104: 183-99.

[87] Kerrigan SW, Clarke N, Loughman A, Meade G, Foster TJ, Cox D. Molecular basis for *Staphylococcus aureus*-mediated platelet aggregate formation under arterial shear in vitro. *Arterioscler Thromb Vasc Biol*. 2008; 28: 335-40.

[88] Cox D, McConkey S. The role of platelets in the pathogenesis of cerebral malaria. *Cellular and Molecular Life Sciences*. 2010; 67: 557-68.

[89] Idro R, Jenkins NE, Newton CR. Pathogenesis, clinical features, and neurological outcome of cerebral malaria. *Lancet Neurol*. 2005; 4: 827-40.

[90] Angchaisuksiri P. Coagulopathy in malaria. *Thromb Res*. 2014; 133: 5-9.

[91] Muley A, Lakhani J, Bhirud S, Patel A. Thrombocytopenia in Plasmodium vivax Malaria: How Significant? *J Trop Med*. 2014; 2014: 567469.

[92] Patel U, Gandhi G, Friedman S, Niranjan S. Thrombocytopenia in malaria. *J Natl Med Assoc*. 2004; 96: 1212-4.

[93] Erhart LM, Yingyuen K, Chuanak N, Buathong N, Laoboonchai A, Miller RS, Meshnick SR, Gasser RA, Jr., Wongsrichanalai C. Hematologic and clinical indices of malaria in a semi-immune population of western Thailand. *Am J Trop Med Hyg*. 2004; 70: 8-14.

[94] Rogier C, Gerardin P, Imbert P. Thrombocytopenia is predictive of lethality in severe childhood falciparum malaria. *Arch Dis Child.* 2004; 89: 795-a-6.

[95] Pain A, Ferguson DJ, Kai O, Urban BC, Lowe B, Marsh K, Roberts DJ. Platelet-mediated clumping of *Plasmodium falciparum*-infected erythrocytes is a common adhesive phenotype and is associated with severe malaria. *Proc Natl Acad Sci U S A.* 2001; 98: 1805-10.

[96] Gerardin P, Rogier C, Ka AS, Jouvencel P, Brousse V, Imbert P. Prognostic value of thrombocytopenia in African children with falciparum malaria. *Am J Trop Med Hyg.* 2002; 66: 686-91.

[97] Facer CA, Theodoridou A. Elevated plasma levels of P-selectin (GMP-140/CD62P) in patients with Plasmodium falciparum malaria. *Microbiol Immunol.* 1994; 38: 727-31.

[98] Scott CS, Van Zyl D, Ho E, Ruivo L, Mendelow B, Coetzer TL. Thrombocytopenia in patients with malaria: automated analysis of optical platelet counts and platelet clumps with the Cell Dyn CD4000 analyser. *Clin Lab Haematol.* 2002; 24: 295-302.

[99] Chang WL, Li J, Sun G, Chen HL, Specian RD, Berney SM, Granger DN, van der Heyde HC. P-selectin contributes to severe experimental malaria but is not required for leukocyte adhesion to brain microvasculature. *Infect Immun.* 2003; 71: 1911-8.

[100] Combes V, Rosenkranz AR, Redard M, Pizzolato G, Lepidi H, Vestweber D, Mayadas TN, Grau GE. Pathogenic role of P-selectin in experimental cerebral malaria: importance of the endothelial compartment. *Am J Pathol.* 2004; 164: 781-6.

[101] Adam C, Geniteau M, Gougerot-Pocidalo M, Verroust P, Lebras J, Gibert C, Morel-Maroger L. Cryoglobulins, circulating immune complexes, and complement activation in cerebral malaria. *Infect Immun.* 1981; 31: 530-5.

[102] Rock G, Clark W, Sternbach M, Kolajova M, McLaine P. Haemolytic uraemic syndrome is an immune-mediated disease: role of anti-CD36 antibodies. *Br J Haematol.* 2005; 131: 247-52.

[103] Ockenhouse CF, Magowan C, Chulay JD. Activation of monocytes and platelets by monoclonal antibodies or malaria-infected erythrocytes binding to the CD36 surface receptor in vitro. *J Clin Invest.* 1989; 84: 468-75.

[104] Kelton JG, Keystone J, Moore J, Denomme G, Tozman E, Glynn M, Neame PB, Gauldie J, Jensen J. Immune-mediated thrombocytopenia of malaria. *J Clin Invest.* 1983; 71: 832-6.

[105] Yamaguchi S, Kubota T, Yamagishi T, Okamoto K, Izumi T, Takada M, Kanou S, Suzuki M, Tsuchiya J, Naruse T. Severe thrombocytopenia suggesting immunological mechanisms in two cases of vivax malaria. *American Journal of Hematology.* 1997; 56: 183-6.

[106] Cooke GS, Aucan C, Walley AJ, Segal S, Greenwood BM, Kwiatkowski DP, Hill AVS. Association Of Fcγ Receptor IIa (CD32) Polymorphism With Severe Malaria In West Africa. *Am J Trop Med Hyg*. 2003; 69: 565-8.

[107] Seka-Seka J, Brouh Y, Yapo-Crezoit AC, Atseye NH. The role of serum immunoglobulin E in the pathogenesis of Plasmodium falciparum malaria in Ivorian children. *Scand J Immunol*. 2004; 59: 228-30.

[108] Grau GE, Mackenzie CD, Carr RA, Redard M, Pizzolato G, Allasia C, Cataldo C, Taylor TE, Molyneux ME. Platelet accumulation in brain microvessels in fatal pediatric cerebral malaria. *J Infect Dis*. 2003; 187: 461-6.

[109] Dorovini-Zis K, Schmidt K, Huynh H, Fu W, Whitten RO, Milner D, Kamiza S, Molyneux M, Taylor TE. The neuropathology of fatal cerebral malaria in malawian children. *Am J Pathol*. 2011; 178: 2146-58.

[110] Tandon NN, Lipsky RH, Burgess WH, Jamieson GA. Isolation and characterization of platelet glycoprotein IV (CD36). *J Biol Chem*. 1989; 264: 7570-5.

[111] Barnwell JW, Asch AS, Nachman RL, Yamaya M, Aikawa M, Ingravallo P. A human 88-kD membrane glycoprotein (CD36) functions in vitro as a receptor for a cytoadherence ligand on Plasmodium falciparum-infected erythrocytes. *J Clin Invest*. 1989; 84: 765-72.

[112] Ockenhouse CF, Tandon NN, Magowan C, Jamieson GA, Chulay JD. Identification of a platelet membrane glycoprotein as a falciparum malaria sequestration receptor. *Science*. 1989; 243: 1469-71.

[113] Biswas AK, Hafiz A, Banerjee B, Kim KS, Datta K, Chitnis CE. Plasmodium falciparum uses gC1qR/HABP1/p32 as a receptor to bind to vascular endothelium and for platelet-mediated clumping. *PLoS pathogens*. 2007; 3: 1271-80.

[114] Treutiger CJ, Heddini A, Fernandez V, Muller WA, Wahlgren M. PECAM-1/CD31, an endothelial receptor for binding Plasmodium falciparum-infected erythrocytes. *Nature medicine*. 1997; 3: 1405-8.

[115] Kilejian A. Characterization of a protein correlated with the production of knob-like protrusions on membranes of erythrocytes infected with Plasmodium falciparum. *Proc Natl Acad Sci U S A*. 1979; 76: 4650-3.

[116] Leech JH, Barnwell JW, Aikawa M, Miller LH, Howard RJ. Plasmodium falciparum malaria: association of knobs on the surface of infected erythrocytes with a histidine-rich protein and the erythrocyte skeleton. *J Cell Biol*. 1984; 98: 1256-64.

[117] Aley SB, Sherwood JA, Howard RJ. Knob-positive and knob-negative Plasmodium falciparum differ in expression of a strain-specific malarial antigen on the surface of infected erythrocytes. *J Exp Med*. 1984; 160: 1585-90.

[118] Baruch DI, Gormley JA, Ma C, Howard RJ, Pasloske BL. Plasmodium falciparum erythrocyte membrane protein 1 is a parasitized erythrocyte receptor for adherence to

CD36, thrombospondin, and intercellular adhesion molecule 1. *PNAS*. 1996; 93: 3497-502.

[119] Smith J, Kyes S, Craig A, Fagan T, Hudson-Taylor D, Miller L, Baruch D, Newbold C. Analysis of adhesive domains from the A4VAR Plasmodium falciparum erythrocyte membrane protein-1 identifies a CD36 binding domain. *Mol Biochem Parasitol*. 1998; 97: 133-48..

[120] Mo M, Lee HC, Kotaka M, Niang M, Gao X, Iyer JK, Lescar J, Preiser P. The C-terminal segment of the cysteine-rich interdomain of Plasmodium falciparum erythrocyte membrane protein 1 determines CD36 binding and elicits antibodies that inhibit adhesion of parasite-infected erythrocytes. *Infect Immun*. 2008; 76: 1837-47.

[121] Baruch DI, Ma XC, Pasloske B, Howard RJ, Miller LH. CD36 Peptides That Block Cytoadherence Define the CD36 Binding Region for Plasmodium falciparum-Infected Erythrocytes. *Blood*. 1999; 94: 2121-7.

[122] Hollestelle MJ, Donkor C, Mantey EA, Chakravorty SJ, Craig A, Akoto AO, O'Donnell J, van Mourik JA, Bunn J. von Willebrand factor propeptide in malaria: evidence of acute endothelial cell activation. *British Journal of Haematology*. 2006; 133: 562-9.

[123] Grau GE, Tacchini-Cottier F, Vesin C, Milon G, Lou JN, Piguet PF, Juillard P. TNF-induced microvascular pathology: active role for platelets and importance of the LFA-1/ICAM-1 interaction. *Eur Cytokine Netw*. 1993; 4: 415-9.

[124] van der Heyde HC, Gramaglia I, Sun G, Woods C. Platelet depletion by anti-CD41 (αIIb) mAb injection early but not late in the course of disease protects against Plasmodium berghei pathogenesis by altering the levels of pathogenic cytokines. *Blood*. 2005; 105: 1956-63.

[125] Bate CA, Taverne J, Kwiatkowski D, Playfair JH. Phospholipids coupled to a carrier induce IgG antibody that blocks tumour necrosis factor induction by toxic malaria antigens. *Immunology*. 1993; 79: 138-45.

[126] Piguet PF, Kan CD, Vesin C. Role of the tumor necrosis factor receptor 2 (TNFR2) in cerebral malaria in mice. *Lab Invest*. 2002; 82: 1155-66.

[127] Lou J, Donati YR, Juillard P, Giroud C, Vesin C, Mili N, Grau GE. Platelets play an important role in TNF-induced microvascular endothelial cell pathology. *Am J Pathol*. 1997; 151: 1397-405.

[128] Wassmer SC, Lepolard C, Traore B, Pouvelle B, Gysin J, Grau GE. Platelets reorient Plasmodium falciparum-infected erythrocyte cytoadhesion to activated endothelial cells. *J Infect Dis*. 2004; 189: 180-9.

[129] Grau G, Tacchini-Cottier F, Vesin C, Milon G, Lou J, Piguet P, Juillard P. TNF-induced microvascular pathology: active role for platelets and importance of the LFA-1/ICAM-1 interaction. *Eur Cytokine Netw*. 1993; 4: 415-9.

[130] Wassmer SC, de Souza JB, Frere C, Candal FJ, Juhan-Vague I, Grau GE. TGF-beta1 released from activated platelets can induce TNF-stimulated human brain endothelium apoptosis: a new mechanism for microvascular lesion during cerebral malaria. *J Immunol*. 2006; 176: 1180-4.

[131] Bridges DJ, Bunn J, van Mourik JA, Grau G, Preston RJS, Molyneux M, Combes V, O'Donnell JS, de Laat B, Craig A. Rapid activation of endothelial cells enables Plasmodium falciparum adhesion to platelet-decorated von Willebrand factor strings. *Blood*. 2010; 115: 1472-4.

[132] Sun G, Chang WL, Li J, Berney SM, Kimpel D, van der Heyde HC. Inhibition of platelet adherence to brain microvasculature protects against severe Plasmodium berghei malaria. *Infect Immun*. 2003; 71: 6553-61.

[133] Wassmer SC, Combes V, Candal FJ, Juhan-Vague I, Grau GE. Platelets potentiate brain endothelial alterations induced by Plasmodium falciparum. *Infect Immun*. 2006; 74: 645-53.

[134] Polack B, Delolme F, Peyron F. Protective role of platelets in chronic (Balb/C) and acute (CBA/J) Plasmodium berghei murine malaria. *Haemostasis*. 1997; 27: 278-85.

[135] Wassmer SC, Taylor T, MacLennan CA, Kanjala M, Mukaka M, Molyneux ME, Grau GE. Platelet-Induced Clumping of *Plasmodium falciparum*-Infected Erythrocytes from Malawian Patients with Cerebral Malaria: Possible Modulation In Vivo by Thrombocytopenia. *The Journal of Infectious Diseases*. 2008; 197: 72-8.

[136] Aggrey AA, Srivastava K, Ture S, Field DJ, Morrell CN. Platelet induction of the acute-phase response is protective in murine experimental cerebral malaria. *J Immunol*. 2013; 190: 4685-91.

[137] McMorran BJ, Marshall VM, de Graaf C, Drysdale KE, Shabbar M, Smyth GK, Corbin JE, Alexander WS, Foote SJ. Platelets Kill Intraerythrocytic Malarial Parasites and Mediate Survival to Infection. *Science*. 2009; 323: 797-800.

[138] Srivastava K, Cockburn IA, Swaim A, Thompson LE, Tripathi A, Fletcher CA, Shirk EM, Sun H, Kowalska MA, Fox-Talbot K, Sullivan D, Zavala F, Morrell CN. Platelet Factor 4 Mediates Inflammation in Experimental Cerebral Malaria. *Cell Host & Microbe*. 2008; 4: 179-87.

[139] McMorran BJ, Wieczorski L, Drysdale KE, Chan JA, Huang HM, Smith C, Mitiku C, Beeson JG, Burgio G, Foote SJ. Platelet factor 4 and Duffy antigen required for platelet killing of Plasmodium falciparum. *Science*. 2012; 338: 1348-51.

[140] Correia MC, Domingues AL, Lacerda HR, Santos EM, Machado CG, Hora V, Neves MA, Brito A, Coelho MR, Silva JL. Platelet function and the von Willebrand factor antigen in the hepatosplenic form of schistosomiasis mansoni. *Trans R Soc Trop Med Hyg*. 2009; 103: 1053-8.

[141] Stanley RG, Ngaiza JR, Wambayi E, Lewis J, Doenhoff MJ. Platelets as an innate defence mechanism againstSchistosoma mansoniinfections in mice. *Parasite Immunology*. 2003; 25: 467-73.

[142] Stanley R, Ngaiza J, Atieno E, Jell G, Francklow K, Jackson C, Parry H, Doenhoff M. Immune-dependent thrombocytopaenia in mice infected with *Schistosoma mansoni. Parasitology*. 2003; 126: 225-9.

[143] Da'dara AA, Skelly PJ. Schistosomes versus platelets. *Thromb Res*. 2014.

[144] Kennedy PGE. Clinical features, diagnosis, and treatment of human African trypanosomiasis (sleeping sickness). *The Lancet Neurology*. 2013; 12: 186-94.

[145] Nunes MC, Dones W, Morillo CA, Encina JJ, Ribeiro AL, Council on Chagas Disease of the Interamerican Society of C. Chagas disease: an overview of clinical and epidemiological aspects. *J Am Coll Cardiol*. 2013; 62: 767-76.

[146] da Silva RV, Malvezi AD, Augusto Lda S, Kian D, Tatakihara VL, Yamauchi LM, Yamada-Ogatta SF, Rizzo LV, Schenkman S, Pinge-Filho P. Oral exposure to Phytomonas serpens attenuates thrombocytopenia and leukopenia during acute infection with Trypanosoma cruzi. *PLoS One*. 2013; 8: e68299.

[147] Cox D, Motoyama Y, Seki J, Aoki T, Dohi M, Yoshida K. Pentamidine: a non-peptide GPIIb/IIIa antagonist--in vitro studies on platelets from humans and other species. *Thrombosis and Haemostasis*. 1992; 68: 731-6.

[148] Cox D, Uga S, Motoyama Y, Yoshida K. Characterization of the fibronectin binding properties of *Trypanasoma cruzi* epimastigotes. *J Protozool Res*. 1992; 2: 149-57.

[149] Tribulatti MV, Mucci J, Van Rooijen N, Leguizamon MS, Campetella O. The trans-sialidase from Trypanosoma cruzi induces thrombocytopenia during acute Chagas' disease by reducing the platelet sialic acid contents. *Infect Immun*. 2005; 73: 201-7.

[150] Varma N, Naseem S. Hematologic changes in visceral leishmaniasis/kala azar. *Indian J Hematol Blood Transfus*. 2010; 26: 78-82.

[151] Cortese L, Terrazzano G, Piantedosi D, Sica M, Prisco M, Ruggiero G, Ciaramella P. Prevalence of anti-platelet antibodies in dogs naturally co-infected by Leishmania infantum and Ehrlichia canis. Vet J. 2011; 188: 118-21.

[152] Greenbaum DC, FitzGerald GA. Platelets, Pyrexia, and Plasmodia. N Engl J Med. 2009; 361: 526-8.

Section 3

# The Role of Platelets in Various Disease States

Chapter 6

# Platelets — Allies of Tumour Cells

Annachiara Mitrugno, Niamh Moran and Pat Metharom

Additional information is available at the end of the chapter

http://dx.doi.org/10.5772/60681

## 1. Introduction

### 1.1. History of platelets and their association with cancer

In 1865, Armand Trousseau observed several cases of severe blood clotting in patients with malignancy [1] but was unable to speculate on the underlying mechanism. In 1882, Bizzozero first demonstrated that blood platelets, or thrombocytes, adhered to damaged blood vessels and hypothesised that these blood components played a central role in haemostasis and experimental thrombosis [2]. Subsequently, Riess reported an association between thrombocytosis (defined as a platelet count of >400x$10^9$/ L of blood) and cancer death [3]. Almost a century later, these preliminary observations were revisited and confirmed [4, 5], initiating a renewed interest in a potential role for platelets in cancer metastasis, invasion and angiogenesis [6-10]. In this chapter, we will explore the evidence demonstrating a wider remit for platelets than simple haemostasis and thrombosis. We will review the data suggesting that platelets facilitate circulating cancer cells to traverse physiological and immunological obstacles and establish as solid tumours in remote places, where they enable a bespoke blood supply. In addition, we will explore the complex molecular mechanisms that underlie the platelet-tumour cell interactions.

## 2. Platelet biology in haemostasis and cancer

The role of platelets in haemostasis and thrombosis is well known. Platelets survey the blood vessels for evidence of damage. Upon detection, platelets undergo a rapid but highly regulated activation which results in dramatic shape change, adhesion to the exposed sub-endothelial matrix, secretion of important effectors from dense granules and/or alpha-granules, formation of a haemostatic platelet aggregate and activation of the coagulation cascade. All of these processes lead to reinforcement of the platelet plug in closing the breech in the vessel wall [11]. Thus, the currently accepted role for platelets is to contribute to haemostasis by their physiological ability to maintain the structural integrity of the blood vessels.

The role of platelets in cancer metastases is less well known. However, numerous experimental studies have shown that thrombocytopenia (defined as a platelet count of <100x$10^9$/L blood) induced in tumour-bearing mice, effectively reduces tumour dissemination and tumour growth [6, 17]. Moreover, thrombocytosis may be an indicator of an advanced stage of cancer and is often associated with poor prognosis. Thus, platelets appear to exert a pro-metastatic function, enabling tumour development.

Metastasis is the dissemination of cancer cells from the primary tumour mass to distant organs and occurs predominantly through the blood stream [12]. It is an intricate multi-step cascade during which cancer cells intravasate from the primary site into the blood vessels, circulate in the blood towards distant anatomical sites, adhere to the luminal wall of micro-vessels (arterioles and capillaries) and penetrate into the surrounding tissue (extravasation) to eventually colonize it [13]. Survival of the newly relocated tumour foci depends on the subsequent establishment of a novel blood supply to support tumour growth, a process termed angiogenesis [14]. Metastasis is responsible for as much as 90% of cancer associated mortality [15].

The pro-metastatic activity of platelets can be explained as the *pathological* capability to prolong tumour cell survival in the circulation and in the new metastatic location. Survival of circulating tumour cells (CTCs) in the circulation is achieved by protecting them from immune destruction, facilitating their adhesion to the vascular endothelium or enabling extravasation of the tumour cells to secondary sites. Moreover, platelets play a role in enabling angiogenesis to provide a necessary blood supply for a growing tumour mass [16-19, 20].

In normal circulation within intact vasculature, most platelets do not undergo significant interactions with the endothelial surface during their entire lifetime. The quiescent state of platelets is protected by the presence of extrinsic regulators, such as nitric oxide (NO) and prostacyclin ($PGI_2$), produced continuously by intact endothelial cells. Moreover, the presence of potential platelet activators such as collagen, adenosine diphosphate (ADP) and thrombin are tightly regulated in the bloodstream. Only strong biological signals such as the exposure of the sub-endothelial matrix components (VWF, collagen, fibrinogen, laminin, fibronectin) following endothelial damage or the generation of thrombin via the coagulation cascade will permit platelet activation to enable a haemostatic or a thrombotic response. Platelets adhere to sub-endothelial molecules via their surface receptors for von Willebrand Factor, VWF (GPIb/IX/V), collagen ($\alpha_2\beta_1$ and GPVI), fibrinogen ($\alpha_{IIb}\beta_3$), fibronectin ($\alpha_5\beta_1$) and laminin ($\alpha_6\beta_1$), resulting in platelet capture, activation, shape change and release of secretory granules. The relative contribution of each receptor-ligand interaction is influenced by blood flow condition, with GpIb-VWF interplay prevailing under high shear conditions observed in arterioles/stenotic arteries [21]. Activated platelets rapidly secrete and produce a number of soluble molecules, mainly ADP and thromboxane ($TXA_2$), triggering activation of surrounding platelets leading to the formation of a platelet-rich clot. Moreover, activated platelets express

http://dx.doi.org/10.5772/60681

negatively charged surface phospholipids that contribute to localised coagulation leading to thrombin generation. Thrombin then further activates platelets *via* protease-activated receptors -1 (PAR-1), -4 (PAR-4) and GPIb-IX-V [22-25] and also enzymatically converts fibrinogen into fibrin [26]. The binding of fibrin results in further reinforcement of the existing platelet plug and of its anchorage to the site of vascular injury [21]. Figure 1 shows an overview of platelet activation responses to wounding and cancer metastasis.

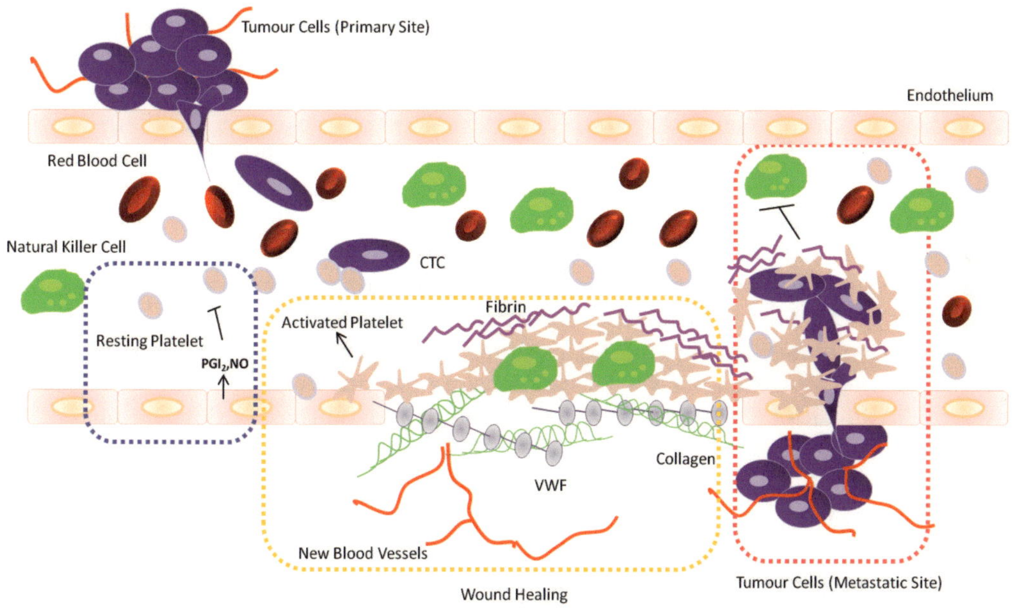


**Figure 1.** Differentiating platelet activity in haemostasis and cancer. *Blue Box*: In physiological condition platelets circulate in the blood stream in a quiescent state. Prostacyclin $I_2$ ($PGI_2$) and nitric oxide (NO) are the main soluble mediators through which the endothelium inhibits platelet reactivity. *Yellow Box*: In response to endothelial injury, highly thrombogenic proteins such as von Willebrand factor (VWF) and collagen are exposed, which synergistically induce platelet activation and haemostatic plug formation. Fibrin consolidates the platelet plug while newly formed blood vessels (angiogenesis) provide nutrients to inflammatory cells and clear cell debris. *Red Box*: Circulating cancer cells (CTC) activate and aggregate platelets *via* paracrine and/or juxtacrine signals to ensure their survival in the bloodstream, and to permit extravasation and proliferation at the metastatic site. Fibrin supports tumour inflammation and provides important scaffolding for tumour cell attachment to the endothelium. Newly formed vessels guarantee nutrients and oxygen for tumour growth and survival.

Importantly, platelet activation, aggregation and secretion, are also triggered in a carcinogenic microenvironment [6, 9, 27] and serve to enable tumour metastasis. The first experimental observation of platelet involvement in cancer metastasis dates back to 1968 when Gasic and colleagues demonstrated an anti-metastatic effect associated with thrombocytopenia in mouse models [6]. Subsequently, several *in vitro* and *in vivo* experimental models provided direct demonstrations of the profound pro-survival influence that platelet activation exerts on three critical stages during blood borne metastasis:

1. cancer dissemination through the blood (haematogenous spread);

2. tissue invasion or extravasation from the vasculature at the metastatic site and

3. Tumour angiogenesis and tumour blood vessels stability.

### 2.1. Platelets enable cancer cell dissemination during haematogenous spread

During their migration through the bloodstream, circulating cancer cells (CTCs) are exposed to an unfavourable environment, characterised by shear forces and innate immune cytotoxicity. In order to escape immune recognition and overcome shear forces, CTCs in the bloodstream attract an entourage of platelets and use them as a cellular shield for their survival [18, 28]. Evidence that platelets prevent natural killer cells (NK) from destroying CTCs, comes from both *in vivo and* in *vitro* studies. Platelet-depletion in mice causes a reduction in tumour colonization when compared to mice with normal platelet counts [29]. In addition, the ability of NK cells to lyse the tumour cells *in vitro* is directly correlated with platelet density [29]. Palumbo and colleagues subsequently demonstrated that platelet-fibrin deposits form a cloak around B16-F10 melanoma cells helping to camouflage the tumour cells to enable them to escape immune recognition and elimination [30]. The mesh of fibrin, induced by tissue factor on the surface of CTCs, envelops the cancer cells [18, 31] permitting them to evade recognition by NK cells [32, 33]. In addition, the coat of platelets enables a mechanism of molecular mimicry resulting in the acquisition of platelet-derived major histocompatibility complex (MHC-I) by cancer cells [34]. Moreover, platelet derived transforming growth factor β ($TGF_{\beta}$) and platelet derived growth factor (PDGF) can impede NK immune surveillance by down-regulating the NK cell activating immune-receptor (NKG2D) [35] and NK cell PDGF receptor- expression [36]. Thus platelets enhance CTC survival, permitting them to traverse the blood vessels to establish a secondary locations.

### 2.2. Platelets support cancer cell extravasation

In order to leave the circulation and metastasize, cancer cells must adhere to the microvasculature of a target organ and penetrate the surrounding tissue [37]. As early as 1985, electron micrographs showed B16 melanoma cells trapped in an intricate network of platelets and fibrin at the lung vasculature site [38]. Indeed, under *in vitro* flow conditions, platelets facilitate tumour cells adhesion to enable the cancer cells to tether and arrest to the subendothelium [39, 40] by using platelet P-selectin and $\alpha_{IIb}\beta_3$ as potential bridging molecules. Tethering and adhesion of colon carcinoma (LS174T, COLO205, and HCT-8) and melanoma cells (M21, M397, M501 and M537) to the subendothelium can be prevented by antagonism of P-selectin or $\alpha_{IIb}\beta_3$, on platelet surfaces [39-41]. Furthermore, platelets adhering to CTCs are activated to release growth factors (including vascular endothelium growth factor (VEGF), TGFβ, and PDGF) and proteases of the matrix metalloprotease (MMP) class at sites of adhesion to the endothelium [42-44]. Once released, platelet-derived cytokines enhance endothelial growth while MMPs will degrade specific component of the extracellular matrix (ECM) encouraging vascular permeability and extravasation of tumour cells, as well as the release of growth factors sequestered in the ECM [45].

Extravasation is also supported by platelet-derived nucleotides. Munc13-4 deficient mice, whose platelets lack the ability to secrete dense granule components such as ADP and ATP, or mice deficient in the $P2Y_2$-ATP receptor on endothelial cells, demonstrate a significant reduction in metastasis in mouse models of melanoma (B16) and breast carcinoma (LCC) [20]. Thus, platelet-bound adhesive molecules and platelet derived soluble molecules synergistically help cancer cells to traverse the endothelial cell barriers, penetrate the parenchyma and establish new lesions.

### 2.3. Platelets promote tumour angiogenesis and safeguard vascular integrity

The assembly of a new vascular network (angiogenesis) is of central importance to the growth of solid tumours beyond 2-3 mm [46]. The role of platelets in angiogenesis and be found in recent comprehensive reviews [14, 47]. An intimate association with the circulation is required for the tumour to acquire necessary nutrients, to shed metabolic waste products and to sustain further tumour growth and invasion [43, 48]. Interestingly, tumour blood vessels display remarkable morphological abnormalities involving permeability and leakiness, and excessive and haphazard branching [45, 49]. This vessel morphology permits the access of CTCs to the circulation, favouring contacts with platelets which, in turn, can function as source of pro-angiogenic factors at the metastatic niche and contribute to tumour survival and progression [50]. Indeed, platelets can stimulate endothelial cell proliferation and augment the formation of capillaries-like tubes *in vitro* [51] and angiogenesis *in vivo* [17, 52, 53]. Brock's finding that tumour-derived vascular endothelial growth factor (VEGF), a molecule that enables angiogenesis by stimulating endothelial cells proliferation and migration, can stimulate endothelial cells to expose VWF is noteworthy [54]. It has in fact been speculated that the release of platelet binding or activating molecules, such as VWF, may favour platelet adhesion to the vascular wall with a consequent activation and release of further pro-angiogenic molecules [50].

Platelets are recognised as major physiological transporters of VEGF in blood of healthy subjects and patients with breast and colorectal cancer [50, 55-59]. The possible rationale underlying this phenomenon became apparent when the ability of platelets to actively and selectively sequester tumour-derived angiogenesis regulators in a carcinogenic microenvironment was shown [60, 61]. Therefore, it was not surprising to observe that platelets isolated from tumour-bearing mice and activated with ADP could induce angiogenesis more efficiently than platelets obtained from cancer-free mice [62].

In addition to VEGF, platelets are carriers of many crucial regulators of angiogenesis (pro- and anti- angiogenic factors), which can be released, in a selective fashion according to the nature of the stimulus [19, 63, 64], a concept that is still somewhat controversial. However in this context, MCF-7 breast cancer cells can orchestrate the preferential release of pro-angiogenic molecules (e.g. VEGF), but not of the anti-angiogenic counterpart (e.g. endostatin), from platelet $\alpha$-granules, to induce angiogenesis *in vitro* [19]. Interestingly, treatment of human platelets with aspirin (COX-1 inhibitor) or antibodies against $\alpha_{IIb}\beta_3$ prior to exposure to breast cancer cells has been shown to inhibit the release of pro-angiogenic factors *in vitro* [19, 65, 66].

In addition to storage and release of angiogenic regulators, platelets can also contribute to maintaining tumour vessel homeostasis by protecting tumour-vasculature from haemorrhaging. In 2008, Wagner's group demonstrated that the metastatic rate of experimental tumours in a thrombocytopenic mouse model was restored when mice were retransfused with platelets from a littermate [17]. However, if the retransfused platelets were rendered incapable of a secretion response, then the growth rate of metastatic tumours was again found to be low. Thus, platelet granular contents, released from activated platelets, was responsible for the greater metastatic potential in platelet-replete mice [17]. The authors noted a tendency for the metastatic tumours to have fragile blood vessels and also demonstrated evidence of haemorrhage in the thrombocytopenic mice. Transfusing these mice with fresh platelets rescued this effect, allowing robust angiogenesis at the secondary lesions and permitting more metastatic colonization of the mouse lungs[17, 53]. However, depletion of platelet granules prior to transfusion into the thrombocytopenic mice limited the angiogenic effect, without eliminating platelet's ability to blood clotting process. Overall, this research suggests that the platelet secretome is responsible for the establishment of a necessary blood supply to the tumour mass and that this ability occurs independently from thrombus formation. In addition to this, a recent study demonstrated impaired blood vessel density and maturation at the tumour niche in platelet-depleted mice [67]. Thus, the pathological role that platelets can play in cancer metastasis has now become more evident. However, the molecular mechanisms underlying these interactions have remained somewhat elusive.

Figure 2 summarises the proposed role for platelets in enabling (A) survival of CTCs, and (B) extravasation and metastatic growth as discussed above.

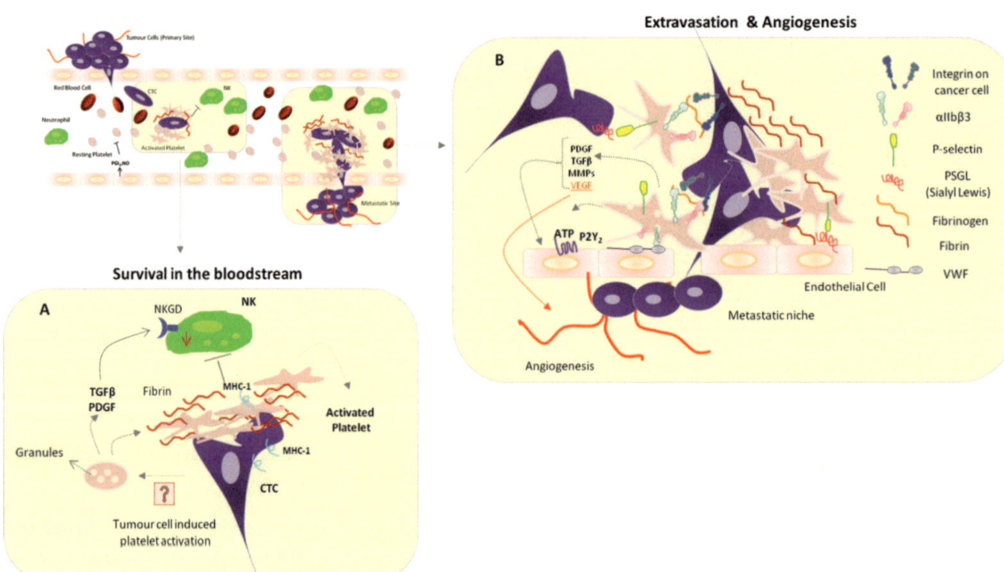


**Figure 2.** Simplified schematic model of platelet-mediated cancer progression. A. *Platelets support cancer cell survival in the bloodstream.* CTC induce platelet aggregation and secretion. Aggregated platelets surround and protect CTC from NK-mediated lysis via physical shielding. Platelets also release $TGF_{\beta}$ and PDGF, which function as downregulators of the NK-activating receptor NKGD. In addition, CTC can escape the immune surveillance through molecular mimicry of platelets (See Section 1.2.1 for further details). B. *Platelets contribute to tumour extravasation and angiogenesis.* Activated platelets interaction with tumour cells is thought to be mediated by P-selectin binding to PSGL-1 (P-selectin glycoprotein ligand-1) and integrin-fibrinogen-integrin bridges. Platelet release of growth and angiogenic factors as well as proteases contributes to cancer cell extravasation and formation of new stable capillaries at the metastatic niche (See section 1.2.2 & 1.2.3 for further details).

## 3. The identity of platelet surface receptors involved in cancer progression

The surface of human platelets contains multiple receptors that help platelets to react in response to a wide range of agonists and adhesive proteins. The roles of these receptors in thrombosis are well established. There is also ample evidence to support the involvement of some platelet receptors in the process of tumour cell induced platelet aggregation (TCIPA) and cancer spreading in the bloodstream [68-72].

### 3.1. G Protein-Coupled Receptors (GPCR)

The seven transmembrane receptors (7TM) are well represented in platelets (Table 1) and constitute both the major checkpoints that maintain platelets in a resting state (e.g.; $PGI_2$ receptor/IP) and the primary mediators of the second phase of platelet activation during thrombosis and haemostasis (e.g.; ADP receptors/$P2Y_1$ and $P2Y_{12}$; Thromboxane $TXA_2$ Receptor/TP) [73].

| LIGANDS | RECEPTORS |
|---|---|
| Thrombin | PAR 1, 4 |
| ADP | $P2Y_{12}$, $P2Y_1$ |
| $TXA_2$ | TP |
| $PGI_2$ | IP |
| $PGE_2$ | $EP_1$/$EP_3$/$EP_4$ |
| Lipids | PAF |
| Lysophospholipids (LPL) | LPL-R |
| C-X-C Chemokines | CXCR-4 |
| CC-Chemokines | CCR1,CCR3,CCR4 |
| Epinephrine/dopamine | β2 Adrenergic |
| Serotonin | $5\text{-}HT_{2A}$ |

**Table 1.** Platelet GPCRs and Ligands

#### *3.1.1. Protease-Activated Receptors (PARs): Thrombin receptors*

In haemostatic conditions, PARs drive platelet activation in response to thrombin. Thrombin is a plasma serine-protease that is generated in response to activation of the blood coagulation system and converts fibrinogen into fibrin, forming a mesh that serves to strengthen the thrombus and support clot retraction. In addition, thrombin directly activates platelets causing platelet aggregation.

Thrombin is both a platelet agonist and a pro-coagulant molecule that is required for some of the molecular strategies used by cancer cells to progress in their lethal journey. Mice deficient in their primary thrombin receptor, PAR-4, have a reduced ability to support metastasis compared to wild-type mice [74].

### *3.1.2. Purinergic receptor $2Y_{12}$ and $2Y_1$: ADP receptors*

$P2Y_1$ and $P2Y_{12}$ receptors are membrane-binding sites for ADP on platelets. ADP can activate platelets in an autocrine fashion, if released from platelet dense granules following a primary wave of activation, or in a paracrine fashion if secreted by damaged cells at sites of vascular injury. Some carcinomas, mainly neuroblastoma, melanoma and breast cancer cells, have been demonstrated to be capable of secreting ADP [75, 76]. ADP scavengers such as apyrase, efficiently impair *in vitro* platelet activation induced by 59M ovarian cancer cells [77], Caco-2 colon cancer cells [78], MCF-7 breast cancer cells, [79] and HeLa human cervical carcinoma cells [80]. Experiments in mouse models of cancer provided even more direct demonstration of the profound influence that ADP-triggered response exerts on tumour progression. When Lewis lung tumour cells were implanted into host mice lacking the expression of $P2Y_{12}$ receptors, their ability to metastasize to the lungs was disrupted [81]. In complementary experiments, ticagrelor, a $P2Y_{12}$ antagonist, succeeded in blocking tumour metastasis of B16-F10 melanoma- and 4T1 breast cancer cells in mouse models of carcinogenesis [82]. In the same study, ticagrelor prevent cancer cell adhesion to platelets and to endothelial cells, further supporting a role for $P2Y_{12}$-mediated platelet activation in tumour progression. Similarly, treatment with clopidogrel, an irreversible antagonist of $P2Y_{12}$ receptors protected the host mice from pathologic osteolysis and bone loss associated with B16-F10 melanoma tumour growth in bone [83]. Some controversy exists on whether tumour cell types generate ADP themselves or stimulate platelets to release ADP. However, Mitrugno et al, 2014 recently demonstrated that many tumour cells induce platelets to release ADP. Arguably, the most impactful evidence for a role for ADP as a secondary mediator of tumour cell-induced platelet activation comes from a study published by Battinelli and colleagues [19] who showed that both ADP and MCF-7 breast cancer cells were separately able to trigger the release of pro-angiogenic factors from platelet $\alpha$-granules. Platelet ADP receptor antagonists reduced the platelet response to MCF-7, suggesting that the tumour activation operates to induce the secretory event. In addition, the impaired ability of cancer cells to transmigrate through the endothelial barrier in Munc 13-4 deficient mice is suggestive of a strong role for ADP in mediating this response [20]. Munc 13-4 deficient mice lack of the ability to secrete platelet dense granules, and thus ADP and ATP release is prevented. The inability of these mice to demonstrate detectable cancer extravasation and metastasis suggests that platelet dense granule release is vital to cancer development.

### *3.1.3. TP: Thromboxane $A_2$ receptor*

Thromboxane $A_2$, the major TP ligand, is a prostanoid generated in platelets following agonist-induced mobilization of arachidonic acid (AA) from platelet membrane [84]. Similar to ADP, $TXA_2$ can activate platelets in an autocrine fashion, if released by platelets themselves, or in a paracrine modality, if liberated in the extracellular microenvironment by malignant cancer cells [85, 86]. Only a limited number of studies have addressed the issue of the role for platelet TP-$TXA_2$ molecular interplay in tumour cell induced platelet activation (TCIPA) and cancer metastasis. However, a role for $TXA_2$ in cancer metastasis is evident. SQ-29548, a TP antagonist, markedly inhibits osteogenic sarcoma cells- (MG-63) induced platelet aggregation [87]. In addition, $TP^{-/-}$ mutant mice injected with B16F1 melanoma cells present with reduced lung colonization and mortality rate compared to wild-type littermates [88]. Finally, inhibitors of thromboxane synthesis such as Ozagrel, BM-567 or aspirin, impair tumour induced platelet aggregation and carcinogenesis in a number of diverse models [85, 89]. In this context, although aspirin fails to inhibit platelet aggregation elicited *in vitro* by various cancer cells [69, 72, 77, 78, 90] it significantly affects platelet $\alpha$-granule release of pro-angiogenic factors in response to breast cancer cells [19].

Numerous studies from clinical trials have accumulating evidence to suggest that aspirin may represent a potential therapeutic strategy to reduce the risk of developing cancer metastasis and the consequent mortality [91, 92]. In a recent large meta-analysis of >17,000 patients, daily usage of low-dose aspirin has been shown to reduce the incidence, growth and metastasis of a number of cancers in a period of 5-6 years [93]. Overall, several platelet-dependent and independent mechanisms of actions of aspirin as a chemo-preventive agent have been proposed but their relevance in the treatment of cancer remains to be established [94].

### 3.2. Platelet Immunoreceptor Tyrosine-Based Activation Motif (ITAM) receptors

Immunoreceptors are ITAM or hemi-ITAM bearing receptors present on the platelet surface with a conserved double (ITAM) or single (hem-ITAM) YxxL-motif in their cytoplasmic tail. Upon receptor engagement or molecular cross-link, associated Src family kinases (SFKs) phosphorylate the tyrosine residues (Y) within the ITAM creating a docking site for Src homology 2 (SH2) domains of the tyrosine kinase Syk. Recruitment of Syk triggers its activation and the formation of a LAT (linker for activation of T-cells)-signalosome localised to lipid rafts. Among the proteins recruited to the signalosome there are cytosolic adaptors proteins (e.g.; Grb2: growth factor receptor bound protein 2; Gads: Grb2 related adaptor protein downstream of Shc; SLP-76: SH2 domain containing leukocyte protein of 76 kDa), and effector proteins (e.g.; PLC$\gamma$2 and PI-3 kinase). The molecular cross-talk culminates in PLC$\gamma$2 activation which will generate, via its lipase activity, $IP_3$ and DAG leading to calcium mobilization and PKC activation. Ultimately this pathway induces measurable platelet responses, including integrin activation, $TxA_2$ formation, and granule release (Reviewed in:[95]). The main ITAM receptors in platelets are glycoprotein VI (GPVI), F$\gamma$RIIa and C-type lectin like receptor (CLEC-2) and their potential role in tumour cell-platelet cross-talk will be discussed below.

#### *3.2.1. GPVI: Collagen receptor*

GPVI, unique to platelets and megakaryocytes, is the primary signalling receptor for collagen. Its ability to activate an intracellular pathway relies on its constitutive association with the ITAM containing Fc receptor gamma receptor Fc$\gamma$R, [96]. GPVI is a binding-target for several diverse fibrillar types of collagen, such as types I and III, as well as synthetic collagen-related peptide (CRP) and snake venom proteins (e.g.; convulxin) [97]. Although GPVI is considered an essential receptor for platelet activation, there is only limited experimental evidence suggesting a potential involvement for this glycoprotein in tumour metastasis. In genetically altered mice devoid of GPVI, the number of metastatic foci to lungs, following challenges with B16F10.1 melanoma or D121 Lewis carcinoma cells, was dramatically reduced compared to wild type littermates [98]. However, the molecular mechanism(s) that lead to this response remain unclear. Platelet pre-treatment with revacept, a GPVI blocker, or cancer cell treatment with inhibitor of galectin-3, an adhesive molecule with "collagen-like" domain, resulted in a dramatic inhibition of platelet-induced COX-2 over-expression in cancer cells [94]. Thus, GPVI may be involved in tumour cell-induced platelet secretion and induction of epithelial mesenchymal transition (EMT) in cancer cells.

#### *3.2.2. FcγRIIa: IgG receptor*

FcγRIIa is a low affinity Immunoglobulin receptor present in humans but not in mice. FcγRIIa in humans is primarily found in platelets [99, 100]. It binds to IgG immune-complexes, immunoglobulin-opsonised bacteria, and to auto-antibodies that target a subset of platelet membrane proteins [101, 102]. FcγRIIa also functions as an accessory receptor of GpIb-IX-V complex and integrin $\alpha_{IIb}\beta_3$ [103, 104]. Its physical association with the GpIb-V-IX complex has been shown to be responsible for tyrosine phosphorylation within ITAM motifs via Src-family Kinases (SFK) [104, 105]. Platelets from transgenic mice engineered to express FcγRIIa have an improved ability to respond to stimuli resembling haemostatic events, including spreading on fibrinogen, phosphorylation of Syk and PLCγ2, clot retraction and thrombus formation [106]. Mitrugno et al, recently demonstrated that this platelet receptor is responsible for mediating binding events between prostate cancer cells and platelets *in vitro* resulting in tumour cell induced platelet aggregation [72].

#### *3.2.3. CLEC-2: Podoplanin receptor*

In 2006, CLEC-2 was identified as a new hemi-ITAM (single YXXL motif) platelet receptor present as a homodimer on the platelet surface, able to activate molecular events resembling ITAM-bearing receptors through the snake venom toxin rhodocytin [107]. Importantly podoplanin, a sialylated transmembrane glycoprotein and the only-known physiological ligand for CLEC-2, has been found to be expressed on certain types of human glioblastoma (e.g.; LN319) and colon carcinoma (Colon-26) where it serves to enable TCIPA *in vitro* [108]. Metastatic events were found to be impaired in podoplanin knockout mice injected with kidney tumour cells [109]. In respect to this last observation, it has been proposed that the motile invasive behaviour of certain cancer cells relies in part on podoplanin-triggered signals. Indeed the ectopic expression of podoplanin in oral squamous cell carcinoma positively correlates with increased cell motility [110]. In addition, epidermal keratinocytes (MCA3D) acquire a malignant phenotype following transfection with podoplanin [110]. All together these observations reveal a potential role for podoplanin and podoplanin-CLEC-2 cross-talk in cancer progression, suggesting that inhibitors of this molecular program might represent an innovative therapeutic strategy for patients affected by certain types of cancer [44].

### 3.3. GPIb-IX-V Complex: VWF receptor

The GPIb-IX-V complex is a member of the leucine-rich repeats (LLRs) family of adhesive multimeric proteins consisting of two GPIbα subunits disulphide-linked to two GPIbβ subunits and associated non-covalently with GPIX and GPV protein on the platelet surface

[111]. This complex plays an essential role in mediating the initial adhesion of platelets to VWF at sites of vascular injury in high shear conditions (above 1000s$^{-1}$), and in triggering activation of integrin $\alpha_{IIb}\beta_3$ [112, 113]. Upon ligand engagement, the GpIb-X-V complex recruits cytoplasmic SFKs and PI3Ks via the GpIbα cytosolic tail, leading to calcium release and integrin activation. Alternatively, it can couple with the FcγRIIa chain to trigger ITAM-like signalling [104, 114]. VWF, a major but not unique GpIbα ligand, is a large multimeric adhesive glycoprotein associated with collagen in the subendothelial matrix. Importantly, following activation, it can also be released by Weibel-Palade bodies in endothelial cells and α-granules in platelets [115].

The role of GpIbα in cancer metastasis has been subject of many studies that converge in contradictory results. GPIbα is present on some cancer cell surfaces and appears to play a role in cancer cell-induced platelet aggregation [116]. However, the expression of GpIbα on the surface of cancer cells is not common [70, 117]. Contradictory results have been reported in *in vivo* studies. Reduced melanoma metastasis to the lungs is observed in mice deficient in GpIb-IX-V complex [118]. In contrast, administration of anti-GPIbα monovalent antibodies in melanoma-bearing mice resulted in a strong enhancement of lung metastasis [119]. Similarly, an increased metastatic potential was observed in mice lacking VWF [120] but not in mice treated with anti-VWF antibodies, which were protected from metastasis [121]. Thus, the role of GpIb in the cancer cell-platelet loop remains unclear, making it object of further investigation.

### 3.4. Platelet integrins: $\alpha_{IIb}\beta_3$

Integrin $\alpha_{IIb}\beta_3$ is the most abundant cell adhesion molecule on the platelet surface (approximately 80,000 receptors per platelet), with an additional pool of protein that can be recruited from internal α-granule membranes upon platelet activation [122]. $\alpha_{IIb}\beta_3$ exists in a low affinity or inactive state in circulating, un-activated platelets and undergoes conformational changes following platelet stimulation by soluble agonists such as thrombin. Conformationally active integrin displays an increased affinity for its endogenous ligands: principally plasma fibrinogen and VWF. This interaction stabilises the adhesion of platelets to the extracellular matrix and permits cross-linking of activated platelets, causing aggregation and haemostatic plug formation. Importantly, ligand binding to $\alpha_{IIb}\beta_3$ enables "outside-in" molecular circuits, which lead to thrombus stability and fibrin clot retraction [123, 124]

Lacking enzymatic activity, integrins must cooperate with other cytoplasmic proteins to trigger intracellular signals. Importantly, recent investigation has revealed the capacity of $\alpha_{IIb}\beta_3$ to associate with molecular mediators of ITAM-bearing receptors. In this scenario, FcγRIIa has been proposed as a key molecular partner or accessory receptor for $\alpha_{IIb}\beta_3$ [102, 103]. FcγRIIa is recruited to activated $\alpha_{IIb}\beta_3$ microclusters enriched in SFK, leading to the phosphorylation of FcγRIIa-ITAM sequence that provides a link to Syk. As yet however, the mechanism and stoichiometry of the interaction between $\alpha_{IIb}\beta_3$ and FcγRIIa remains obscure.

Integrin $\alpha_{IIb}\beta_3$ is the adhesive molecule which has been most explored in *in vivo* models of haematogenous metastasis and in *in vitro* models of TCIPA [70]. A monoclonal antibody (10E5) directed against $\alpha_{IIb}\beta_3$ inhibits the ability of tumour cells to bind to platelets [121]. The same antibody is also able to reduce the number of metastatic foci to lungs in a mouse model of tumour metastasis using colon carcinoma CT26 cells [125]. Similarly, a reduction in the extent of tumour cell colonisation of the lungs was also observed in integrin $\beta 3^{-/-}$ mice injected with B16F10 melanoma cells [126]. These findings have then been confirmed in a number of additional studies [70]. In addition, $\alpha_{IIb}\beta_3$ inhibitors modulate TCIPA elicited by diverse human tumour cells, including colon carcinoma, cervical and vaginal melanoma and breast cancer [72, 90, 116, 127]. Moreover, abciximab (anti-$\alpha_{IIb}\beta_3$ monoclonal blocking antibody) inhibits the release of pro-angiogenic factors such as VEGF, from the platelet $\alpha$-granules by MCF-7 breast cancer cells [66] indicating that integrin $\alpha_{IIb}\beta_3$ activation is necessary to support platelet activation and platelet secretion. Taken together these results highlight $\alpha_{IIb}\beta_3$ as attractive target for future anti-metastatic therapies.

## 4. Platelet granules and their role in cancer progression

Although considerable progress has been made in understanding how platelets interact with cancer cells to initiate an interdependent relationship, little is known about how that relationship develops. Following platelet association with tumour cells, platelet secretion of dense granules [72], and $\alpha$-granules [19, 66] ensues and the resulting platelet releasates contribute to tumour progression. As yet, however, very little is known about the potential "intrinsic" ability of cancer cells to induce platelet granule release. Moreover, the precise molecular orchestrators of this phenomenon remain completely unknown. It is likely that, like platelet interactions with bacterial micro-organisms, different cancer cell types may interact in different ways with platelets [128]. Ultimately, however, the ability of tumour cells to engineer the release of platelet-stored cytokines and bioactive molecules appear to be a key component of the critical interaction that remains to be elucidated.

### 4.1. $\alpha$-granules

$\alpha$-granules are the most abundant granule population in platelets (50-80 per platelet) presenting a heterogeneous morphology, size and luminal content as well as protein repertoire [64, 129, 130]. Electron tomography of platelet cryo-sections revealed the presence of 3 major different subtypes of $\alpha$-granules based on average size and contents: 1) 200-500 nm spherical $\alpha$-granules featuring an electron dense core and eccentrically localised multimeric VWF tubules; 2) multivesicular 100-200 nm granules displaying a multitude of free luminal membrane vesicles; and 3) 50 nm- tubular $\alpha$-granules rich in fibrin-like structures [129]. Importantly, there seems to be also two further dimension of complexity with regard to (i) $\alpha$-granules protein content and (ii) speed of release.

Immunofluorescence and immuno-electron microscopy data from certain laboratories show distinct localizations for pro- and anti-angiogenic factors in platelet $\alpha$-granules, indicating that proteins are segregated among $\alpha$-granules during their initial synthesis, according to their biological function [60, 130]. This separate packaging then permits a differential secretory behaviour, in terms of type of protein released in response to different stimuli [19, 64, 130]. Ma and colleagues first demonstrated the ability of platelets to release their content in a "thematic" way [131]. VEGF (pro-angiogenic), but not endostatin (anti-angiogenic) was selectively released upon platelet stimulation with PAR-4 agonist while an opposite response was observed following platelet exposure to a thrombin receptor ligand [131]. However, to date, the knowledge of the molecular mechanism(s) orchestrating the selective platelet release remains elusive [129]. It must be noted that recent studies show activation of different PARs elicit similar releasate patterns and cargoes within the $\alpha$-granules are randomly packaged, however there are indications that spreading platelets are capable of sorting and separating $\alpha$-granules subtypes [132-134]. Either way, it will be intriguing to address whether this classification of granules is physiologically meaningful and if it changes during pathological events such as cancer.

$\alpha$-granules are functionally pleiotropic, meaning that they can serve different and significant functions [135]. Thus, the release of their contents can be pivotal in establishing the nature of the surrounding microenvironment [135]. More than 300 molecules have been shown to be released from activated platelets [136], which differ in their origin. Some components may be synthesized in the megakaryocyte whereas others are scavenged from plasma [135]. The contents of platelet $\alpha$-granules also differ in their function [10, 135, 137]. Functionally, $\alpha$-granule contents can be divided in the following categories: 1) adhesive molecules (e.g.; fibrinogen, fibronectin, vitronectin, thrombospondin, VWF, P-selectin, $\alpha_{IIb}\beta_3$) which mediate homotypic (platelet-platelet) and heterotypic (platelet-endothelial cells) interactions and subsequent clot formation (primary heamostasis) ; 2) coagulation factors (e.g.; fibrinogen, pro-thrombin, Factor V, Factor VII) which play a crucial role in the stabilization of the haemostatic clot; 3) fibrinolytic agents (e.g. plasminogen activator inhibitor-1 (PAI-1)) which are important for clot remodelling; 4) growth factors (e.g.; PDGF, VEGF, EGF, TGF$\beta$) which can contribute to wound healing, angiogenesis, chemotaxis and cell proliferation; 5) pro-angiogenic and anti-angiogenic factors (e.g.; angiopoietin, VEGF, endostatin, angiogenin, angiostatin; and tissue inhibitors of metalloproteases 1 and 4 (TIMP1 and TIMP-4) which regulate the *de novo* formation of blood vessels; 6) tissue-remodelling factors (e.g. MMPs, TIMPs and disintegrin metalloproteinases (ADAMs)) which allow structural remodelling of the ECM and the solubilisation and activation of a variety of growth factors tethered in an inactive form to the proteoglycans of the ECM ; 7) pro-inflammatory factors which include a pool of chemokines (e.g.; CXCL1 (GRO-$\alpha$), CXCL4, CXCL5 (ENA-78), CXCL7 (NAP-2), CXCL8 (IL-8), CXCL12 (SDF-1a), CCL2 (MCP-1), CCL3 (MIP-1a), CCL5 (RANTES), CCL17 (TARC)), which induce recruitment, activation, chemokine secretion and differentiation of other cells, involved in wound healing, from the circulation [10, 135].

Importantly, all these molecules have the potential to contribute to the progression of cancer. Moreover, the platelet granule contents may change as a consequence of the host being infected with a cancer [61]. This leads to the intriguing possibility that certain cancer cells can prime circulating platelets with active cytokines, tailored to permit tumour cell survival at a metastatic site. Alternatively, tumour cells may upregulate the levels of select platelet cytokines to enable avoidance of an immune response and thus enhance CTC survival in a host. A more complete understanding of the platelet-tumour cell interdependence will be critical for the design of therapeutic interventions to supress cancer progression.

### 4.2. Platelet dense granules

Each platelet contains just 3 - 8 dense granules, which measure approximately 250 nm in diameter [138]. They concentrate a number of small molecules including: 1) ions (e.g.; calcium, magnesium, phosphate, pyrophosphate); 2) nucleotides (e.g.; ADP, ATP, GTP and GDP). 3) transmitters (e.g.; serotonin, epinephrine, histamine), and 4) membrane proteins which are also found in lysosomes (e.g.; LAMP-2). Serotonin and ADP function as secondary mediators, or positive enhancers of the platelet aggregation response. Interestingly, about 50% of platelet ADP is stored in platelet dense granules and cannot be refilled following platelet activation. In contrast, the metabolic pool of adenine nucleotides, housed in the platelet cytosolic compartment, can be synthesized but not released [139]. Serotonin, is instead sequestered by platelets from plasma and released into the circulation upon activation where it can act as both an autocrine and a paracrine mediator [140]. The autocrine function serves to amplify the platelet response through engagement of the Gq-coupled 5HT2A receptor on platelet surface, whereas the paracrine effect contribute to the modulation of the vascular tone, normally inducing vasoconstriction to limit the blood flow and reduce blood loss at sites of vascular injury [138]. Calcium found in dense granules constitutes from 60 to 70% of total calcium mobilised in platelets. [140-142]. The function of the calcium released by platelets into the extracellular space is uncertain, however it has been speculated that it may play a role in facilitating the binding of the extracellular adhesive proteins to their receptors on platelets [138].

### 4.3. Lysosomes

Lysosomes constitute a less characterised granule type present in platelets in marginal number (0-1 per platelet). They are packaged with cathepsins, carboxypeptidases, β-hexosaminidase, acid phosphatases, enzymes for hydrolyzing various sugars and aryl sulfatases. CD63 and LAMP2 are membrane-bound molecules normally used as markers of lysosomes [138]. Though the exact function of lysosomes in platelets is not known, they are thought to be involved in dissolution of the clot [10].

## 5. Platelet secretion and the progression of cancer

In 1984 Boneu et al., first reported the presence of degranulated platelets, characterised by low levels of ADP and serotonin, in patients with malignant solid tumours [143] suggesting that platelet secretion was a critical event in tumour growth. Wagner's research group subsequently showed that platelet secretions continuously support tumour vascular homeostasis by regulating the stability of tumour vessels [17]. However, the exact identity of platelet-derived factors responsible for tumour vessel protection remains unknown.

A potential role for ADP and serotonin, released by platelet dense granules, has been proposed [63, 72]. Platelet dense granule secretion of adenine nucleotides in a tumorigenic microenvironment may be key to tumour cell extravasation and to the formation of metastatic foci. One mechanism downstream from this phenomenon has been uncovered [20]. Platelet-derived

ATP binds to $P2Y_2$ receptors on endothelial cells triggering a signalling cascade that culminates in the disaggregation of the endothelial barrier. Moreover, platelet-derived ADP can also participate in tumour cell-induced platelet aggregation [144], a strategy adopted by several tumour cell lines to evade the immune system and overcome high arterial shear stress during the haematogenous journey [28].

Cancer cells can also induce platelet release of matrix metalloproteinases (MMPs) and cytokines from $\alpha$-granules [145]. These bioactive molecules can destroy the extracellular matrix barrier and promote invasion and tumour extravasation. Among the MMPs, MMP-2 has been shown to be autocrine mediator of TCIPA elicited by human fibrosarcoma HT-1080, lung carcinoma A549, breast adenocarcinoma MCF7 and colon adenocarcinoma Caco-2 cells [68, 69, 78].

Platelet release of adhesive proteins such as $\alpha_{IIb}\beta_3$, P-selectin, and fibrinogen can also potentially support and stabilise adhesive interaction of tumour cells with both platelets (platelet-cancer aggregate) and endothelial cells, favouring tumour cells transmigration across the endothelial barrier. Similarly, the release of coagulation factors can prompt the conversion of fibrinogen into fibrin which will strengthen the heterotypic platelet-cancer aggregate and ensure its survival and safe docking at the metastatic site [146, 147]. As discussed previously, platelets contain both pro- and anti-angiogenic factors that can be differentially released to ensure optimal tumour angiogenesis [19, 63]. Moreover, in animals bearing malignant tumours, platelets can be conditioned to selectively store and release regulators of angiogenesis [60]. Importantly, it has been shown that platelets are not just simply transporters of tumour-derived pro-angiogenic molecules. In a mouse model of metastasis, Kerr and colleagues have demonstrated the ability of platelet to sequester diverse tumour-derived cytokines and to safely transport them to a distant metastatic niche for release [61]. This excellent strategy seems to be engineered by cancer cells to hijack important pro-metastatic and pro-inflammatory proteins and impede their degradation in plasma. It is noteworthy that this emerging concept of platelets as carriers of tumour-derived proteins can provide a window to the needs of cancer cells and guide the clinician towards an optimal therapeutic approach. Interestingly, in the study by Kerr and colleagues [61], granulocyte colony-stimulating factor (G-CSF) was found to be abundantly released in the plasma of tumour-bearing mice by both platelets and cancer cells. The same result was also separately observed by Wagner's group who subsequently uncovered a potential role for G-CSF in the formation of neutrophil extracellular traps (NETs) and cancer-associated thrombosis [148]. NETs are suggested to facilitate tumour metastasis by trapping circulating tumour cells [149].

Once recruited by the circulating tumour cells, platelets can release a plethora of growth factors including platelet derived growth factor (PDGF-BB) and transforming growth factor beta (TGFβ), which can contribute to the inflammatory state often associated with cancer [10]. In this context, TGF-β derived from platelet $\alpha$-granules profoundly impacts tumour metastasis and survival by enhancing an epithelial-to-mesenchymal transition (EMT), *via* activation of the TGFβ/Smad and NF-KB signalling pathways in tumour cells, and suppressing tumour cell NK-mediated lysis [16, 35]. EMT is a program which enables cancer invasiveness and dissemination [150].

A summary flowchart of platelet secretion events in cancer is presented in Figure 3 summarizing 30 years of the causal evidence linking secretion and tumour survival characteristics. Despite these recent discoveries of platelet secretion affecting cancer cells, and vice versa, the precise molecular mediators at play between tumour cells and platelets are not yet fully understood. The use of anti-platelet agents is currently emerging as potential treatment of malignancy and tumour-derived thrombosis [63, 151]. However, this use of platelet inhibitors to improve cancer prognosis and reduce the risk of fatal metastasis must take into account the delicate balance between inhibiting platelet activation and the associated risk of bleeding. The identification of the precise molecular pathways in platelets in response to activation by cancer cells may permit greater progress in this area.

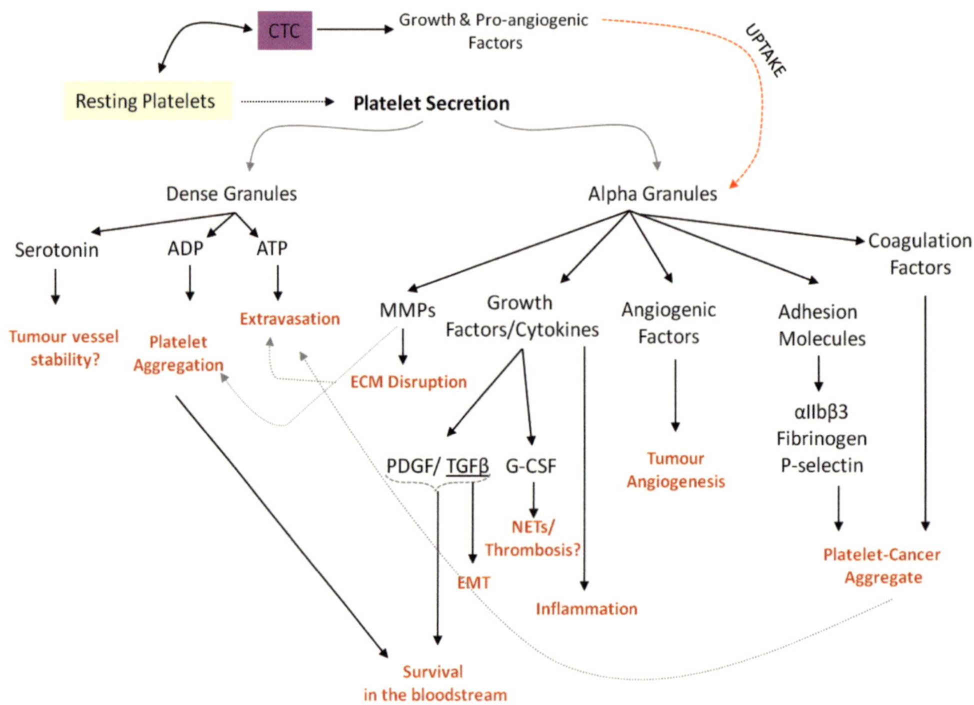


**Figure 3.** Flowchart highlighting the potential role of platelet-released molecular mediators in neoplastic progression.

## Author details

Annachiara Mitrugno[1], Niamh Moran[1*] and Pat Metharom[2]

*Address all correspondence to: nmoran@rcsi.ie

1 Molecular & Cellular Therapeutics, Royal College of Surgeons in Ireland, Dublin, Ireland

2 Faculty of Health Sciences,Curtin Health Innovation Research Institute, Perth, Australia

## References

[1] Varki, A., *Trousseau's syndrome: multiple definitions and multiple mechanisms.* Blood, 2007. 110(6): p. 1723-9.

[2] Bizzozero, G., *Ueiber einen neuen frombestandheil des blutes un dessen rolle bei der thrombose und der blutgerrinnung.* Arch Pathol Anat Physiol, 1882: p. 261-332.

[3] Riess, *Zur pathologischen anatomie des blutes.* Arch Anat Physiol Wissensch Med, 1872. 39: p. 237-49.

[4] Levin, J. and C.L. Conley, *Thrombocytosis Associated with Malignant Disease.* Arch Intern Med, 1964. 114: p. 497-500.

[5] Tranum, B.L. and A. Haut, *Thrombocytosis: platelet kinetics in neoplasia.* J Lab Clin Med, 1974. 84(5): p. 615-9.

[6] Gasic, G.J., T.B. Gasic, and C.C. Stewart, *Antimetastatic effects associated with platelet reduction.* Proc Natl Acad Sci U S A, 1968. 61(1): p. 46-52.

[7] Gasic, G.J., et al., *Platelet-tumor-cell interactions in mice. The role of platelets in the spread of malignant disease.* Int J Cancer, 1973. 11(3): p. 704-18.

[8] Hilgard, P., *The role of blood platelets in experimental metastases.* Br J Cancer, 1973. 28(5): p. 429-35.

[9] Gasic, G.J., et al., *Thrombogenic activity of mouse and human tumors: effects on platelets, coagulation, and fibrinolysis, and possible significance for metastases.* Z Krebsforsch Klin Onkol Cancer Res Clin Oncol, 1976. 86(3): p. 263-77.

[10] Menter, D.G., et al., *Platelets and cancer: a casual or causal relationship: revisited.* Cancer Metastasis Rev, 2014.

[11] Broos, K., et al., *Platelets at work in primary hemostasis.* Blood Rev, 2011. 25(4): p. 155-67.

[12] Hanahan, D. and R.A. Weinberg, *The hallmarks of cancer.* Cell, 2000. 100(1): p. 57-70.

[13] Chambers, A.F., A.C. Groom, and I.C. MacDonald, *Dissemination and growth of cancer cells in metastatic sites.* Nat Rev Cancer, 2002. 2(8): p. 563-72.

[14] Walsh, T.G., P. Metharom, and M.C. Berndt, *The functional role of platelets in the regulation of angiogenesis.* Platelets, 2014: p. 1-13.

[15] Chaffer, C.L. and R.A. Weinberg, *A perspective on cancer cell metastasis.* Science, 2011. 331(6024): p. 1559-64.

[16] Labelle, M., S. Begum, and R.O. Hynes, *Direct signaling between platelets and cancer cells induces an epithelial-mesenchymal-like transition and promotes metastasis.* Cancer Cell, 2011. 20(5): p. 576-90.

[17] Ho-Tin-Noe, B., et al., *Platelet granule secretion continuously prevents intratumor hemorrhage.* Cancer Res, 2008. 68(16): p. 6851-8.

[18] Gay, L.J. and B. Felding-Habermann, *Contribution of platelets to tumour metastasis.* Nat Rev Cancer, 2011. 11(2): p. 123-34.

[19] Battinelli, E.M., B.A. Markens, and J.E. Italiano, Jr., *Release of angiogenesis regulatory proteins from platelet alpha granules: modulation of physiologic and pathologic angiogenesis.* Blood, 2011. 118(5): p. 1359-69.

[20] Schumacher, D., et al., *Platelet-Derived Nucleotides Promote Tumor-Cell Transendothelial Migration and Metastasis via P2Y2 Receptor.* Cancer Cell, 2013. 24(1): p. 130-7.

[21] McFadyen, J.D. and S.P. Jackson, *Differentiating haemostasis from thrombosis for therapeutic benefit.* Thromb Haemost, 2013. 110(5): p. 859-67.

[22] Coughlin, S.R., *Protease-activated receptors in hemostasis, thrombosis and vascular biology.* J Thromb Haemost, 2005. 3(8): p. 1800-14.

[23] Adam, F., et al., *Thrombin-induced platelet PAR4 activation: role of glycoprotein Ib and ADP.* J Thromb Haemost, 2003. 1(4): p. 798-804.

[24] Covic, L., A.L. Gresser, and A. Kuliopulos, *Biphasic kinetics of activation and signaling for PAR1 and PAR4 thrombin receptors in platelets.* Biochemistry, 2000. 39(18): p. 5458-67.

[25] Dubois, C., et al., *Thrombin binding to GPIbα induces integrin alphaIIbbeta3 dependent platelet adhesion to fibrin in ex vivo flowing whole blood.* Thromb Haemost, 2004. 91(2): p. 233-7.

[26] Berndt, M.C., P. Metharom, and R.K. Andrews, *Primary haemostasis: newer insights.* Haemophilia, 2014. 20 Suppl 4: p. 15-22.

[27] Karpatkin, S. and E. Pearlstein, *Role of platelets in tumor cell metastases.* Ann Intern Med, 1981. 95(5): p. 636-41.

[28] Egan, K., N. Cooke, and D. Kenny, *Living in shear: platelets protect cancer cells from shear induced damage.* Clin Exp Metastasis, 2014.

[29] Nieswandt, B., et al., *Lysis of tumor cells by natural killer cells in mice is impeded by platelets.* Cancer Res, 1999. 59(6): p. 1295-300.

[30] Palumbo, J.S., et al., *Platelets and fibrin(ogen) increase metastatic potential by impeding natural killer cell-mediated elimination of tumor cells.* Blood, 2005. 105(1): p. 178-85.

[31] van Es, N., et al., *Effects of cancer on platelets.* Semin Oncol, 2014. 41(3): p. 311-8.

[32] Lipinski, B. and L.G. Egyud, *Resistance of cancer cells to immune recognition and killing.* Med Hypotheses, 2000. 54(3): p. 456-60.

[33] Egyud, L.G. and B. Lipinski, *Significance of fibrin formation and dissolution in the pathogenesis and treatment of cancer.* Med Hypotheses, 1991. 36(4): p. 336-40.

[34] Placke, T., H.G. Kopp, and H.R. Salih, *Modulation of natural killer cell anti-tumor reactivity by platelets.* J Innate Immun, 2011. 3(4): p. 374-82.

[35] Kopp, H.G., T. Placke, and H.R. Salih, *Platelet-derived transforming growth factor-beta down-regulates NKG2D thereby inhibiting natural killer cell antitumor reactivity.* Cancer Res, 2009. 69(19): p. 7775-83.

[36] Gersuk, G.M., et al., *Inhibition of human natural killer cell activity by platelet-derived growth factor (PDGF). III. Membrane binding studies and differential biological effect of recombinant PDGF isoforms.* Scand J Immunol, 1991. 33(5): p. 521-32.

[37] Steeg, P.S., *Tumor metastasis: mechanistic insights and clinical challenges.* Nat Med, 2006. 12(8): p. 895-904.

[38] Crissman, J.D., et al., *Arrest and extravasation of B16 amelanotic melanoma in murine lungs. A light and electron microscopic study.* Lab Invest, 1985. 53(4): p. 470-8.

[39] McCarty, O.J., et al., *Immobilized platelets support human colon carcinoma cell tethering, rolling, and firm adhesion under dynamic flow conditions.* Blood, 2000. 96(5): p. 1789-97.

[40] Dardik, R., et al., *Platelets mediate tumor cell adhesion to the subendothelium under flow conditions: involvement of platelet GPIIb-IIIa and tumor cell alpha(v) integrins.* Int J Cancer, 1997. 70(2): p. 201-7.

[41] Felding-Habermann, B., et al., *Role of beta3 integrins in melanoma cell adhesion to activated platelets under flow.* J Biol Chem, 1996. 271(10): p. 5892-900.

[42] Poggi, A., M. Stella, and M.B. Donati, *The importance of blood cell-vessel wall interactions in tumour metastasis.* Baillieres Clin Haematol, 1993. 6(3): p. 731-52.

[43] Nash, G.F., et al., *Platelets and cancer.* Lancet Oncol, 2002. 3(7): p. 425-30.

[44] Lowe, K.L., L. Navarro-Nunez, and S.P. Watson, *Platelet CLEC-2 and podoplanin in cancer metastasis.* Thromb Res, 2012. 129 Suppl 1: p. S30-7.

[45] Weinberg, R.A., *The biology of Cancer.* Second Edition ed. 2012.

[46] Folkman, J., *Tumor angiogenesis: therapeutic implications.* N Engl J Med, 1971. 285(21): p. 1182-6.

[47] Yan, M., et al., *Pharmacological regulation of platelet factors that influence tumor angiogenesis.* Semin Oncol, 2014. 41(3): p. 370-7.

[48] Kerbel, R.S., *Tumor angiogenesis.* N Engl J Med, 2008. 358(19): p. 2039-49.

[49] Coussens, L.M. and Z. Werb, *Inflammation and cancer.* Nature, 2002. 420(6917): p. 860-7.

[50] Pinedo, H.M., et al., *Involvement of platelets in tumour angiogenesis?* Lancet, 1998. 352(9142): p. 1775-7.

[51] Pipili-Synetos, E., E. Papadimitriou, and M.E. Maragoudakis, *Evidence that platelets promote tube formation by endothelial cells on matrigel.* Br J Pharmacol, 1998. 125(6): p. 1252-7.

[52] Iba, O., et al., *Angiogenesis by implantation of peripheral blood mononuclear cells and platelets into ischemic limbs.* Circulation, 2002. 106(15): p. 2019-25.

[53] Kisucka, J., et al., *Platelets and platelet adhesion support angiogenesis while preventing excessive hemorrhage.* Proc Natl Acad Sci U S A, 2006. 103(4): p. 855-60.

[54] Brock, T.A., H.F. Dvorak, and D.R. Senger, *Tumor-secreted vascular permeability factor increases cytosolic Ca2+ and von Willebrand factor release in human endothelial cells.* Am J Pathol, 1991. 138(1): p. 213-21.

[55] Goubran, H.A., et al., *Platelets effects on tumor growth.* Semin Oncol, 2014. 41(3): p. 359-69.

[56] Peterson, J.E., et al., *Normal ranges of angiogenesis regulatory proteins in human platelets.* Am J Hematol, 2010. 85(7): p. 487-93.

[57] Verheul, H.M., et al., *Platelet: transporter of vascular endothelial growth factor.* Clin Cancer Res, 1997. 3(12 Pt 1): p. 2187-90.

[58] Gisterek, I., et al., *Serum vascular endothelial growth factors a, C and d in human breast tumors.* Pathol Oncol Res, 2010. 16(3): p. 337-44.

[59] Peterson, J.E., et al., *VEGF, PF4 and PDGF are elevated in platelets of colorectal cancer patients.* Angiogenesis, 2012. 15(2): p. 265-73.

[60] Klement, G.L., et al., *Platelets actively sequester angiogenesis regulators.* Blood, 2009. 113(12): p. 2835-42.

[61] Kerr, B.A., et al., *Comparison of tumor and microenvironment secretomes in plasma and in platelets during prostate cancer growth in a xenograft model.* Neoplasia, 2010. 12(5): p. 388-96.

[62] Kuznetsov, H.S., et al., *Identification of luminal breast cancers that establish a tumor-supportive macroenvironment defined by proangiogenic platelets and bone marrow-derived cells.* Cancer Discov, 2012. 2(12): p. 1150-65.

[63] Bambace, N.M. and C.E. Holmes, *The platelet contribution to cancer progression.* J Thromb Haemost, 2011. 9(2): p. 237-49.

[64] Italiano, J.E., Jr., et al., *Angiogenesis is regulated by a novel mechanism: pro- and antiangiogenic proteins are organized into separate platelet alpha granules and differentially released.* Blood, 2008. 111(3): p. 1227-33.

[65] Battinelli, E.M., et al., *Anticoagulation inhibits tumor cell-mediated release of platelet angiogenic proteins and diminishes platelet angiogenic response*. Blood, 2014. 123(1): p. 101-12.

[66] Amirkhosravi, A., et al., *Blockade of GpIIb/IIIa inhibits the release of vascular endothelial growth factor (VEGF) from tumor cell-activated platelets and experimental metastasis*. Platelets, 1999. 10(5): p. 285-92.

[67] Li, R., et al., *Presence of intratumoral platelets is associated with tumor vessel structure and metastasis*. BMC Cancer, 2014. 14: p. 167.

[68] Jurasz, P., et al., *Matrix metalloproteinase 2 in tumor cell-induced platelet aggregation: regulation by nitric oxide.* Cancer Res, 2001. 61(1): p. 376-82.

[69] Alonso-Escolano, D., et al., *Membrane type-1 matrix metalloproteinase stimulates tumour cell-induced platelet aggregation: role of receptor glycoproteins.* Br J Pharmacol, 2004. 141(2): p. 241-52.

[70] Erpenbeck, L. and M.P. Schon, *Deadly allies: the fatal interplay between platelets and metastasizing cancer cells.* Blood, 2010. 115(17): p. 3427-36.

[71] Stegner, D., S. Dutting, and B. Nieswandt, *Mechanistic explanation for platelet contribution to cancer metastasis.* Thromb Res, 2014. 133 Suppl 2: p. S149-57.

[72] Mitrugno, A., et al., *A novel and essential role for FcgammaRIIa in cancer cell-induced platelet activation*. Blood, 2014. 123(2): p. 249-60.

[73] Offermanns, S., *Activation of platelet function through G protein-coupled receptors*. Circ Res, 2006. 99(12): p. 1293-304.

[74] Camerer, E., et al., *Platelets, protease-activated receptors, and fibrinogen in hematogenous metastasis*. Blood, 2004. 104(2): p. 397-401.

[75] Boukerche, H., et al., *Human melanoma cell lines differ in their capacity to release ADP and aggregate platelets.* Br J Haematol, 1994. 87(4): p. 763-72.

[76] Bastida, E., et al., *Platelet activation induced by a human neuroblastoma tumor cell line is reduced by prior administration of ticlopidine.* Thromb Haemost, 1986. 55(3): p. 333-7.

[77] Egan, K., et al., *Platelet adhesion and degranulation induce pro-survival and pro-angiogenic signalling in ovarian cancer cells.* PLoS One, 2011. 6(10): p. e26125.

[78] Medina, C., et al., *Platelet aggregation-induced by caco-2 cells: regulation by matrix metalloproteinase-2 and adenosine diphosphate.* J Pharmacol Exp Ther, 2006. 317(2): p. 739-45.

[79] Heinmoller, E., et al., *Studies on tumor-cell-induced platelet aggregation in human lung cancer cell lines.* J Cancer Res Clin Oncol, 1996. 122(12): p. 735-44.

[80] Sheu, J.R., et al., *Triflavin, an Arg-Gly-Asp-containing peptide, inhibits tumor cell-induced platelet aggregation*. Jpn J Cancer Res, 1993. 84(10): p. 1062-71.

[81] Wang, Y., et al., *Platelet P2Y12 is involved in murine pulmonary metastasis.* PLoS One, 2013. 8(11): p. e80780.

[82] Gebremeskel, S., et al., *The reversible P2Y12 inhibitor ticagrelor inhibits metastasis and improves survival in mouse models of cancer.* Int J Cancer, 2014.

[83] Uluckan, O., et al., *APT102, a novel adpase, cooperates with aspirin to disrupt bone metastasis in mice.* J Cell Biochem, 2008. 104(4): p. 1311-23.

[84] Kramer, R.M., et al., *Thrombin-induced phosphorylation and activation of Ca(2+)-sensitive cytosolic phospholipase A2 in human platelets.* J Biol Chem, 1993. 268(35): p. 26796-804.

[85] de Leval, X., et al., *Pharmacological evaluation of the novel thromboxane modulator BM-567 (II/II). Effects of BM-567 on osteogenic sarcoma-cell-induced platelet aggregation.* Prostaglandins Leukot Essent Fatty Acids, 2003. 68(1): p. 55-9.

[86] Ogletree, M.L., *Overview of physiological and pathophysiological effects of thromboxane A2.* Fed Proc, 1987. 46(1): p. 133-8.

[87] Mehta, P., et al., *Effects of thromboxane A2 inhibition on osteogenic sarcoma cell-induced platelet aggregation.* Cancer Res, 1986. 46(10): p. 5061-3.

[88] Matsui, Y., et al., *Thromboxane A(2) receptor signaling facilitates tumor colonization through P-selectin-mediated interaction of tumor cells with platelets and endothelial cells.* Cancer Sci, 2012. 103(4): p. 700-7.

[89] Yokoyama, I., et al., *Prevention of experimental hepatic metastasis with thromboxane synthase inhibitor.* Res Exp Med (Berl), 1995. 195(4): p. 209-15.

[90] Lian, L., et al., *Inhibition of MCF-7 breast cancer cell-induced platelet aggregation using a combination of antiplatelet drugs.* Oncol Lett, 2013. 5(2): p. 675-680.

[91] Flahavan, E.M., et al., *A cohort study investigating aspirin use and survival in men with prostate cancer.* Ann Oncol, 2014. 25(1): p. 154-9.

[92] Barron, T.I., et al., *Recent prediagnostic aspirin use, lymph node involvement, and 5-year mortality in women with stage I-III breast cancer: a nationwide population-based cohort study.* Cancer Res, 2014. 74(15): p. 4065-77.

[93] Rothwell, P.M., et al., *Effect of daily aspirin on risk of cancer metastasis: a study of incident cancers during randomised controlled trials.* Lancet, 2012. 379(9826): p. 1591-601.

[94] Dovizio, M., et al., *Mechanistic and pharmacological issues of aspirin as an anticancer agent.* Pharmaceuticals (Basel), 2012. 5(12): p. 1346-71.

[95] Boulaftali, Y., et al., *Platelet immunoreceptor tyrosine-based activation motif (ITAM) signaling and vascular integrity.* Circ Res, 2014. 114(7): p. 1174-84.

[96] Watson, S.P. and J. Gibbins, *Collagen receptor signalling in platelets: extending the role of the ITAM.* Immunol Today, 1998. 19(6): p. 260-4.

[97] Nieswandt, B. and S.P. Watson, *Platelet-collagen interaction: is GPVI the central receptor?* Blood, 2003. 102(2): p. 449-61.

[98] Jain, S., S. Russell, and J. Ware, *Platelet glycoprotein VI facilitates experimental lung metastasis in syngenic mouse models.* J Thromb Haemost, 2009. 7(10): p. 1713-7.

[99] Daniels, A.B., et al., *Analysis of FcgammaRIIA cytoplasmic tail requirements in signaling for serotonin secretion: evidence for an ITAM-dependent, PI3K-dependent pathway*. Scand J Immunol, 2010. 71(4): p. 232-9.

[100] Anderson, C.L., et al., *The Fc receptor for immunoglobulin G (Fc gamma RII) on human platelets.* Semin Thromb Hemost, 1995. 21(1): p. 1-9.

[101] Fitzgerald, J.R., T.J. Foster, and D. Cox, *The interaction of bacterial pathogens with platelets.* Nat Rev Microbiol, 2006. 4(6): p. 445-57.

[102] Gao, C., et al., *Eptifibatide-induced thrombocytopenia and thrombosis in humans require FcgammaRIIa and the integrin beta3 cytoplasmic domain.* J Clin Invest, 2009. 119(3): p. 504-11.

[103] Boylan, B., et al., *Identification of FcgammaRIIa as the ITAM-bearing receptor mediating alphaIIbbeta3 outside-in integrin signaling in human platelets.* Blood, 2008. 112(7): p. 2780-6.

[104] Sullam, P.M., et al., *Physical proximity and functional interplay of the glycoprotein Ib-IX-V complex and the Fc receptor FcgammaRIIA on the platelet plasma membrane.* J Biol Chem, 1998. 273(9): p. 5331-6.

[105] Canobbio, I., et al., *Platelet activation by von Willebrand factor requires coordinated signaling through thromboxane A2 and Fc gamma IIA receptor.* J Biol Chem, 2001. 276(28): p. 26022-9.

[106] Zhi, H., et al., *Cooperative integrin/ITAM signaling in platelets enhances thrombus formation in vitro and in vivo.* Blood, 2013. 121(10): p. 1858-67.

[107] Suzuki-Inoue, K., et al., *A novel Syk-dependent mechanism of platelet activation by the C-type lectin receptor CLEC-2.* Blood, 2006. 107(2): p. 542-9.

[108] Suzuki-Inoue, K., et al., *Involvement of the snake toxin receptor CLEC-2, in podoplanin-mediated platelet activation, by cancer cells.* J Biol Chem, 2007. 282(36): p. 25993-6001.

[109] Suzuki-Inoue, K., *Essential in vivo roles of the platelet activation receptor CLEC-2 in tumour metastasis, lymphangiogenesis and thrombus formation.* J Biochem, 2011. 150(2): p. 127-32.

[110] Martin-Villar, E., et al., *Characterization of human PA2.26 antigen (T1alpha-2, podoplanin), a small membrane mucin induced in oral squamous cell carcinomas.* Int J Cancer, 2005. 113(6): p. 899-910.

[111] Lopez, J.A. and J.F. Dong, *Structure and function of the glycoprotein Ib-IX-V complex.* Curr Opin Hematol, 1997. 4(5): p. 323-9.

[112] Kasirer-Friede, A., et al., *Signaling through GP Ib-IX-V activates alpha IIb beta 3 independently of other receptors.* Blood, 2004. 103(9): p. 3403-11.

[113] Berndt, M.C., et al., *The vascular biology of the glycoprotein Ib-IX-V complex.* Thromb Haemost, 2001. 86(1): p. 178-88.

[114] Canobbio, I., C. Balduini, and M. Torti, *Signalling through the platelet glycoprotein Ib-V-IX complex.* Cell Signal, 2004. 16(12): p. 1329-44.

[115] Ruggeri, Z.M., *Von Willebrand factor: looking back and looking forward.* Thromb Haemost, 2007. 98(1): p. 55-62.

[116] Grossi, I.M., et al., *Role of tumor cell glycoproteins immunologically related to glycoproteins Ib and IIb/IIIa in tumor cell-platelet and tumor cell-matrix interactions.* FASEB J, 1988. 2(8): p. 2385-95.

[117] Jain, S., J. Harris, and J. Ware, *Platelets: linking hemostasis and cancer.* Arterioscler Thromb Vasc Biol, 2010. 30(12): p. 2362-7.

[118] Jain, S., et al., *Platelet glycoprotein Ib alpha supports experimental lung metastasis.* Proc Natl Acad Sci U S A, 2007. 104(21): p. 9024-8.

[119] Erpenbeck, L., et al., *Inhibition of platelet GPIb alpha and promotion of melanoma metastasis.* J Invest Dermatol, 2010. 130(2): p. 576-86.

[120] Terraube, V., et al., *Increased metastatic potential of tumor cells in von Willebrand factor-deficient mice.* J Thromb Haemost, 2006. 4(3): p. 519-26.

[121] Karpatkin, S., et al., *Role of adhesive proteins in platelet tumor interaction in vitro and metastasis formation in vivo.* J Clin Invest, 1988. 81(4): p. 1012-9.

[122] Wagner, C.L., et al., *Analysis of GPIIb/IIIa receptor number by quantification of 7E3 binding to human platelets.* Blood, 1996. 88(3): p. 907-14.

[123] Coller, B.S. and S.J. Shattil, *The GPIIb/IIIa (integrin alphaIIbbeta3) odyssey: a technology-driven saga of a receptor with twists, turns, and even a bend.* Blood, 2008. 112(8): p. 3011-25.

[124] Cox, D., M. Brennan, and N. Moran, *Integrins* as *therapeutic targets: lessons and opportunities.* Nat Rev Drug Discov, 2010. 9(10): p. 804-20.

[125] Karpatkin, S., C. Ambrogio, and E. Pearlstein, *The role of tumor-induced platelet aggregation, platelet adhesion and adhesive proteins in tumor metastasis.* Prog Clin Biol Res, 1988. 283: p. 585-606.

[126] Bakewell, S.J., et al., *Platelet and osteoclast beta3 integrins are critical for bone metastasis.* Proc Natl Acad Sci U S A, 2003. 100(24): p. 14205-10.

[127] Kitagawa, H., et al., *Involvement of platelet membrane glycoprotein Ib and glycoprotein IIb/IIIa complex in thrombin-dependent and -independent platelet aggregations induced by tumor cells.* Cancer Res, 1989. 49(3): p. 537-41.

[128] Kerrigan, S.W. and D. Cox, *Platelet-bacterial interactions.* Cell Mol Life Sci, 2010. 67(4): p. 513-23.

[129] van Nispen tot Pannerden, H., et al., *The platelet interior revisited: electron tomography reveals tubular alpha-granule subtypes.* Blood, 2010. 116(7): p. 1147-56.

[130] Sehgal, S. and B. Storrie, *Evidence that differential packaging of the major platelet granule proteins von Willebrand factor and fibrinogen can support their differential release.* J Thromb Haemost, 2007. 5(10): p. 2009-16.

[131] Ma, L., et al., *Proteinase-activated receptors 1 and 4 counter-regulate endostatin and VEGF release from human platelets.* Proc Natl Acad Sci U S A, 2005. 102(1): p. 216-20.

[132] van Holten, T.C., et al., *Quantitative proteomics analysis reveals similar release profiles following specific PAR-1 or PAR-4 stimulation of platelets.* Cardiovasc Res, 2014. 103(1): p. 140-6.

[133] Kamykowski, J., et al., *Quantitative immunofluorescence mapping reveals little functional coclustering of proteins within platelet alpha-granules.* Blood, 2011. 118(5): p. 1370-3.

[134] Peters, C.G., A.D. Michelson, and R. Flaumenhaft, *Granule exocytosis is required for platelet spreading: differential sorting of alpha-granules expressing VAMP-7.* Blood, 2012. 120(1): p. 199-206.

[135] Whiteheart, S.W., *Platelet granules: surprise packages.* Blood, 2011. 118(5): p. 1190-1.

[136] Coppinger, J.A., et al., *Characterization of the proteins released from activated platelets leads to localization of novel platelet proteins in human atherosclerotic lesions.* Blood, 2004. 103(6): p. 2096-104.

[137] Blair, P. and R. Flaumenhaft, *Platelet alpha-granules: basic biology and clinical correlates.* Blood Rev, 2009. 23(4): p. 177-89.

[138] McNicol, A. and S.J. Israels, *Platelet dense granules: structure, function and implications for haemostasis.* Thromb Res, 1999. 95(1): p. 1-18.

[139] Jurk, K. and B.E. Kehrel, *Platelets: physiology and biochemistry.* Semin Thromb Hemost, 2005. 31(4): p. 381-92.

[140] White, J.G., *The dense bodies of human platelets. Origin of serotonin storage particles from platelet granules.* Am J Pathol, 1968. 53(5): p. 791-808.

[141] Nesbitt, W.S., et al., *Intercellular calcium communication regulates platelet aggregation and thrombus growth.* J Cell Biol, 2003. 160(7): p. 1151-61.

[142] White, J.G., *The dense bodies of human platelets: inherent electron opacity of the serotonin storage particles.* Blood, 1969. 33(4): p. 598-606.

[143] Boneu, B., et al., *Exhausted platelets in patients with malignant solid tumors without evidence of active consumption coagulopathy*. Eur J Cancer Clin Oncol, 1984. 20(7): p. 899-903.

[144] Jurasz, P., D. Alonso-Escolano, and M.W. Radomski, *Platelet--cancer interactions: mechanisms and pharmacology of tumour cell-induced platelet aggregation.* Br J Pharmacol, 2004. 143(7): p. 819-26.

[145] Santos-Martinez, M.J., et al., *Role of metalloproteinases in platelet function.* Thromb Res, 2008. 121(4): p. 535-42.

[146] Biggerstaff, J.P., et al., *Fibrin monomer increases platelet adherence to tumor cells in a flowing system: a possible role in metastasis?* Thromb Res, 1998. 92(6 Suppl 2): p. S53-8.

[147] Im, J.H., et al., *Coagulation facilitates tumor cell spreading in the pulmonary vasculature during early metastatic colony formation.* Cancer Res, 2004. 64(23): p. 8613-9.

[148] Demers, M. and D.D. Wagner, *Neutrophil extracellular traps: A new link to cancer-associated thrombosis and potential implications for tumor progression.* Oncoimmunology, 2013. 2(2): p. e22946.

[149] Cools-Lartigue, J., et al., *Neutrophil extracellular traps sequester circulating tumor cells and promote metastasis.* The Journal of Clinical Investigation, 2013. 123(8): p. 3446-3458.

[150] Radisky, D.C., Epithelial-mesenchymal transition. J Cell Sci, 2005. 118(Pt 19): p. 4325-6.

[151] Buller, H.R., et al., Cancer and thrombosis: from molecular mechanisms to clinical presentations. J Thromb Haemost, 2007. 5 Suppl 1: p. 246-54.

Chapter 7

# Platelets, Inflammation and Respiratory Disease

Brian P. O'Sullivan and Steven W. Kerrigan

Additional information is available at the end of the chapter

http://dx.doi.org/10.5772/60569

## 1. Introduction

The lungs have several characteristics that separate them from other organs; they receive the total cardiac output, they have two sources of perfusion, pulmonary and bronchial arteries, and they are exposed to the external environment, making them vulnerable to damage caused by inhaled microorganisms and airborne particulates. Chronic obstructive pulmonary disease (COPD), consisting of both chronic bronchitis and emphysema, is caused by inhalation of tobacco combustion products that cause inflammatory changes that overwhelm the body's natural anti-inflammatory defense mechanisms. Inhaled bacteria and viruses lead to infection and infiltration of polymorphonucleocytes (PMN) whose exo-products including superoxides, hyopchlorous acid, and elastases damage lung tissue even as they repel the infecting organisms. Additionally, events such as sepsis and shock can set off a systemic inflammatory cascade involving the lungs.

Virtually all lung diseases (with the exception of congenital malformations) involve some degree of inflammation of the airways, the alveoli, or the parenchyma. Given the increasing recognition of the role of platelets in inflammation, it is not surprising that platelet biology has become an active area of interest for respirologists around the world. Evidence of this is the publication in the last several years of comprehensive reviews of platelet and lung biology, platelets and innate immunity, and the contribution of platelets to specific disorders such as asthma, acute lung injury, and cystic fibrosis.[1-6] In this chapter we will review the basic biology of the platelet-lung interaction and work that demonstrates the important part these cell-like structures play both in maintenance of lung health and in multiple pulmonary diseases.

## 2. Platelet genesis in the lung

Megakaryocytes emerge from the bone marrow and travel to the lung where they are trapped in the microvasculature and form elongated processes known as proplatelets. Shear forces or other factors then cause proplatelets to release individual platelets.[7] Platelet release occurs in bone marrow, but there is mounting evidence that much platelet release from proplatelets occurs in the pulmonary circulation, making the lungs the birthplace of the platelet.[1] Evidence supporting this includes the observation of megakaryocytes in pulmonary vascular beds and an increased number of platelets in pulmonary venous blood as compared to pulmonary arterial blood. The presence of a large pool of newly formed platelets in the pulmonary circulation means that there is ample opportunity for interaction with other blood cells. PMN, which like megakaryocytes have trouble navigating the pulmonary microvasculature due to their resistance to deformation, accumulate in the pulmonary circuit creating a pool of marginated white blood cells. This leads to intimate contact between these cells and the potential for cell-cell interactions.

## 3. Platelets in Inflammation

Platelets are anucleate cytoplasts that for many years were felt to play a role exclusively in hemostasis. More recent studies suggest that platelets also play an important role in inflammation, including promoting the inflammatory response to influenza virus.[8, 9] Platelets are derived from the same myeloid stem cell as traditional inflammatory cells and therefore have retained the ability to serve as inflammatory cells. For example they can undergo chemotaxis, contain and release adhesive proteins, activate other inflammatory cells, release vasoactive substances, and have the capacity to express or release pro-inflammatory mediators such as thromboxane (TX) $A_2$,, platelet activating factor (PAF), brain derived neurotrophic factor (BDNF), and platelet factor 4 (PF4, also known as, CXCL4), as well as a host of other chemokines and chemokine receptors (Table 1).[10-13] Platelets contain the largest amount of transforming growth factor-β (TGFβ) in the body and express pattern recognition toll-like receptors.[14] Furthermore, direct cell-cell contact by specific adhesion molecules facilitates transcellular metabolism of arachidonic acid (AA) by both PMN and platelets.[15, 16] Platelets provide free AA to PMN, which enhances production of PMN-derived leukotriene (LT) $B_4$ and the cysteinyl leukotrienes, $LTC_4$, $LTD_4$, and $LTE_4$. At the same time, platelet-derived enzymes such as 12-lipoxygenase act on PMN eicosanoid products to produce other lipid mediators, including the anti-inflammatory lipoxins (LXs).[17] Although platelets do not have nuclei, they do contain substantial amounts of mRNA and are recognized as being capable of *de novo* synthesis of a growing number of proteins including adhesion molecules, CD40L, and interleukin-1β.[14, 18, 19]

Platelets are a linking element between hemostasis, inflammation, and tissue repair.[12, 14] Not only are they activated via traditional pathways (thrombin, adenosine diphosphate (ADP), $TXA_2$), they can be stimulated by antigens, antigen-antibody complexes, microorganisms, and bacterial endotoxins, including lipopolysaccharide from gram negative bacteria such as, *Pseudomonas aeruginosa*.[20] Platelet granules store a large number of biologically active substances that can be released upon activation. It has been suspected that platelets can undergo differential granule release of pro- or anti-inflammatory mediators depending on specific circumstances.[14] Release of mediators stored in platelet granules and *de novo* platelet production of other mediators can enhance the inflammatory response. Histamine and serotonin increase vascular permeability; ADP increases the agonist-induced oxidative burst in PMN; platelet-derived growth factor (PDGF) stimulates chemotaxis for monocytes and primes eosinophils to produce superoxide anion; and, PF4 induces PMN to adhere to unstimulated vascular endothelium, induces the release of histamine from basophils, and stimulates the adherence of eosinophils to vascular walls.[11] Platelets can also release RANTES (regulated upon activation, normal T-cell expressed and secreted), which plays an important role in recruitment and adhesion of monocytes to activated endothelium.[21] Once leukocytes are recruited to tissue, platelets potentiate the inflammatory process by inhibiting apoptosis of PMN, monocytes, and eosinophils.[22, 23]

| Inflammatory mediator | Platelet location | Mediator type | Inflammatory role |
|---|---|---|---|
| **$TXA_2$** | Synthesized | Eicosanoid | Platelet amplification, Monocyte activation & T-cell differentiation |
| **IL-1β** | Synthesized | Cytokine | Endothelial cell activation |
| **PDGF** | α-granules | Growth factor | Neutrophil, monocyte and macrophage recruitment |
| **PF4** | α-granules | Chemokine | Eosinophil, neutrophil and T- cell recruitment, |
| **TGF-β** | α-granules | Growth factor | Fibroblast and monocyte recruitment |
| **PDHRF** | α-granules | Chemokine | Eosinophil recruitment |
| **P-selectin** | α-granules | Selectin receptor | Adhesion of platelets to monocytes, neutrophils, lymphocytes; complement activation |
| **CD63** | α-granules | Tetraspanin receptor | Neutrophil, monocyte recruitment |
| **MIP-1α** | α-granules | Cytokine | Eosinphil and Neutrophil activation, B-cell immunoglobulin production |
| **VEGF** | α-granules | Growth factor | Lymphocyte & endothelial cell activation |
| **RANTES** | α-granules | Chemokine | T-celll & monocyte migration and recruitment |
| **5-HT** | δ-granules | Transmitter | Dendritic cell & lymphocyte activation |
| **ADP** | δ-granules | Nucleotide | Leukocyte, platelet & endothelial cell activation |
| **Histamine** | δ-granules | Transmitter | Activation of the endothelial cells; increase in permeability |
| **Glutamate** | δ-granules | | Lymphocyte trafficking |

Platelets metabolize arachidonic acid (AA) via the cyclooxygenase and lipoxygenase pathways to produce inflammatory mediators, the most abundant of which are $TXA_2$, via the cyclooxygenase pathway, and 12-S-HETE, via the 12-lipoxygenase pathway.[24] Platelet 12-lipoxygenase interacts with the products of AA metabolism by other cells (notably PMN) to produce lipoxins.[17] In addition, PMN stimulated by endotoxin release PAF, which activates platelets,[25] that in turn recruit more PMN to the inflamed area. Platelets also provide positive feedback mechanisms for their own activation. ADP secreted from dense granules and $TXA_2$ formed from AA bind to P2Y and TP receptors on the platelet surface, complete initial platelet activation, and recruit additional platelets into the activated fraction. Thus, once the inflammatory cascade has been initiated, leukocytes and platelets combine to propagate and amplify it.

In addition to the active role platelets play in producing inflammatory mediators – and perhaps even more important – is the role they play in the process of migration of WBC from the vascular compartment to the site of tissue injury or inflammation. In order for leukocytes to invade inflamed or infected tissue, the white blood cell must first be tethered to the vessel wall and roll along the endothelial surface, then attach firmly to the endothelium, and finally migrate through the endothelium into the tissue. The final two steps, firm attachment and diapedesis, are the result of up regulation of integrin molecules, particularly integrin $\alpha_M\beta_2$ (Mac-1, CD11b/CD18). However, tethering and rolling are dependent upon the function of selectins, especially P-selectin.[26] P-selectin is stored in $\alpha$-granules of platelets and Weibel-Palade bodies of endothelial cells, from which it is translocated to the cell surface membrane upon activation of the cell. Once expressed, P-selectin binds to leukocytes via P-selectin glycoprotein ligand-1 (PSGL-1).[27] P-selectin glycoprotein ligand-1 is constitutively expressed on leukocytes and allows for formation of neutrophil-platelet, monocyte-platelet, and eosinophil-platelet aggregates if P-selectin is trafficked to platelet cell membranes. Although endothelial expression of P-selectin alone can lead to leukocyte rolling, this process (which is a necessary precursor to firm attachment and diapedesis) is much more efficient in the presence of platelet P-selectin in part due to platelet-leukocyte aggregates which amplify the ability of WBC to be recruited to the endothelial surface by cross-linking (figure 1).[28] Expression of platelet membrane P-selectin and release of their chemoattractants enhances leukocyte recruitment into the lung tissue. The number of platelets adherent to pulmonary vessels (the marginated pool) need not be large in order to affect vascular permeability and PMN recruitment. A small number of activated platelets can signal PMN-platelet and platelet-platelet interactions that lead to an increased number of platelet-PMN aggregates, which can become tethered to the pulmonary vascular endothelium.

Thus, platelets fit the definition of traditional inflammatory cells in many ways -- they are capable of phagocytosis and elaboration of pro-inflammatory cytokines, chemokines, and lipid mediators, and are vital for the process of leukocyte tethering and rolling, which are necessary fist steps in recruitment of leukocytes to areas of inflammation. Animals made deficient in platelets or in whom platelet P-selectin is blocked or deficient are less capable of mounting an inflammatory response and have fewer white blood cells in target organs and humans with inflammatory processes have increased numbers of platelet-leukocyte aggregates and

http://dx.doi.org/10.5772/60569

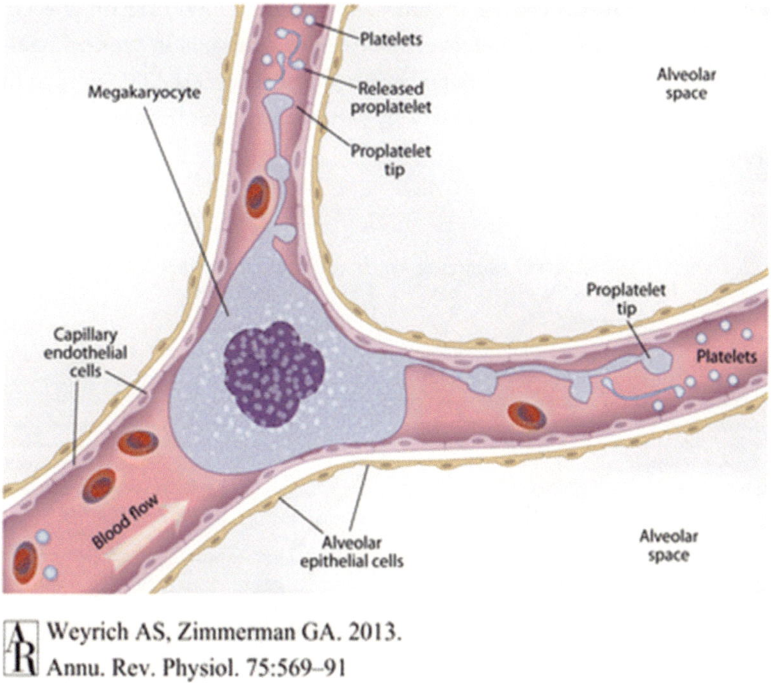


**Figure 1.** Megakaryocytes are found in human lung microvessels and may spawn platelets and platelet precursors in this location. Reproduced from Weyrich and Zimmerman 2013. Platelets in Lung Biology. Annu. Rev. Physiol. 75:569-91 with permission from Annual Review of Physiology, Volume 75 © 2013 by Annual Reviews.

increased expression of platelet P-selectin, both markers of platelet activation.[29, 32] In summary, platelets are a key component of the inflammatory response in pulmonary tissue.

## 4. Platelets and lung health

In addition to the pro-inflammatory properties of platelets outlined above, these tiny blood constituents are essential effector cells in lung hemorrhage and in vascular barrier function. As reviewed by Weyrich and Zimmerman, platelets play at least 5 roles in maintaining endothelial barrier function in the pulmonary circulation: release of soluble molecules that enhance barrier function, physical obstruction of gaps, maintenance of structural features of endothelial cells, stimulation of endothelial growth, and neutralization of agents that might enhance endothelial permeability.[1] Thrombocytopenia, therefore, can have a detrimental effect on barrier function beyond simple hemorrhage. Among the secreted products that enhance endothelial cell-cell interactions and promote vascular integrity are shingosine-1-phosphate (S1P), serotonin, and angiopoietin-1. S1P appears to be particularly important in stabilizing pulmonary endothelium by enhancing adherens junctions and tight junctions.[8] There is evidence that a critical number of platelets are necessary for basal barrier integrity. Platelets are also important for vascular repair and remodeling. The vasoactive substances that platelets release may play protective or damaging roles depending on the circumstances surrounding platelet activation. Platelets are active effector cells in wound healing and can also play roles in angiogenesis and vascular repair and remodeling.[33] Some of these actions, when dysregulated, may lead to pulmonary hypertension, smooth muscle proliferation, and pathological remodeling of lung tissue.

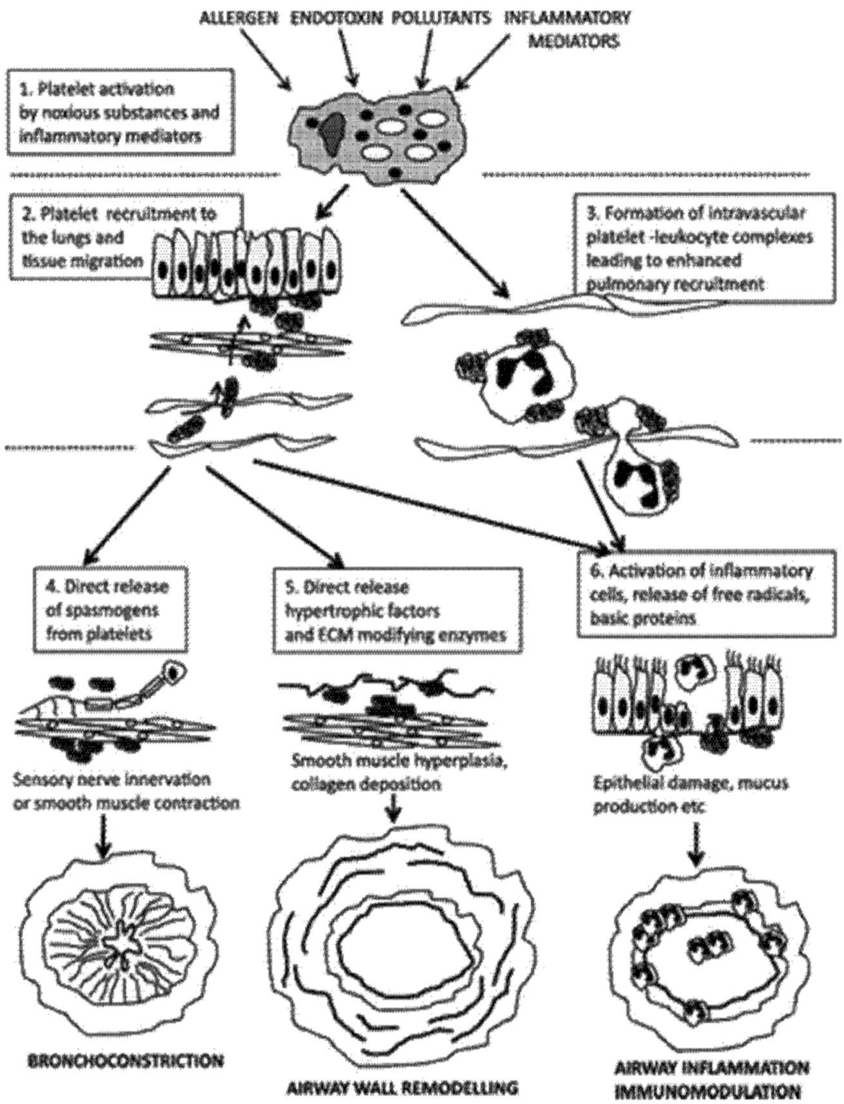


**Figure 2.** Platelet activation leading to airway inflammation. 'Reproduced from Page & Pitchford, Platelets Coming of Age: Implications for Our Understanding of Allergic Inflammation, Am J Respir Crit Care Med 2013;187:459-460, with permission of the American Thoracic Society. Copyright © 2015 American Thoracic Society.

http://dx.doi.org/10.5772/60569

## 5. Platelets and asthma

Over a century ago Sir William Osler recognized that asthma was an inflammatory disease. Much work has been done since then looking for causes and treatments of airway inflammation in patients with asthma.[34] However, despite the fact that as long ago as 1967 it was recognized that platelets could release the vasoactive substance serotonin in response to a hypersensitivity challenge[35] it is only recently that the importance of platelets in this disease process has been recognized and explored in detail.

In a series of elegant animal and human experiments spanning more than a decade, investigators have shown that platelets play a fundamental role in the recruitment of leucocytes to the lungs following exposure to allergens and play a key role in the onset and perpetuation of airway inflammation in asthma.[2] Studies have shown that animals deficient in platelets, platelet receptors, or factors activating platelets have abrogation of responses to allergic challenges.[29, 32, 36, 37] De Sanctis et al[38] looked at ovalbumin sensitized mice that were P-selectin deficient and found reduced numbers of eosinophils and lymphocytes in lung lavage fluid compared to wild type mice, indicating the importance of this platelet-expressed adhesion molecule in mediating allergen induced pulmonary inflammation. Following this work, Ulfman and colleagues[39] showed that P-selectin bearing platelets were integral in tethering of eosinophils to activated endothelium in an ex-vivo perfusion model. Further studies have shown the importance of platelet P-selectin and soluble P-selectin in eosinophil attachment to VCAM-1.[40] These authors concluded that their findings were, "...compatible with a scenario whereby P-selectin, on eosinophil-associated activated platelets or acquired from plasma or from prior interactions with endothelial cells or platelets, activates eosinophil $\alpha4\beta1$ integrin and stimulates eosinophils to adhere to VCAM-1 and move to the airway in asthma."[40] Antibodies that block P-selectin have been shown to decrease leukocyte recruitment in animal models of asthma and inflammation.[2] P-selectin appears to be a necessary component of the allergic response in sensitized animals. Platelets also appear to play a role in causing disease in the lung parenchyma itself, with evidence of platelet diapedesis into lungs in animals sensitized to allergens.[41] Platelets that have trans-migrated into tissue can then release their abundant pro-inflammatory mediators and exacerbate allergic inflammation, a possibility that could explain non-eosinophilc airway inflammation that has been reported in some human asthmatic patients.

Human studies substantiate the finding of the importance of platelets seen in allergic animal models. There is a decreased half-life of platelets in atopic patients, implying increased platelet activation and turnover. Increased circulating neutrophil-platelet aggregates and monocyte-platelet aggregates have been seen in atopic humans and up to 25% of eosinophils may be attached to platelets in such subjects.[40] As noted in animal studies, these attachments increase expression of surface markers (integrins), which enhance leukocyte adhesion to blood vessels. Moritani and colleagues[42] were able to demonstrate an association between platelet activation as assessed by P-selectin expression and RANTES release with an asthmatic diathesis in humans. Similarly, Durk and colleagues[43] have shown increased serotonin in segmental lavage fluid from asthmatic subjects when challenged locally, implying a role for

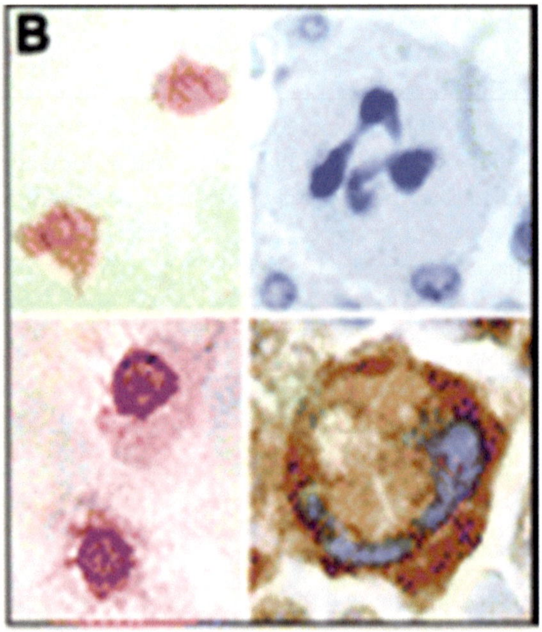


**Figure 3.** Immunocytochemical detection of CFTR in human PLTs (top left: irrelevant antibody; bottom left: anti-CFTR antibody) and bone marrow megakaryoblasts (top right: irrelevant antibody; bottom right: anti-CFTR antibody). Reproduced from Mattosccio et al., Cystic fibrosis transmembrane conductance regulator (CFTR) expression in human platelets: impact on mediators and mechanisms of the inflammatory response. FASEB J 2010;24:3970-3980. with permission of the Federation of American Societies for Experimental Biology. © 2010 FASEB

activated platelets, the major source of serotonin in the human lung, in allergic inflammation. These authors suggest that peripheral serotonin production could be a viable target for future asthma therapy. Others have shown a temporal relationship between circulating platelet-derived factors (included soluble P-selectin) and early and late asthmatic response in allergic subjects. Lommatzsch, et al[10] have looked at another, less well-studied platelet secretion, brain-derived neurotrophic factor (BDNF). This group found that patients with asthma had higher levels of BDNF in serum, platelets, and plasma compared to non-asthmatic matched controls. BNDF levels correlated with parameters of airway obstruction and hyper-reactivity, making this mediator of neuronal plasticity one more platelet product capable of affecting the asthmatic airways.

Associations between platelets and metabolites of arachidonic acid have been identified in asthma patients. Lipoxins play a role in the resolution phase of inflammation and are the product of interaction between PMN-associated arachidonic acid and platelet-derived 12-lipoxygenase. Oxidative stress in asthma is correlated with decreased $LXA_4$ in patients with severe asthma and reflects a loss of anti-inflammatory balance in these patients. In this group of patients ex-vivo incubation of cells with an inhibitor of LX degradation significantly inhibited the PAF-induced platelet-leukocyte aggregates in peripheral blood that contribute to persistent airway inflammation.[44] It is conceivable that drugs that increase LXs or other pro-resolution mediators could offer an alternative or adjunct to corticosteroid therapy in asthma.

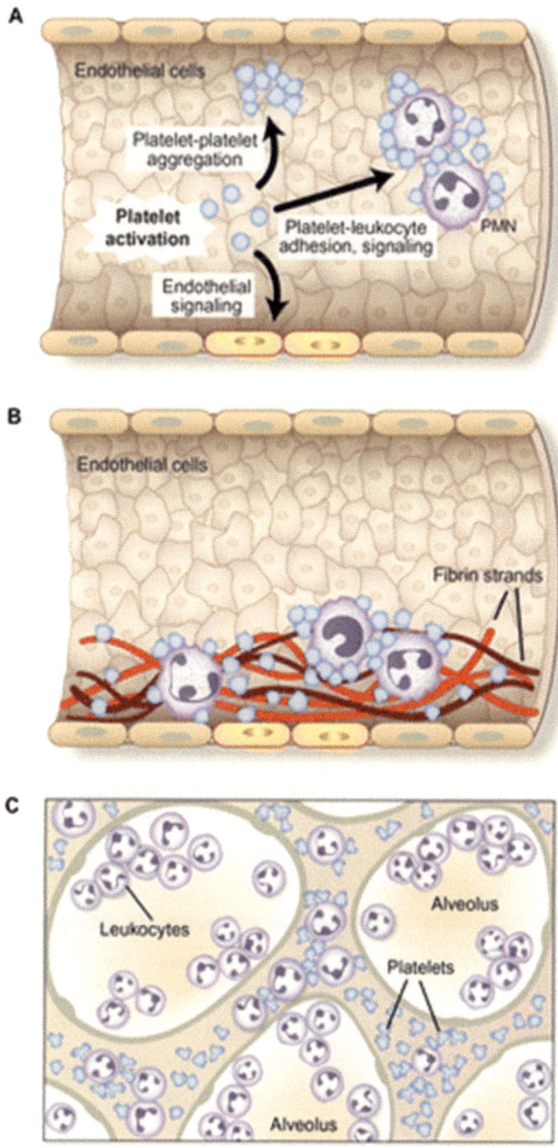


**Figure 4.** Platelet-leukocyte interactions in respiratory endothelium in acute lung Injury. Platelet activation upregulates adhesion molecules. (B) Platelets and PMN accumulation in microvasculature is enhanced by fibrin deposition in response to enodthelial injury. (C) Platelets facilitate accumulation of PMN in alveoli and interstitial spaces and contribute to alveolar leak syndromes. 'Reproduced from Bozza et al., Amicus or adversary: platelets in lung biology, acute injury, and inflammation. Am J Respir Cell Mol Biol 2009;40:123-134, with permission of the American Thoracic Society. Copyright © 2015 American Thoracic Society.'

In a series of human studies specifically looking at aspirin exacerbated respiratory disease, examination of nasal polyps from aspirin sensitive subjects demonstrated extravascular platelets adjacent to leukocytes. Platelets appeared to contribute an inordinate amount of $LTC_4$ synthase activity in these subjects compared to non-aspirin sensitive subjects.[45] $LTC_4$ synthase converts AA-derived $LTA_4$ to the bioactive bronchospastic $LTC_4$. Further mouse studies by this group have shown a potential role for anti-platelet drugs in aspirin induced asthma. Reduced production of melatonin by platelets also has been seen in aspirin-sensitive asthmatics.[46] This deficit could, through several mechanisms, lead to increased platelet activation and be a factor in these patients' intolerance to aspirin.

It is possible that the coagulation cascade may also play a role in the airway remodeling seen in chronic asthmatic patients.[47] Although some early studies using selectin inhibitors have been reported, human studies of the role of anti-platelet agents in the control of asthma are lacking. Growing evidence in human and non-human models clearly makes this a promising area to pursue.

## 6. Platelets and cystic fibrosis

Cystic fibrosis (CF) is an autosomal-recessive illness that is the most common lethal inherited disease in the Caucasian population. CF is caused by a mutation in the cystic fibrosis transmembrane conductance regulator (CFTR) gene on the long arm of chromosome 7.[48] The CFTR protein acts as a chloride and bicarbonate channel, among other functions. Loss of chloride channel function leads to dehydration of the airway surface liquid, which leads to thickened airway secretions, chronic respiratory infection, neutrophilic lung infection, pulmonary destruction, and premature death.[48] The majority of CF patients also have pancreatic insufficiency, predisposing them to malnutrition and fat-soluble vitamin deficiency. The CFTR protein acts predominantly as a chloride channel, but plays multiple other roles in cellular metabolism, including influencing long chain fatty acid synthesis.[49] A hyper-inflammatory state – whether innately due to CFTR dysfunction or a result of chronic infection – contributes to lung destruction over time in CF patients. This inflammatory process is characterized by PMN infiltration of airways and pulmonary parenchyma with elaboration of free neutrophil elastase and pro-inflammatory cytokines.[50] Platelets play a crucial role in facilitating the recruitment of PMN into the CF lung, and as active members of the innate immunity family release their own pro- and anti-inflammatory agents. The process of PMN recruitment in CF is similar to that described above for asthma.

By the end of the 1980s a number of studies had been performed assessing the function of platelets from CF patients. These studies were done prior to the discovery of the CFTR gene and with an incomplete understanding of the underlying molecular defect in these patients. A better picture of the role of platelets in CF has emerged with improved techniques for evaluating platelet function and a more complete knowledge of CFTR function.[5, 51] Cross-sectional studies showing an inverse relationship between platelet activation and pulmonary function provide evidence for a role for platelets in CF lung disease. These studies have shown that: 1) increased platelet numbers correlate with decreased arterial blood oxygen tension ($P_aO_2$),[52] 2) an increase in urinary concentration of thromboxane metabolites (a marker of platelet activation *in vivo*) correlates with decreased forced expiratory volume ($FEV_1$),[53, 54] and 3) increased plasma concentrations of soluble CD40 ligand (sCD40L).[55]

Several groups have demonstrated increased reactivity of CF platelets. Ciabattoni and colleagues[54] showed enhanced lipid peroxidation, which contributes to platelet activation in CF patients. They documented increased urinary excretion of $TxB_2$ metabolites and iso-prostanes, consistent with oxidative stress and increased arachidonic acid turnover in CF patients and hypothesized that these factors led to platelet aggregation and activation and contributes to lung disease in CF patients. O'Sullivan and co-workers[56] showed that washed platelets from CF subjects express increased agonist-induced surface P-selectin expression (a marker of platelet activation) compared to those from control subjects. Also, platelets from CF patients incubated in plasma from non-CF subjects were more reactive to agonists than control platelets in the same plasma. Even though CF plasma upregulated function of both CF and non-CF derived platelets, CF patients' platelets were more reactive than their matched controls.[56] In addition, McGivern and colleagues demonstrated that CF patients' platelets were defective in release of their dense granules. This observation was critical as platelet dense granules contain many mediators responsible for the recruitment of inflammatory cells. Thus CF patients may have a muted inflammatory cell mobilization.[57] Together these studies support platelet activation in CF. Given the known interaction between platelets and leuko-cytes in the pulmonary circulation and the abundance of PMN in CF bronchoalveolar lavage and biopsy/autopy specimens, it is apparent that platelet activation mediates the inflammatory cell infiltration to at least some degree.

CFTR protein expression was first described in epithelial cells from nasal epithelium and sweat glands in humans. Since that time, CFTR expression has been identified in circulating blood cells including PMN, leukocytes, and monocytes. It is feasible that platelets also express CFTR and that its absence might explain some of the abnormalities in platelet function seen in CF patients. There have been reports of indirect evidence of loss of CFTR function in CF platelets. Agam et al.[58] demonstrated abnormal platelet volume changes in response to $PGE_1$, reflecting down regulation of a cAMP-regulated channel, of which CFTR is one. In another indirect evaluation of CFTR function in CF platelets, Ulane and collaborators [59] demonstrat-ed an intrinsic increase in turnover of platelet membrane phospholipids (specifically, phos-phatidylcholine), which they ascribed to CFTR dysfunction. Although CFTR protein and mRNA have not been detected in control or CF platelets by some investigators,[56] Mattoscio et al[51] did find evidence of CFTR in platelets and megakaryocytes using flow-cytometry, immunohistochemical stains, Western blot, and RT-PCR. Elegant studies by this group on CF platelet proteomics has shown distinct characteristics of CF platelets that predispose them to promoting pulmonary inflammation. In particular, they showed constitutive overexpression of beta-3 integrin, which contributes to platelet activation and which can activate the NF-KB pathway in PMN.[60]

Platelets have been found to contain an excess of the long-chain polyunsaturated fatty acid known as Mead acid.[56] When Mead acid is metabolized by platelet 12-lipoxygenase an end-product is generated with $PGE_2$-like activity, which enhances platelet aggregation.[61, 62] Platelet 12-lipoxygenase also acts on arachidonic acid released from PMN cell membranes to form members of the anti-inflammatory lipoxin family. CF patients have a defect in lipoxin synthesis that appears to be directly related to a lack of normal function of CFTR in platelets. [51] In addition to their anti-inflammatory properties LXs also contribute to maintenance of normal airway surface liquid depth.[63] Loss of this normal airway lubrication is one of the fundamental pathogenic features of CF and appears to be exacerbated by the lack of normally functioning CFTR protein in platelets. Furthermore, cells from respiratory epithelium of CF patients have a decreased amount of another long chain polyunsaturated fatty acid, docosahexaenoic acid (DHA).[49] DHA is a precursor to a group of anti-inflammatory compounds known as resolvins, which are important in leading to the resolution of the normal host response to infection or injury.[64] Thus, intrinsic defects in CF platelets enhance the inflammatory process, inhibit its resolution, and contribute to the underlying defect in airway surface liquid. It appears that when normal CFTR function is lost in those with CF results in patients with CF it results in upregulation of inflammation and a corresponding loss of the counterbalancing resolution phase of inflammation.

In addition to intrinsic platelet abnormalities, there is abundant evidence of the presence of pro-inflammatory mediators in CF patients' plasma. Increased levels of sCD40L, $LTB_4$, immune complexes, interleukins, ATP, and tumor necrosis factor-$\alpha$ have all been documented. [55, 65, 67] It is possible that platelet activation in CF is merely an "innocent bystander" effect due to the fact that the platelets are immersed in a pool of platelet-activating substances. In fact, there is evidence that platelets from non-CF subjects are activated when incubated in CF plasma.[56] Many of these mediators both come from and activate platelets; therefore, it is hard to know if platelet activation causes inflammation or if inflammation causes platelet activation. In summary, loss of normal CFTR function can indirectly increase platelet activation through its affect on plasma factors such as specific cytokines, fatty acids, ATP, and vitamin E, and loss of CFTR function specifically in platelets can directly increase platelets activation. The final result, irrespective of cause of activation, is increased recruitment and activation of leukocytes into the CF lung, elaboration of mediators that cause tissue damage, and enhanced loss of lung function

## 7. Platelets and acute lung injury

The acute respiratory distress syndrome (ARDS) is defined as acute onset of hypoxemia in response to insults including sepsis, trauma, aspiration, and toxins. In 1994 the American-European Consensus Conference defined ARDS as acute onset of hypoxemia with bilateral infiltrates on chest roentgenogram and no evidence of left atrial hypertension.[68] The American-European group defined another entity, acute lung injury (ALI), as similar lung disease but with a lesser degree of hypoxemia. Although a 2012 task force[68] did not include ALI as a distinct entity, instead subsuming it in a sub-category of ARDS, many still use the combined term ALI/ARDS to describe those suffering from acute, severe respiratory distress.

http://dx.doi.org/10.5772/60569

Despite multiple new therapeutic interventions based on well done clinical trials, mortality in the most severe category of ARDS still hovers around 50%.[69]

A hallmark of ARDS is increased capillary leak and influx of neutrophils and fluid into the lung interstitium. Recent reviews have emphasized the role of platelets in instigating this pulmonary vascular leak.[3, 8] Sepsis and trauma in particular lead to systemic inflammation and vascular permeability. Interestingly, several of the strategies employed in critical care units that have led to decreased mortality from ALI/ARDS include interventions that decrease platelet activation; these include low volume ventilation, nitric oxide administration, and anti-inflammatory/anti-platelet medications.[3] This insight has led to a trial of the anti-platelet agent aspirin in ARDS, the Lung Injury Prevention Study with Aspirin.[70]

The interplay between coagulation and inflammation has become an increasingly active area of investigation in acute lung injury. Activation of the coagulation pathway, including platelet activation, and decreased fibrinolysis contributes to ALI/ARDS. The maintenance of a normal endothelial cell barrier is a critical component of the fluid and protein diffusion balance in the pulmonary circulation. In health, platelets play an important role in systemic and pulmonary vascular integrity (see above). A number of studies show that platelet depletion can lead to vascular leakage and that reconstitution with infused platelets can correct the barrier defect (reviewed in reference 1). Platelets may take up radical oxygen species and release preformed mediators such as serotonin, which contribute to endothelial barrier stability. Among these mediators is sphingosine 1-phosphate (S1P), a lipid growth factor that promotes endothelial integrity and which may be a therapeutic agent in capillary leak syndromes.[71, 72] Thus, platelets – by direct thrombotic action and through release of specific mediators – can provide protection of respiratory function by decreasing the likelihood of capillary leak in response to injurious effectors.

Platelets may provide a degree of protection for the injured lung through their hemostatic mechanisms; however, observations suggest a negative role for platelets in experimental alveolar injury. A hallmark of ALI/ARDS pathology is the presence of microthrombi in the pulmonary circulation. Studies have shown increased numbers of platelets and leukocytes in pulmonary capillaries and platelet-fibrin thrombi have been detected in autopsy specimens from patients dying of ALI/ARDS.[3] Thrombocytopenia is a poor prognostic factor in sepsis and may represent sequestering of activated platelets in the microcirculation.[3] Post-mortem and biopsy samples have shown thrombi within pulmonary arteries, arterioles, and capillaries from patients suffering from ALI/ARDS and can explain in part the ventilation-perfusion mismatching that contributes to the severe hypoxemia seen clinically.[73] These thrombi are the result of activation of platelet hemostatic mechanisms, which have the capability to be both beneficial and harmful to an ill patient. Activated human platelets synthesize tissue factor and provide signals that induce tissue factor production by monocytes.[8] Tissue factor then leads to formation of microthrombi and clots that then occlude pulmonary vessels. The ability to inhibit thrombus formation may explain some of the clinical effect of inhaled nitric oxide (NO) in critically ill patients. NO has been shown to decrease platelet aggregation and improve oxygenation in a small cohort of ALI/ARDS patients, which the investigators attributed to its anti-thrombotic effect[74] and in vitro studies by another group showed an NO dose-dependent decrease in ADP and collagen induced platelet aggregation, P-selectin expression, and fibrinogen binding.[75] NO administration to ALI/ARDS patients demonstrated similar reductions in platelet aggregation and P-selecting expression. It is possible that the transient in oxygenation seen with NO administration lies in part in its anti-platelet action and not just as a vasodilator.

Systemic inflammation caused by sepsis activates circulating cells and leads to formation of heterotypic aggregates.[76] These platelet-leukocyte interactions lead to production and release of factors that can disrupt vascular integrity. The major effector cell in ALI/ARDS is the PMN, which causes endothelial damage, plasma leakage, and hypoxemia.[77] The importance of neutrophils in syndromes of acute alveolar damage is underscored by animal studies where lung injury is abolished by induction of neutropenia. Since platelets play such a key role in PMN tethering and rolling it is not surprising that they play an active role in the inflammatory process accompanying ALI/ARDS. Since platelets are integral to PMN tethering and rolling it is not surprising that they play an active role in sepsis. Using a mouse model of sepsis-induced ALI caused by inhaled lipopolysaccharide (LPS) Grommes and colleagues[78] demonstrated that animals deficient in either platelets or neutrophils had marked reduction in neutrophilic infiltration and protein/fluid leak into alveoli. In separate experiments these investigators depleted either platelets or neutrophils. Further work showed that treatment with monoclonal antibodies to the platelet-derived chemokines CCL5 and CXCL4 led to decreased neutrophil recruitment, plasma exudation, and protease release. The mechanism for this pulmonary protection appeared to be disruption of the platelet-leukocyte heteromers formed by these chemokines. Surprisingly, these authors did not find that blocking adhesion molecules commonly associated with platelet-neutrophil aggregation, specifically P-selectin and GPIIb/IIIa, led to decreased diffuse alveolar damage.

Although the work by Grommes et al implicated CCL5 and CXCL4 and not P-selectin as the critical surface markers in heterotypic aggregate formation, others found that selective disruption of platelet P-selectin led to decreased platelet-PMN aggregates, decrease $TXA_2$ release, and decreased lung injury in an acid-induced model of ALI.[79] Further evidence of the fundamental role of platelet-leukocyte aggregates in ALI/ARDS comes from work by Ortiz-Munoz and colleagues[80] who showed that the aspirin-induced LX, 15-epi-lipoxin $A_4$, has a protective effect in LPS induced lung injury through its ability to disrupt heterotypic aggregate formation. Using intravital microscopy they were able to show formation of platelet-neutrophil aggregates in response to LPS administration and a sharp decline in aggregate formation, platelet activation, and lung injury following aspirin administration.[80] Thus a large number of studies indicate the importance of activated platelets and platelet-leukocyte aggregates in the development of ALI/ARDS in animal models. Evidence of P-selectin upregulation on the surface of circulating platelets in humans with ALI/ARDS supports the theory that these cytoplasts play and active role in human disease, too.[3, 30] Patients with sepsis have been shown to have increased surface P-selectin expression on platelets and increased plasma levels of products of $\alpha$-granule release.[76] It is well recognized that expression of P-selectin is a marker of platelet activation and, the animal study of Grommes et al[78] not withstanding, leads to formation of platelet-leukocytes heterotypic aggregates. Although this likely represents an adaptive mechanism of enhancing leukocyte recruitment to areas of infection or injury, a maladaptive consequence of platelet activation is the tissue injury and alveolar leakage that results from release of their cytoplasmic contents and recruitment of activated PMN.

LPS from gram-negative bacteria is a potent activator of platelets and platelet-leukocyte aggregates. In addition to producing mediators that can trigger platelet activation, both gram-negative and gram-positive bacteria can interact directly with platelets. In their thrombotic role, platelets adhere to exposed sub-endothelial matrix at the site of vascular injury as the first line of defense against hemorrhage. This places them in perfect position to act as sentinels against invading microorganisms. In fact, platelets are now recognized as part of the innate immune system patrolling the endothelium and capable of rapid release of an array of immunomodulatory cytokines.[6] Furthermore, platelets express toll-like receptors and interactions with bacteria through these pattern recognition receptors can lead to aggregation and/or activation of platelets directly, or indirectly through the action of plasma proteins.[4, 81] Infected thrombi formed by bacterial-platelet adhesion can seed the microcirculation of the lung or stick to exposed surfaces such as damaged heart valves.[82] Human platelets can engulf, but do not kill bacteria due to a lack of myeloperoxidase and their inability to form "killing chambers" isolated from the cytoplasm and the cell's exterior.[83] However, upon activation at the site of endothelial injury, platelet granules release thrombin-inducible platelet microbiocidal proteins, which act against a broad range of microbes. The released anti-microbial proteins include platelet activating factor-4 (CXCL4), RANTES, and β-defensins.[6, 82] Platelets then have a Janus-like character acting either for the betterment or detriment of the host; which it is depends on the timing and location of the stimulus. Platelet activation and release of anti-microbial proteins may halt invasion by bacteria or may cause tissue damage by upregulating inflammation by recruiting and activating more platelets, leukocytes, and heterotypic aggregates. Recent work implicates a specific single nucleotide polymorphism linked to platelets, which is associated with ARDS risk at least partially mediated via effects on platelet count. [84]

There is growing evidence implicating the role of neutrophil extracellular traps (NETs) in the genesis of lung damage in sepsis.[81, 85] NETs are extracellular lattices, which are capable of capturing and killing bacteria. Clark et al[81] were able to show that NETs are released from PMN in response to binding of platelet TLR4 to neutrophil TLR4 ligand but that stimulation of PMN with bacterial LPS in the absence of platelets did not induce NET release. Presumably an aspect of the innate immune system that protect organisms from bacterial infection, NETs are primarily released in small capillaries and are capable of causing damage to endothelial tissue. Whereas platelets contribute to the integrity of the endothelial barrier and promote bacterial killing, they also promote endothelial damage directly by release of their own pre-formed and rapidly transcripted mRNA products and from activation of leukocytes, whose inflammatory products and NETs have adverse effects on the pulmonary parenchyma.

Transfusion related acute lung injury (TRALI) is the leading cause of transfusion-related mortality and is defined as acute lung injury that occurs during or within 6 hours of transfusion of one or more units of blood or blood components.[86] Known risk factors for developing TRALI include several recipient factors indicative of severity of underlying illness (including high pressure mechanical ventilation, a trigger for platelet activation) and donor factors such as female sex, HLA class II antibodies, and volume of anti-human neutrophil antigens.[86] Patients with TRALI have evidence of systemic inflammation with increases in circulating neutrophils and a decrease in platelets compared with controls, similar to those with the systemic inflammatory response syndrome seen in sepsis.[87] It is likely that TRALI is caused by infusion of anti-neutrophil antibodies and/or biologically active lipids (potentially platelet derived) that interact with recipient neutrophils that are already primed by the underlying illness.[8, 88] Activation of platelets and neutrophils then leads to the cascade of endothelial injury and permeability seen in other forms of acute lung injury. A study showed that infusion of stored platelet concentrates, rich in lipid mediators, could cause ALI when infused into rats pretreated with LPS.[88] Treatment with aspirin, which induces lipid mediator such as LXs with antagonistic actions on platelet activation and platelet-neutrophil aggregation, abrogated the TRALI response in a murine model of TRALI.[80]

## 8. Platelets and chronic obstructive pulmonary disease

The vast majority of studies on chronic bronchitis and emphysema have focused on the role of tobacco smoke exposure as the causative agent. Clinical trials tend to look at the effect of various bronchodilators or antibiotics in the treatment of COPD exacerbations. However, dampening the response to the inciting constituents of tobacco smoke has the potential to alleviate many of the downstream consequences of cigarette smoking. A handful of studies have examined platelet counts and platelet volumes in COPD, with sometimes contradictory results.[89, 90] PMN have been shown to play a fundamental role in the development and progression of COPD and their transmigration across pulmonary endothelium is critical to their function in COPD.[91, 92] The process of activation of platelets and adherence of inflammatory cells to pulmonary endothelium is enhanced by cigarette smoke.[93] Given the role of PMN in the destructive nature of COPD and the known role of platelets in facilitating transmigration of these cells in the pulmonary circulation, it is intuitive to believe that platelets must play a role in COPD just as they do in asthma and CF.

## 9. Summary

Platelets clearly play a major role in the development of multiple acute lung injury syndromes including transfusion-related pulmonary problems. Activation and aggregation of platelets plays a crucial role in the recruitment and activation of leukocytes to the site of lung injury/ infection. Additionally, platelets are part of the innate immune system and are capable of triggering immune responses via release of pro-inflammatory cytokines and chemokines. It is not surprising, therefore, that they are an integral part of the inflammatory cascade in a host of pulmonary diseases. In addition to the specific processes discussed in detail in this chapter, platelets are undoubtedly active participants in a myriad of other lung processes that involve cellular infiltration and tissue destruction. The platelet is ubiquitous in pulmonary disease

http://dx.doi.org/10.5772/60569

genesis and sustainability. Further work with platelet inhibitors, specific and non-specific, may lead to novel approaches to therapy of chronic and acute lung disease.

## Author details

Brian P. O'Sullivan[1*] and Steven W. Kerrigan[2]

*Address all correspondence to: osullivb@hitchcock.org

1 Geisel School of Medicine at Dartmouth, Hanover, NH, USA

2 Royal College of Surgeons in Ireland, Dublin, Ireland

## References

[1] Weyrich AS, Zimmerman GA. Platelets in lung biology. *Ann Rev Physiol.* 2013;75:569-591.

[2] Page C, Pitchford S. Platelets and allergic inflammation. *Clin Exper Allergy.* 2014;44:901-913.

[3] Katz JN, Kolappa KP, Becker RC. Beyond thombosis: The versatile platelet in critical illness. *Chest.* 2011;139:658-668.

[4] Cox D, Kerrigan SW, Watson SP. Platelets and the innate immune system: Mechanisms of bacterial-induced platelet activation. *J Thromb Haemost.* 2011;9:1097-1107.

[5] O'Sullivan BP, Michelson AD. The inflammatory role of platelets in cystic fibrosis. *Am J Respir Crit Care Med.* 2006;173(5):483-490.

[6] Duerschmied D, Bode C, Aherns I. Immune functions of platelets. *Thromb Haemost.* 2014;112:678-691.

[7] Geddis AE, Kaushansky K. The root of platelet production. *Science.* 2007;317:1689-1691.

[8] Bozza F, Shah A, Weyrich A, Zimmerman G. Amicus or adversary: Platelets in lung biology, acute injury, and inflammation. *Am J Respir Cell Mol Biol.* 2009;40:123-134.

[9] Le V,Ba, Schneider J,G., Boergeling Y, Berri F, Ducatez M, Guerin J, Adrian I, Errazuriz-Cerda E, Frasquilho S, Antunes L, Lina B, Bordet J, Jandrot-Perrus M, Ludwig S, Riteau B. Platelet activation and aggregation promote lung inflammation and influenza virus pathogenesis. *Am J Respir Crit Care Med.* 2015;Online first 09-FEB-2015(10.1164/rccm.201406-1031OC).

[10] Lommatzsch M, Schloetcke K, Klotz J, Schuhbaeck K, Zingler D, Zingler C, Schulte-Herbruggen O, Gill H, Schuff-Werner P, Virchow JC. Brain-derived neurotrophic factor in platelets and airflow limitation in asthma. *Am J Respir Crit Care Med.* 2005;171(2):115-120.

[11] Herd CM, Page CP. Pulmonary immune cells in health and disease: Platelets. *Eur Respir J.* 1994;7:1145-1160.

[12] Gear AR, Camerini D. Platelet chemokines and chemokine receptors: Linking hemostasis, inflammation, and host defense. *Microcirculation.* 2003;10(3-4):335-50.

[13] Klinger MHF. Inflammation. In: Michelson AD, ed. *Platelets.* San Diego: Academic Press; 2002:459-467.

[14] Semple J, Italiano J, Freedman J. Platelets and the immune continuum. *Nat Rev Immunol.* 2011;11:264-274.

[15] Maclouf JA, Murphy RC. Transcellular metabolism of neutrophil-derived leukotriene A4 by human platelets. A potential cellular source of leukotriene C4. *J Biol Chem.* 1988;263:174-181.

[16] de Gaetano G, Cerletti C, Evangelista V. Recent advances in platelet-polymorphonuclear leukocyte interaction. *Haemostasis.* 1999;29(1):41-9.

[17] Serhan CN, Sheppard KA. Lipoxin formation during human neutrophil-platelet interactions. evidence for the transformation of leukotriene A4 by platelet 12-lipoxygenase in vitro. *J Clin Invest.* 1990;85(3):772-80.

[18] Lindemann S, Tolley ND, Dixon DA, McIntyre TM, Prescott SM, Zimmerman GA, Weyrich AS. Activated platelets mediate inflammatory signaling by regulated interleukin 1beta synthesis. *J Cell Biol.* 2001;154(3):485-90.

[19] Weyrich AS, Schwertz H, Kraiss LW, Zimmerman GA. Protein synthesis by platelets: Historical and new perspectives. *J Thromb Haemost.* 2009(2):241-246.

[20] Konig B, Jaeger K, Sage A, Vasil M, Konig W. Role of pseudomonas aeruginosa lipase in inflammatory mediator release from human inflammatory effector cells (platelets, granulocytes, and monocytes). *Infect Immun.* 1996;64(8):3252-3258.

[21] von Hundelshausen P, Weber KSC, Huo Y, Proudfoot AEI, Nelson PJ, Ley K, Weber C. RANTES deposition by platelets triggers monocyte arrest on inflamed and atherosclerotic endothelium. *Circulation.* 2001;103(13):1772-1777.

[22] Brunetti M, Martelli N, Manarini S, Mascetra N, Musiani P, Cerletti C, Aiello FB, Evangelista V. Polymorphonuclear leukocyte apoptosis is inhibited by platelet-released mediators, role of TGFb-1. *Thromb Haemost.* 2000;84:478-483.

[23] Raiden S, Schettini J, Salamone G, Trevani A, Vermeulen M, Gamberale R, Giordano M, Geffner J. Human platelets produce granulocyte-macrophage colony-stimulating factor and delay eosinophil apoptosis. *Lab Invest.* 2003;83:589-598.

[24] Weber A. Aspirin and activated platelets. In: Curtis-Prior P, ed. *The eicosanoids*. West Sussex, England: John Wiley & Sons, Ltd.; 2004:373-385.

[25] Watanabe J, Marathe GK, Neilsen PO, Weyrich AS, Harrison KA, Murphy RC, Zimmerman GA, McIntyre TM. Endotoxins stimulate neutrophil adhesion followed by synthesis and release of platelet-activating factor in microparticles. *J Biol Chem*. 2003;278(35):33161-33168.

[26] Ma Y, Plow EF, Geng J. P-selectin binding to P-selectin glycoprotein ligand-1 induces an intermediate state of {alpha}M{beta}2 activation and acts cooperatively with extracellular stimuli to support maximal adhesion of human neutrophils. *Blood*. 2004;104(8):2549-2556.

[27] Mayadas T, Johnson R, Rayburn H, Hynes R, Wagner D. Leukocyte rolling and extravasation are severely compromised in P-selectin deficient mice. *Cell*. 1993;74:541-554.

[28] Burger PC, Wagner DD. Platelet P-selectin facilitates atherosclerotic lesion development. *Blood*. 2003;101(7):2661-6.

[29] Pitchford SC, Yano H, Lever R, Riffo-Vasquez Y, Ciferri S, Rose MJ, Giannini S, Momi S, Spina D, O'Connor B, Gresele P, Page CP. Platelets are essential for leukocyte recruitment in allergic inflammation. *J Allerg Clin Immunol*. 2003;112(1):109-18.

[30] George J, Pickett E, Saucerman S, McEver R, Kunicki T, Kieffer N, Newman P. Platelet surface glycoproteins: Studies on resting and activated platelets and platelet membrane microparticles in normal subjects, and observations in patients during adult respiratory distress syndrome adn cardiac surgery. *J Clin Invest*. 1986;78:340-348.

[31] Pitchford SC, Riffo-Vasquez Y, Sousa A, Momi S, Gresele P, Spina D, Page CP. Platelets are necessary for airway wall remodeling in a murine model of chronic allergic inflammation. *Blood*. 2004;103(2):639-47.

[32] Pitchford SC, Momi S, Giannini S, Casali L, Spina D, Page CP, Gresele P. Platelet P-selectin is required for pulmonary eosinophil and lymphocyte recruitment in a murine model of allergic inflammation. *Blood*. 2005;105:2074-81.

[33] Ho-Tin-Noe B, Demers M, Wagner DD. How platelets safeguard vascular integrity. *J Thromb Haemost*. 2011;9(Suppl 1):56-65.

[34] Holgate ST. Lessons learnt from the epidemic of asthma. *Quart J Med*. 2004;97:247-257.

[35] Caspary EA, Comaish JS. Release of serotonin from human platelets in hypersensitivity states. *Nature*. 1967;214:286-287.

[36] Lellouch-Tubiana A, Lefort J, Simon M, Pfister A, Vargaftig B. Eosinophil recruitment into guinea pig lungs after PAF-acether and allergen administration: Modula-

tion by prostacycline, platelet depletion, and selective antagonists. *Am Rev Respir Dis*. 1988;137:948-954.

[37] Coyle A, Page C, Atkinson L, Flanagin R, Metzger W. The requirement for platelets in allergin-induced late asthmatic airway obstruction: Eosinophil infiltration and heightened airway responsiveness in allergic rabbits. *Am Rev Respir Dis*. 1990;142:587-593.

[38] De Sanctis GT, Wolyniec WW, Green FH, Qin S, Jiao A, Finn PW, Noonan T, Joetham AA, Gelfand E, Doerschuk CM, Drazen JM. Reduction of allergic airway responses in P-selectin-deficient mice. *J Appl Physiol*. 1997;83(3):681-687.

[39] Ulfman LH, Joosten DP, van Aalst CW, Lammers JW, van de Graaf EA, Koenderman L, Zwaginga JJ. Platelets promote eosinophil adhesion of patients with asthma to endothelium under flow conditions. *American Journal of Respiratory Cell & Molecular Biology*. 2003;28(4):512-9.

[40] Johansson MW, Mosher DF. Activation of beta-1 integrins on blood eosinophils by P-selectin. *Am J Respir Cell Mol Biol*. 2011;45:889-897.

[41] Pitchford SC, Momi S, Baglioni S, Casali L, Giannini S, Rossi R, Page CP, Gresele P. Allergen induces the migration of platelets to lung tissue in allergic asthma. *Am J Respir Crit Care Med*. 2008;177:604-612.

[42] Moritani C, Ishioka S, Haruta Y, Kambe M, Yamakido M. Activation of platelets in bronchial asthma. *Chest*. 1998;113(2):452-458.

[43] Dürk T, Duerschmied D, Müller T, Grimm M, Reuter S, Vieira RP, Ayata K, Cicko S, Sorichter S, Walther DJ, Virchow JC, Taube C, Idzko M. Production of serotonin by tryptophan hydroxylase-1 and release via platelets contribute to allergic airway inflammation. *Am J Respir Crit Care Med*. 2013;187:476-485.

[44] Ono E, Dutile S, Kazani S, Wechsler ME, Yang J, Hammock BD, Douda DN, Tabet Y, Khaddaj-Mallat R, Sirois M, Sirois C, Rizcallah E, Rousseau E, Martin R, Sutherland ER, Castro M, N Jarjour N, Israel E, Levy BD, National Heart, Lung, and Blood Institute's Asthma Clinical Research Network. Lipoxin generation is related to soluble epoxide hydrolase activity in severe asthma. *Am J Respir Crit Care Med*. 2014;190:886-897.

[45] Laidlaw TM, Kidder MS, Bhattacharyya N, Xing W, Shen S, Milne GL, Castells MC, Chay H, Boyce JA. Cysteinyl leukotriene overproduction in aspirin-exacerbated respiratory disease is driven by platelet-adherent leukocytes. *Blood*. 2012;119(16): 3790-3798.

[46] Evsyukova HV. Expression of melatonin in platelets of patients with aspirin-induced asthma. *Eur J Clin Invest*. 2011;41:781-784.

[47] Brims FJH, Chauhan AJ, Higgins B, Shute JK. Coagulation factors in the airways in moderate and severe asthma and the effect of inhaled steroids. *Thorax*. 2009;64:1037-1043.

[48] O'Sullivan BP, Freedman SD. Cystic fibrosis. *Lancet*. 2009;373:1891-1904.

[49] Freedman SD, Blanco PG, Zaman MM, Shea JC, Ollero M, Hopper IK, Weed DA, Gelrud A, Regan MM, Laposata M, Alvarez JG, O'Sullivan BP. Association of cystic fibrosis with abnormalities in fatty acid metabolism. *N Engl J Med*. 2004;350:560-9.

[50] Cantin AM. Cystic fibrosis lung inflammation: Early, sustained, and severe. *Am J Respir Crit Care Med*. 1995;151:939-41.

[51] Mattoscio D, Evangelista V, De Cristofaro R, Recchiuti A, Pandolfi A, Di Silvestre S, Manarini S, Martelli N, Rocca B, Petrucci G, Angelini DF, Battistini L, Robuffo I, Pensabene T, Pieroni L, Furnari ML, Pardo F, Quattrucci S, Lancellotti S, Davì G, Romano M. Cystic fibrosis transmembrane conductance regulator (CFTR) expression in human platelets: Impact on mediators and mechanisms of the inflammatory response. *FASEB J*. 2010;24:3970-3980.

[52] Gross S, Luckey C. The oxygen tension-platelet relationship in cystic fibrosis. *Am Rev Respir Dis*. 1969;100:513-7.

[53] Davi G, Iapichino L, Balsamo V, Ganci A, Giammarresi C, Patrignani P, Patrono C. Thromboxane biosynthesis and pulmonary function in cystic fibrosis. *Adv Prostaglandin Thromboxane Leukot Res*. 1995;23:369-71.

[54] Ciabattoni G, Davi G, Collura M, Iapichino L, Pardo F, Ganci A, Romagnoli R, Maclouf J, Patrono C. In vivo lipid peroxidation and platelet activation in cystic fibrosis. *Am J Respir Crit Care Med*. 2000;162(4 Pt 1):1195-201.

[55] Falco A, Romano M, Lapichino L, Collura M, Davi G. Increased soluble CD40 ligand levels in cystic fibrosis. *J Thromb Haemost*. 2004;2:557-560.

[56] O'Sullivan BP, Linden MD, Frelinger LA, Barnard MR, Spencer-Manzon M, Morris JE, Salem RO, Laposata M, Michelson AD. Platelet activation in cystic fibrosis. *Blood*. 2005;105:4635-4641.

[57] McGivern TJP, Molloy K, Bahar M, McElvaney NG, Moran N, Kerrigan SW. A platelet dense-granule secretion defect may lead to a muted inflammatory cell mobilization response in cystic fibrosis patients. *J Thromb Haemost*. 2013;11:1939-1942.

[58] Agam G, Aviram M, Zilberman-Kaufman M, Rothstein A, Livne AA. Cyclic AMP-related and cation-affected human platelet chloride transport regulation. *Eur J Clin Chem Clin Biochem*. 1995;33(6):329-35.

[59] Ulane MM, Butler JD, Peri A, Miele L, Ulane RE, Hubbard VS. Cystic fibrosis and phosphatidylcholine biosynthesis. *Clin Chim Acta*. 1994;230(2):109-16.

[60] Pieroni L, Finamore F, Ronci M, Mattoscio D, Marzano V, Mortera SL, Quattrucci S, Federici G, Romano M, Urbani A. Proteomics investigation of human platelets in

healthy donors and cystic fibrosis patients by shotgun nUPLC-MSE and 2DE: A comparative study. *Mol Biosyst.* 2011;7:630-639.

[61] Lagarde M, Burtin M, Sprecher H, Dechavanne M, Renaud S. Potentiating effect of 5,8,11-eicosatrienoic acid on human platelet aggregation. *Lipids.* 1983;18:291-4.

[62] Lagarde M, Burtin M, Rigaud M, Sprecher H, Dechavanne M, Renaud S. Prostaglandin $E_2$-like activity of 20:3n-9 platelet lipoxygenase end-product. *FEBS Lett.* 1985;181(1):53-6.

[63] Verriere V, Higgins G, Al-Alawi M, Costello RW, McNally P, Chiron R, Harvey BJ, Urbach V. Lipoxin A4 stimulates calcium-activated chloride currents and increases airway surface liquid height in normal and cystic fibrosis airway epithelia. *PLoS One.* 2012;7(5):e37746. doi: 10.1371/journal.pone.0037746 [doi].

[64] Serhan CN, Hong S, Gronert K, Colgan SP, Devchand PR, Mirick G, Moussignac RL. Resolvins: A family of bioactive products of omega-3 fatty acid transformation circuits initiated by aspirin treatment that counter proinflammation signals. *J Exp Med.* 2002;196(8):1025-37.

[65] Carpagnano GE, Barnes PJ, Geddes DM, Hodson ME, Kharitonov SA. Increased leukotriene B4 and interleukin-6 in exhaled breath condensate in cystic fibrosis. *Am J Respir Crit Care Med.* 2003;167(8):1109-12.

[66] Church JA, Jordan SC, Keens TG, Wang C. Circulating immune complexes in patients with cystic fibrosis. *Chest.* 1981;80:405-411.

[67] Berger M. Lung inflammation early in cystic fibrosis: Bugs are indicted, but the defense is guilty. *Am J Respir Crit Care Med.* 2002;165(7):857-8.

[68] Anon T. Acute respiratory distress syndrome: The berlin definition. *JAMA.* 2012;307:2526-2533.

[69] Beitler JR, Schoenfeld DA, Thompson BT. Preventing ARDS: Progress, promise, pitfalls. *Chest.* 2014;146:1102-1113.

[70] Kor DJ, Talmor DS, Banner-Goodspeed VM, Carter RE, Hinds R, Park PK, Gajic O, Gong MN. Lung injury prevention with aspirin (LIPS-A): A protocol for a multicentre randomised clinical trial in medical patients at high risk of acute lung injury. *BMJ Open.* 2012(5).

[71] Garcia JG, Liu F, Verin AD, Birukova A, Dechert MA, Gerthoffer WT, Bamberg JR, English D. Sphingosine 1-phosphate promotes endothelial cell barrier integrity by edg-dependent cytoskeletal rearrangement. *J Clin Invest.* 2001;108:689-701.

[72] Bhattacharya J. Lung injury: Sphingosine-1-phosphate to the rescue. *Am J Respir Crit Care Med.* 2004;170(9):928-929. doi: 170/9/928 [pii].

[73] Bone RC, Francis PB, Pierce AK. Intravascular coagulation associated wit the adult respiratory distress syndrome. *Am J Med.* 1976;61:585-589.

[74] Samama CM, Diaby M, Fellahi JL, Mdhafar A, Eyraud D, Arock M, Guillosson JJ, Coriat P, Rouby JJ. Inhibition of platelet aggregation by inhaled nitric oxide in patients with acute respiratory distress syndrome. *Anesthesiology*. 1995;83(1):56-65.

[75] Gries A, Bode C, Peter K, Herr A, Böhrer H, Motsch J, Martin E. Inhaled nitric oxide inhibits human platelet aggregation, P-selectin expression, and fibrinogen binding in vitro and in vivo. *Circulation*. 1998;97(15):1481-1487. doi: 10.1161/01.CIR.97.15.1481.

[76] de Stoppelaar SF, van 't Veer C, der Poll T. The role of platelets in sepsis. *Thromb Haemost*. 2014;112:666-677.

[77] Grommes J, Soehnlein O. Contribution of neutrophils to acute lung injury. *Mol Medicine*. 2011;17:293-307.

[78] Grommes J, Alard JE, Drechsler M, Wantha S, Morgelin M, Kuebler WM, Jacobs M, von Hundelshausen P, Markart P, Wygrecka M, Preissner KT, Hackeng TM, Koenen RR, Weber C, Soehnlein O. Disruption of platelet-derived chemokine heteromers prevents neutrophil extravasation in acute lung injury. *Am J Respir Crit Care Med*. 2012;185:628-636.

[79] Zarbock A, Singbartl K, Ley K. Compete reversal of acid-induced acute lung injury by blocking of platetel-neutrophil aggregation. *J Clin Invest*. 2006;116:3211-3219.

[80] Ortiz-Munoz G, Mallavia B, Bins A, Headley M, Krummel MF, Looney MR. Aspirin-triggered 15-epi-lipoxin A4 regulates neutrophil-platelet aggregation and attenuates acute lung injury in mice. *Blood*. 2014;124:2625-2634.

[81] Clark SR, Ma AC, Tavener SA, McDonald B, Goodarzi Z, Kelly M, Patel KD, Chakrabarti S, McAvoy E, Sinclair GD, Keys EM, Allen-Vercoe E, DeVinney R, Doig CJ, Green F, Kubes P. Platelet TLR4 activates neutrophil extracellular traps to ensnare bacteria in septic blood. *Nat Med*. 2007;13:463-469.

[82] Fitzgerald JR, Foster TJ, Cox D. The interaction of bacterial pathogens with platelets. *Nat Rev Microbiol*. 2006;4:445-457.

[83] White JG. Why human platelets fail to kill bacteria. *Platelets*. 2006;17:191-200.

[84] Wei,Yongyue, Wang,Zhaoxi, Su,Li, Chen,Feng, Tejera,Paula, Bajwa E,K., Wurfel M,M., Lin,Xihong, Christiani D,C..

[85] Andrews RK, Arthur JF, Gardiner EE. Neutrophil extracellular traps (NETs) and the role of platelets in infection. *Thromb Haemost*. 2014;112:659-665.

[86] Toy P, Gajic O, Bacchetti P, Looney MR, Gropper MA, Hubmayr R, Lowell CA, Norris PJ, Murphy EL, Weiskopf RB, Wilson G, Koenigsberg M, Lee D, Schuller R, Wu P, Grimes B, Gandhi MJ, Winters JL, Mair D, Hirschler N, Sanchez Rosen R, Matthay MA, TRALI Study Group. Transfusion-related acute lung injury: Incidence and risk factors. *Blood*. 2012;119(7):1757-1767. doi: 10.1182/blood-2011-08-370932 [doi].

[87] Looney MR, Roubinian N, Gajic O, Gropper MA, Hubmayr RD, Lowell CA, Bacchetti P, Wilson G, Koenigsberg M, Lee DC, Wu P, Grimes B, Norris PJ, Murphy EL, Gan-

dhi MJ, Winters JL, Mair DC, Schuller RM, Hirschler NV, Rosen RS, Matthay MA, Toy P, Transfusion-Related Acute Lung Injury Study Group. Prospective study on the clinical course and outcomes in transfusion-related acute lung injury*. *Crit Care Med*. 2014;42:1676-1687.

[88] Silliman CC, Bjornsen AJ, Wyman TH, Kelher M, Allard J, Bieber S, Voelkel NF. Plasma and lipids from stored platelets cause acute lung injury in an animal model. *Transfusion*. 2003;43(5):633-640. doi: 10.1046/j.1537-2995.2003.00385.x.

[89] Wang R, Li J, Cao Z, Li Y. Mean platelet volume is decreased during an acute exacerbation of chronic obstructive pulmonary disease. *Respirology*. 2013;18(8):1244-1248. doi: 10.1111/resp.12143.

[90] Biljak VR, Pancirov D, Cepelak I, Popovic-Grle S, Stjepanovic G, Grubisic TZ. Platelet count, mean platelet volume and smoking status in stable chronic obstructive pulmonary disease. *Platelets*. 2011;22:466-470.

[91] Gane J, Stockley R. Mechanisms of neutrophil transmigration across the vascular endothelium in COPD. *Thorax*. 2011. doi: 10.1136/thoraxjnl-2011-200088.

[92] Hoenderdos K, Condliffe A. The neutrophil in chronic obstructive pulmonary disease. too little, too late or too much, too soon?<br /><br />. *Am J Respir Cell Mol Biol*. 2012;48:531-539.

[93] Sharma J, Young DM, Marentette JO, Rastogi P, Turk J, McHowat J. Lung endothelial cell platelet-activating factor production and inflammatory cell adherence are increased in response to cigarette smoke component exposure. Am J Physiol Lung Cell Mol Physiol. 2012;302:L47-55.

Chapter 8

# A Role for Platelets in Normal Pregnancy

Maryam Al Obaidly, Carmen Regan, Bashir Lwaleed and Niamh Moran

Additional information is available at the end of the chapter

http://dx.doi.org/10.5772/61210

## 1. Introduction

### 1.1. Haemostasis in pregnancy

Normal haemostasis is a complex equilibrium involving a balance between blood-borne pro-coagulant proteins, the natural anticoagulation system and the fibrinolytic system. Normal human pregnancy is associated with profound alterations to the haemostatic balance wherein the pro-coagulant effects become dominant. A marked progressive increase in the concentration of pro-coagulant proteins (Factors VII, VIII, X, Von Willebrand factor, Fibrinogen) is observed in blood plasma at all stages of pregnancy. These changes coincide with decreases in natural anticoagulants and lower levels of natural fibrinolytic agents and are more pronounced in the uteroplacental circulation than in the systemic circulation during pregnancy [7]. In parallel, markers of platelet activation are markedly elevated throughout normal pregnancy suggestive of a functional role for platelet activation during normal gestation.

It is often argued that this altered haemostatic status is required as the maternal coagulation system prepares for the challenges of parturition, and aims to minimize intrapartum blood loss. However, the alterations in the haemostatic system begin as early as the first trimester, suggesting a requirement for such changes in the proper progression of the early stages of pregnancy, in addition to their role in regulation of post-partum bleeding. For example, alterations in haemostasis enable the necessary changes in the uteroplacental vasculature to support the establishment of the trophoblast invasion of the spiral arteries of the uterus early in gestation [12].

The altered haemostatic status during normal pregnancy presents a number of physiological challenges in the vasculature and results in an increased risk of excessive thrombosis, especially within the uteroplacental circulation. This enhanced pregnancy-associated thrombotic risk may provide the mechanistic basis for many of the major pregnancy complications, such as pre-eclampsia, HELLP syndrome (Hemolysis, Elevated Liver enzymes and Low Platelet count) and intrauterine growth retardation (IUGR) [13].

Pre-eclampsia (PE) is a multifaceted disorder that complicates between 2 and 8% of all pregnancies. It is the most common causes of morbidity and mortality in mothers and babies in the Western world [14]. Clinical signs of disease, such as an elevated maternal blood pressure and proteinuria, become apparent as early as gestation week-20 [9]. Such symptoms can dictate urgent delivery of a preterm baby (<40 weeks). The underlying pathology appears to be a complex interaction of the placental and maternal tissues [15] that leads to generalized endothelial dysfunction. This heightens the normal shift of haemostatic equilibrium toward hypercoagulability. As part of this generalized hypercoagulability status in pregnancy, evidence for enhanced platelet activation, observed in normotensive pregnancies [18], are further increased in women with preeclampsia giving rise to the formation of platelet-derived microthrombi in smaller vessels [20] and an associated disseminated intravascular coagulation [21]. Similar to changes in the coagulation parameters, changes in platelet activation status are recorded before gestational week 13 in PE. Intrauterine growth retardation is often associated with PE, and is correlated with reduced uteroplacental blood flow caused by platelet-rich microthrombi.

## 2. Changes in platelet parameters during pregnancy

The normal blood platelet count in healthy non-pregnant individuals varies between 150-400 X $10^9$/L. Early studies into platelet parameters in normotensive pregnant women reported a progressive drop in the normal platelet count [22]. Indeed mild, non clinical, thrombocytopenia (platelets 100-150 x $10^9$/L), is observed in up to 10% of all pregnancies [6]. It is likely that this is largely a haemodilution effect that results from the maternal blood volume expansion [23]. The decrease in platelet count is accompanied by an increase in mean platelet volume [24] and a notable change in the granule content [25].

Changes in platelet function, and platelet activation status, have been widely reported during pregnancy. However, measurement of platelet activation is complex. There is no one accepted index of platelet activation, although a number of tests and assays are used as surrogate markers of platelet activation in studies on gestational platelet activation. Usually a blood sample is collected from the patient and mixed with an appropriate anticoagulant before being transported to a laboratory for analysis. Platelets are assayed either in whole blood samples or are processed to remove red blood cells and plasma to yield platelet-rich plasma (PRP) or washed platelets (WP), respectively. Thereafter standard or high throughput assays are utilized as appropriate. Platelet aggregation assays are used frequently (Light Transmission Aggregometry; LTA) and can be performed in PRP or WPs [27]. Alternatively high throughput assays of platelet function can be used to assess multiple samples, or multiple agonists, simultaneously. The Moran group have recently developed a high throughput assay of platelet dense-granule secretion to permit extensive assessment of a dose-range of agonists on a relatively small blood sample. In addition, mobile diagnostic analysers of platelet function, such as the PFA-100, have been developed to assess the acute capacity of platelets to form thrombotic aggregates and can be performed in whole blood [31].

In addition to standard assays of platelet function, platelet activation may be inferred, from the presence of activated cell adhesion molecules on the surface of isolated platelets. Such markers include the activated platelet integrin αIIbβ3 (assessed by the monoclonal antibody PAC-1 or fibrinogen-binding) or the enhanced surface expression of the α-granule protein P-Selectin (CD62P) or dense-granule derived protein, CD63 on the surface of circulating platelets.

Platelet granules are rich sources of bioactive agents that are selectively released in response to diverse platelet activating stimuli. Thus, evidence of the presence of secreted platelet-derived bioactive agents in plasma or urine can be used to determine if platelet activation has occurred *in vivo*. Typically, elevated levels of plasma β -thromboglobulin (βTG) and Platelet Factor-4 (PF4) are an indication that platelet release of the contents of platelet α-granules has occurred [36]. Similarly, plasma adenosine or ATP levels reflect release from dense granules. Finally, elevated concentrations of plasma or urinary 11-dehydro Thromboxane $B_2$, a stable metabolite of platelet-generated Thromboxane $A_2$, reflect recent platelet activation. One concern with the use of secreted proteins as markers of platelet activation is the fact that, once released from platelets, biomolecules will have variable half-lives and sensitivity to storage conditions [39], making it difficult to determine how recently the sampled platelets were activated. The use of thromboxane as a marker is also complicated, as this eicosanoid, previously presumed to be only synthesized in platelets, can also be produced by fetal and maternal macrophages in the uteroplacental unit [40].

Proteins that are shed from the surface of activated platelets are also used as surrogate markers of platelet activation. These include soluble P-Selectin (CD62-P) and soluble CD40 Ligand (CD154). Activated platelets also release microparticles (MPs) [43]. However, MPs found in blood may originate from a number of different sources in addition to platelet α-granules. Hence they have not been widely used in assessments of platelet function in pregnancy.

Basal levels of P-Selectin and αIIbβ3 are progressively elevated on the surface of platelets during gestation, suggesting that an inherent activation of platelets occurs during normal pregnancy. In addition, the capacity of platelets to aggregate [31] and adhere [32] in response to various stimuli is enhanced in normotensive pregnant women but is somewhat reduced in platelets from women with preeclampsia [45]. Enhanced fibrinogen binding to circulating platelets, indicative of platelet activation, is also observed in pregnant women compared to non-pregnant subjects [34]. Plasma levels of βTG and PF4, secreted from platelet α-granules, and ADP/ adenosine, secreted from platelet dense granules are elevated during pregnancy.

Many indices of platelet activation have been shown to correlate with gestational age [32], though some, such as platelet responsiveness to agonist stimulation, peak at weeks 30-36 and decline thereafter (Table 1). Only a few studies have assessed platelet function at multiple time points throughout pregnancy and so, information is limited regarding the absolute indices of platelet activation and their temporal relationship to gestational events. However, in general it can be concluded that platelets are hyperactivated from as early as gestational week 10, in the first trimester of pregnancy.

## 3. Changes in platelet parameters in preeclampsia

The gestational changes in haemostatic and platelet responses are altered in women with PE. Accordingly, β-TG and PF4 are elevated in PE above levels observed in normotensive pregnancy. CD63 and P-Selectin levels are increased on the surface of platelets from patients with PE, indicative of recent secretion of dense and $\alpha$-granules, respectively. However, the lack of elevated plasma levels of adenosine or ATP suggest that the secretory events were not acute [26]. The half-life of adenosine is less than 1 minute in plasma in contrast to β-TG, which has a half-life > 120 minutes. Thus, the data suggests that a slow sustained secretion from platelet granules occurs. This is distinct from the pattern that is expected following a thrombotic event where markers of dense granules and $\alpha$-granule release occur acutely and simultaneously. Furthermore, the capacity of platelets from PE patients to acutely aggregate *ex vivo* appears to be attenuated compared to normotensive subjects. This is indeed consistent with the evidence, reported by Janes & Goodall [34] that although activated, degranulated platelets are observed in the circulation in PE, and no evidence for platelet thrombi or platelet aggregates are observed. Together this data shows strong evidence for widespread and sustained platelet secretion in PE. Although platelet thrombi are not observed, activated circulating platelets are observed that contain bound fibrinogen[20]; a strong indication of a thrombotic tendency.

| Marker of platelet activation | Normotensive pregnancy | Preeclampsia |
|---|---|---|
| Platelet Aggregation (LTA; PFA-100) | Responsiveness is greater in normotensive pregnant women than in non pregnant . Platelet hyperaggragation peaks at weeks 20 & 30; declines at week 36 | Platelet aggregation is decreased in both mildly and severely preeclamptic women in comparison with non-pregnant women . Increased numbers of platelets binding to fibrinogen are observed [20]. |
| Surface expression of CD62P on Platelets | Increases with gestational age | Evidence of activated, degranulated platelets in the circulation [34]. CD62P expression is accentuated in PIH<PE<severe PE |
| Surface expession of CD63 on Platelets | elevated in normotensive women | Further elevated in women with non-proteinuric and proteinuric pre-eclampsia [34]. Increased first-trimester CD63 expression is an independent risk factor for development of preeclampsia |
| ATP Secretion | Increases with gestational age [26]. Adenosine in plasma is elevated [46] | Significantly lower in PE than in normotensive pregnant subjects [26] |
| Thromboxane metabolites in plasma or Urine | Increased in normotensive pregnancies . Elevated at 20 weeks and continues to increase thereafter | An imbalance between the production of two metabolites of arachidonic acid, thromboxane and prostacyclin, that favors thromboxane. [53] Greater enhancement of $TxA_2$ production in PIH than in normotensive pregnancies |
| Plaasma levels of β-Tg/ PF4 (secreted from platelet $\alpha$-granules) | Elevatedin normotensive pregnancy; Peaks at gestational weeks 30, & 36 | Greater than in normotensive pregnancy |
| Soluble CD62P in plasma | Elevated by 24 weeks | No difference vs normotensive pregnancy |

**Table 1.** Please add caption

Other haemostatic changes that occur in systemic and uteroplacental circulations during normotensive pregnancies appear to be accentuated in patients with preeclampsia [7]. For example, thromboxane $A_2$ biosynthesis is increased in PE above that observed in normotensive pregnancy and appears to correlate with disease severity. It is preceded by a decreased endogenous production of the endothelial-derived eicosanoid, Prostaglandin $I_2$ ($PGI_2$) [55]. The altered ratio of these thrombo-regulatory eicosanoids appears to play a critical pathological role in preeclampsia. In addition, blood-borne microparticles (MPs) are elevated in preeclampsia and have demonstrable adverse effects on endothelial function. Isolated MPs from preeclamptic women, though not those from normotensive pregnant women, have been shown to downregulate endothelial NO production. NO is a critical regulator of platelet activation, and a regulator of the sensitivity of vascular endothelial cells to trophic agents. By altering the endothelial response and reducing the endogenous production of NO in preeclamptic vascular beds, MPs in preeclamptic women can markedly affect platelet activation and vascular remodeling. Thus in preeclamptic women, many elements of the delicate balance governing platelet activation appear to be dysregulated, predisposing towards premature and excessive platelet secretion. It is tempting to suggest that this dysregulation underlies the pathophysiological mechanisms in PE.

It is postulated therefore that platelets are hyper-reactive in normal pregnancy, and are primed to undergo granule-release at appropriate times and vascular locations. Thus, platelet passage through the placental vasculature can cause acute platelet activation and secretory events, which result in the release of bioactive mediators from platelet $\alpha$-granules. The nature of these bioactive mediators and their functional roles in normal, and preeclamptic, pregnancies remain to be elucidated. Women at risk of developing preeclampsia may have an abnormality in their platelet activation or a temporal dysregulation of these events resulting in atypical vascular events. In fact, increased first-trimester CD63 expression on platelets is an independent risk factor for development of preeclampsia, confirming that early subclinical platelet defects occur in this population.

## 4. Mechanisms of platelet activation during pregnancy

It has been strongly suggested that platelets contribute to protective mechanisms against excessive bleeding during childbirth. Whilst this is indeed relevant, it seems premature to start such thrombotic preparations as early is gestational week 10-12. Thus, platelets must play a role into other gestational requirements. Any roles for platelets are likely to result from their activation in the circulation. However, the mechanisms underlying platelet activation in pregnancy remain largely unknown.

A number of studies have indicated that platelets are hyperresponsive during pregnancy. This may be explained by the increased gestational production of the platelet-activating prostaglandin, thromboxane $A_2$ ($TXA_2$] by platelets. $TXA_2$ can enhance platelet responsiveness to low levels of physiological activation. Thus increases in ambient $TXA_2$ may prime platelets for activation by other agonists. Indeed platelets generate more intracellular calcium in response to standard pro-thrombotic stimuli as pregnancy progresses. In parallel, a reduced synthesis of inhibitory cyclic AMP is observed in platelets from pregnant donors. This reduced production of platelet cAMP may be secondary to altered endothelial function during pregnancy whereby endothelial cells release less of the inhibitory regulators of platelet function (Nitric Oxide and $PGI_2$). Overall, the sensitivity of platelets to activation is enhanced during pregnancy by a parallel increase in ambient pro-thrombotic agents, $TxA_2$ and calcium, and a decrease in anti-thrombotic influences such as intraplatelet cAMP. It is possible that such changes may be initiated by the elevated progesterone level extant during pregnancy, as it has previously been noted that cyclical changes in progesterone during the luteal phase of the ovarian cycle similarly affects platelet function and activation status. Platelets are therefore 'primed' to response to stimulation by various gestational adaptions.

The molecular mechanisms underlying the direct activators of platelets in the placental beds remain unclear, but two independent activators have been identified. Firstly, circulating primed, platelets adhere to the extracellular matrix in the uteroplacental vascular beds and are activated to release various soluble factors to regulate trophoblastic vascular infiltration and differentiation. Secondly, local generation of thrombin, and its interaction with platelet thrombin receptors (PARs) is critical for efficient gestation [62]. However, although generated locally from the plasma coagulation cascade, this thrombin does not participate in fibrin cross-linking, the usual culmination step in blood coagulation. Instead, it directly activates platelet PAR receptors and induces platelets to release their stored contents.

The capacity and sensitivity of platelets to secrete their granular contents therefore is enhanced as pregnancy progresses. Indeed, substantial evidence that this occurs is presented in Table 1. Moreover, data from the Moran laboratory confirms that alterations in platelet function are evident as early as 10-12 gestational weeks (unpublished data; MAO, NM).

## 5. Functional roles for platelet activation during normotensive pregnancy

As discussed above, the gestational role of platelets in pregnancy is likely to be mediated via the secretion of the cargo from platelet $\alpha$-granules. This cargo is comprised of cytokines and other bioactive agents, stored in the abundant platelet granules and includes coagulation proteins such as Fibrinogen and Factors V and XIII. Up to 800 different proteins have been identified in the platelet $\alpha$-granule proteome. Moreover, the contents of platelet $\alpha$-granules can be selectively released in response to discrete activation signals.

In normotensive pregnancy, maternal platelets adhere to the extracellular matrix in the uteroplacental vasculature and are activated in the spiral arteries. As a consequence of this activation of maternal platelets, elevated levels of platelet derived cytokines and bioactive agents are released, that assist and enable trophoblastic arterial infiltration. In addition, platelet derived biomolecules drive morphological changes of trophoblasts and enable angiogenesis in the placental beds. This enables localized physiological vascular remodeling to ensure the appropriate development of embryonic and maternal placental circulations. The precise nature of the platelet releasate in these circumstances has not been fully explored to date. However, there is some evidence that the nature of the releasate differs between normotensive and pre-eclamptic subjects,

Thus, the platelet activation detected in pregnancy (Table 1) is an indicative record of $\alpha$-granule secretion events in the placental vasculature. Importantly, no overt thrombosis is observed in normotensive pregnancies, despite the localized platelet activation and secretion. The requirement for localized platelet regulation of vascular remodeling probably underlies the need for platelets to be primed at early gestational stages in normal pregnancy. The consequent elevation in markers of platelet activation, as shown in Table 1, is simply a confirmation that platelet secretion events have occurred, rather than being suggestive of a pro-thrombotic role for platelets during normal gestation.

## 6. Non-thrombotic roles of platelets in pregnancy

Platelets serve as mobile stores of active biomolecules that can be transported around the body via the vasculature. This function of platelets is well defined in cancer, where platelet stored biomolecules can be released in a bespoke manner by circulating tumour cells to enable the development of a novel, bespoke network of new blood vessels to supply a growing metastatic tumour with suitable nutrients and waste removal functions (See Chapter 6: Mitrugno et al). It is tempting to speculate therefore, that platelets store a relevant and bespoke collection of bioactive compounds during pregnancy. Thus platelet $\alpha$-granules serve as vectors of biological messages for vascular homeostasis during pregnancy. Similarly, platelet-derived MPs may serve to deliver bespoke cocktails of bioactive molecules to uteroplacental vascular beds to facilitate the required vascular changes to support gestation. In support of this, MPs from women with preeclampsia, compared to those from normotensive pregnant women, showed greater pro-inflammatory effects on the vascular wall, inducing vascular hyporeactivity in small blood vessels [65].

However, the key question then becomes one of how the body balances the dual needs of requiring primed platelets to release their cargo at relevent vascular beds in the dynamic, fast-flowing environment of the uteroplacental vasculature, whilst preventing inappropriate thrombosis from occurring; yet maintaining the potential to respond to thrombotic needs should they arise elsewhere in the body.

## 7. Regulation of prothrombotic responses in platelets during normotensive pregnancy

Pregnancy-specific glycoproteins (PSGs) are a family of soluble cell adhesion proteins found in the plasma at various stages of pregnancy. They are largely derived from trophoblastic cells during pregnancy and are abundantly expressed in maternal blood [66]. There are ten human PSG genes (PSG1 - PSG9, PSG11). Several recent studies have indicated that individual PSGs have immunoregulatory, pro-angiogenic, and anti-platelet functions, though their precise functions during pregnancy remain largely speculative.

Recently Shanley et al demonstrated that PSG1 had a high affinity for binding to the major platelet integrin $\alpha IIb\beta 3$. It competes with fibrinogen for binding to this integrin, thereby inhibiting local platelet aggregation [27]. However, the capacity of platelets to secrete the contents of their $\alpha$-and dense granules is unaffected by PSG1. Thus PSG1 enables the secretory responses of circulating platelets, whilst attenuating their thrombotic tendencies.

In parallel, a role for PSG1 in the activation of the anti-inflammatory cytokine, transforming growth factor-beta (TGF) has recently been established. TGF-β regulates many biological events essential for the successful completion of pregnancy including trophoblast invasion and proliferation, angiogenesis, and tolerance to the fetal to the fetal allograft during pregnancy. Of note, platelets serve as a major storage site for TGF-β and release it in response to platelet-activating stimuli. Plasma concentrations of active TGF-β are significantly higher in pree-clamptic women than in normotensive pregnant women [70]. In the presence of a high concentration of PSG1, TGF-β, released from primed platelets in the maternal uteroplacental circulation, is activated and enabled to exert its vascular remodeling effects. Yet due to the high locally-produced concentrations of PSG1, aggregation of platelets does not occur.

Thus PSG1 can simultaneously inhibit platelet aggregation and enable the release of platelet granular-contents including TGF-β, to promote vascular remodeling. This strongly supports the contention that the role of platelet activation during pregnancy is to permit the local delivery of cytokines, via the secretion of $\alpha$-granule contents, rather than the more widely accepted role of inducing thrombotic events. It is likely that complications of pregnancy such as preeclampsia arise when the balance between the thrombotic function of platelets and their secretory functions is disturbed.

## 8. The 'priming' of platelets may contribute to complications of pregnancy

As discussed previously, platelets are primed for activation at early gestational stages. One of the mechanisms of platelet priming is their enhanced ability to synthesize the platelet-specific prothrombotic eicosanoid $TxA_2$, in an environment where opposing antithrombotic influences, namely $PGI_2$ and NO, are downregulated. Measuring $TxA_2$ levels during pregnancy can therefore yield important information on platelet status during gestation.

The concentrations of $TxA_2$ observed in normotensive pregnancy are significantly raised above levels seen in normal healthy non-pregnant donors. In fact, gestational $TxA_2$ levels equate to pathological concentrations identified in cardiovascular patients (Table 2). Yet, despite these pathological levels of circulating prothrombotic eicosanoids, there is little evidence for enhanced platelet-rich thrombotic events during normotensive pregnancy, confirming therefore, that the intended physiological purpose of the elevated platelet activation is not thrombotic in nature. Together, these studies suggest an underlying physiological balance during pregnancy to prime platelets for activation whilst regulating thrombosis.

The need to understand the physiological and molecular mechanisms underlying the enhanced gestational platelet activation is underscored by observations that platelet activation is further accentuated in patients with PE and that pathological thrombotic events can occur if the balance is disturbed.

| **Population** | **[urinary 11-dehdro $TXB_2$]** | **Reference** |
|---|---|---|
| Non-pregnant, healthy subjects | Basal levels approx. 275 pg/mg creatinine | |
| Normotensive, pregnant subjects | 3 fold ↑ over basal levels | |
| Patients with Preeclampsia | ↑ ↑ 1.3 fold increase relative to normotensive pregnant subjects | |
| Patients with Ischemic disease | ↑ donors; similar to normotensive pregnant women | |

**Table 2.** Please add caption

Thus, bioactive agents are released from platelets in a controlled, systematic way during pregnancy to enable required hemostatic changes in the uteroplacental vasculature. However, platelet aggregation and thrombus formation are not required, or could be contraindicated during pregnancy, and are therefore suppressed by PSG1 [27] or similar soluble proteins.

Our limited knowledge of how platelets might contribute to complications of pregnancy evolves from our understanding of the nature of the delicate balance between platelet-activating forces during normotensive pregnancy and the need to prevent thrombosis in the uteroplacental vascular beds. Thus, under the influence of gestational progesterone, endothelial cells produce less NO and $PGI_2$ and platelets produce more $TXA_2$. This tilts the haemostatic balance towards platelet activation and thrombosis. Exposed extracellular matrix proteins in the placental vascular beds bind and activate the primed platelets inducing secretion of their $\alpha$-granule contents. Any tendency for platelets to aggregate is however balanced by the local production of high concentrations of PSG1 [27], which prevents integrin mediated platelet aggregation. In parallel, local generation of Thrombin, the procoagulant, proteolytic enzyme of the coagulation cascade, occurs in normotensive pregnancy [7]. Yet its function is not to generate fibrin, as would be expepcted in the coagulation cascade. Instead, thrombin in the placental beds acts directly on platelet thrombin receptors to induce platelet release from $\alpha$-granules. The fibrinogenic actions of thrombin are moderated by Thrombomodulin (TM) and are essential for successful development of the placenta [62]. Interestingly, TM is also stored in platelet $\alpha$-granules, comprising up to 10% of total granule stores, and is released in response to platelet activation [74]. Absence of TM causes fatal arrest of placental morphogenesis in mice, but this action is not related to its ability to affect fibrin formation, leading the authors to conclude that TM regulates the capacity of thrombin to activate platelets [62]. Moreover, the experiments of Sood and coleagues demonstrate that the delicate balance between the required functions of platelets in pregnancy and their regulation, to prevent unwanted thrombosis, can all-too-easily be shifted to cause placental failure and complications of pregnancy.

## 9. Summary

Therefore we suggest that platelets are not minor participants in the gestational events of pregnancy. Instead, they are active mediators of the complex regulatory system which has several, as yet uncharacterized mechanisms. They serve as vectors for vascular homeostasis during pregnancy, that co-ordinate a delicate balance between delivering relevant and potent biological messages through their granule-delivery system, whilst avoiding platelet-related thrombotic events.

## Author details

Maryam Al Obaidly[1*], Carmen Regan[2], Bashir Lwaleed[3] and Niamh Moran[1]

*Address all correspondence to: maryamalobaidly@rcsi.ie

1 Molecular & Cellular Therapeutics, Royal College of Surgeons in Ireland, Ireland

2 Coombe Women's Hospital, Dublin 8 and Royal College of Surgeons in Ireland, Dublin, Ireland

3 Faculty of Health Sciences, University of Southampton, Southampton General Hospital, UK

## References

[1] Szecsi PB, Jorgensen M, Klajnbard A, Andersen MR, Colov NP, Stender S. Haemostatic reference intervals in pregnancy. Thrombosis and haemostasis. 2010 Apr; 103(4):718-27. PubMed PMID: 20174768.

[2] Franchini M. Haemostasis and pregnancy. Thrombosis and haemostasis. 2006 Mar; 95(3):401-13. PubMed PMID: 16525566.

[3] Howie PW. Blood clotting and fibrinolysis in pregnancy. Postgraduate medical journal. 1979 May;55(643):362-6. PubMed PMID: 382169. Pubmed Central PMCID: 2425447.

[4] Hellgren M. Hemostasis during normal pregnancy and puerperium. Seminars in thrombosis and hemostasis. 2003 Apr;29(2):125-30. PubMed PMID: 12709915.

[5] Brenner B. Haemostatic changes in pregnancy. Thrombosis research. 2004;114(5-6): 409-14. PubMed PMID: 15507271.

[6] Holmes VA, Wallace JM. Haemostasis in normal pregnancy: a balancing act? Biochemical Society transactions. 2005 Apr;33(Pt 2):428-32. PubMed PMID: 15787621.

[7] Higgins JR, Walshe JJ, Darling MR, Norris L, Bonnar J. Hemostasis in the uteroplacental and peripheral circulations in normotensive and pre-eclamptic pregnancies. American journal of obstetrics and gynecology. 1998 Aug;179(2):520-6. PubMed PMID: 9731863.

[8] Hayashi M, Inoue T, Hoshimoto K, Hirabayashi H, Negishi H, Ohkura T. The levels of five markers of hemostasis and endothelial status at different stages of normotensive pregnancy. Acta obstetricia et gynecologica Scandinavica. 2002 Mar;81(3):208-13. PubMed PMID: 11966476.

[9] Bramham K, Parnell B, Nelson-Piercy C, Seed PT, Poston L, Chappell LC. Chronic hypertension and pregnancy outcomes: systematic review and meta-analysis. Bmj. 2014;348:g2301. PubMed PMID: 24735917. Pubmed Central PMCID: 3988319.

[10] Konijnenberg A, Stokkers EW, van der Post JA, Schaap MC, Boer K, Bleker OP, et al. Extensive platelet activation in preeclampsia compared with normal pregnancy: enhanced expression of cell adhesion molecules. American journal of obstetrics and gynecology. 1997 Feb;176(2):461-9. PubMed PMID: 9065199.

[11] Perneby C, Vahter M, Akesson A, Bremme K, Hjemdahl P. Thromboxane metabolite excretion during pregnancy--influence of preeclampsia and aspirin treatment. Thrombosis research. 2011 Jun;127(6):605-6. PubMed PMID: 21316743.

[12] Jaffe R. First trimester utero-placental circulation: maternal-fetal interaction. Journal of perinatal medicine. 1998;26(3):168-74. PubMed PMID: 9773374.

[13] Sibai B, Dekker G, Kupferminc M. Pre-eclampsia. Lancet. 2005 Feb 26-Mar 4;365(9461):785-99. PubMed PMID: 15733721.

[14] Carty DM, Delles C, Dominiczak AF. Preeclampsia and future maternal health. Journal of hypertension. 2010 Jul;28(7):1349-55. PubMed PMID: 20467325.

[15] Roberts JM, Taylor RN, Musci TJ, Rodgers GM, Hubel CA, McLaughlin MK. [Preeclampsia: a disorders of the endothelial cells?]. Der Gynakologe. 1992 Feb;25(1):2-6. PubMed PMID: 1547977. Praeklampsie: Eine Storung der Endothelzellen.

[16] Sargent IL, Borzychowski AM, Redman CW. Immunoregulation in normal pregnancy and pre-eclampsia: an overview. Reproductive biomedicine online. 2007;14 Spec No 1:111-7. PubMed PMID: 20483406.

[17] Romero R, Nien JK, Espinoza J, Todem D, Fu W, Chung H, et al. A longitudinal study of angiogenic (placental growth factor) and anti-angiogenic (soluble endoglin and soluble vascular endothelial growth factor receptor-1) factors in normal pregnancy and patients destined to develop preeclampsia and deliver a small for gesta-

tional age neonate. The journal of maternal-fetal & neonatal medicine. 2008 Jan;21(1): 9-23. PubMed PMID: 18175241. Pubmed Central PMCID: 2587364.

[18] Holthe MR, Lyberg T, Staff AC, Berge LN. Leukocyte-platelet interaction in pregnancies complicated with preeclampsia. Platelets. 2005 Mar;16(2):91-7. PubMed PMID: 15823865.

[19] Holthe MR, Staff AC, Berge LN, Lyberg T. Different levels of platelet activation in preeclamptic, normotensive pregnant, and nonpregnant women. American journal of obstetrics and gynecology. 2004 Apr;190(4):1128-34. PubMed PMID: 15118653.

[20] Bharucha K, Kulkarni S, Nair S, Ghosh K, Mohanty D, Walvekar V, et al. Functional and fibrinogen receptor studies in platelets in pre-eclamptic toxaemia of pregnancy. Platelets. 1999 Jul;10(4):197-202. PubMed PMID: 16801092.

[21] McKillop C, Forbes CD, Howie PW, Prentice CM. Soluble fibrinogen/fibrin complexes in pre-eclampsia. Lancet. 1976 Jan 10;1(7950):56-8. PubMed PMID: 54580.

[22] Janes SL. Thrombocytopenia in pregnancy. Postgraduate medical journal. 1992 May; 68(799):321-6. PubMed PMID: 1630974. Pubmed Central PMCID: 2399429.

[23] Costantine MM. Physiologic and pharmacokinetic changes in pregnancy. Frontiers in pharmacology. 2014;5:65. PubMed PMID: 24772083. Pubmed Central PMCID: 3982119.

[24] Valera MC, Parant O, Vayssiere C, Arnal JF, Payrastre B. Physiologic and pathologic changes of platelets in pregnancy. Platelets. 2010;21(8):587-95. PubMed PMID: 20873962.

[25] Swanepoel AC, Pretorius E. Ultrastructural analysis of platelets during three phases of pregnancy: a qualitative and quantitative investigation. Hematology. 2015 Jan; 20(1):39-47. PubMed PMID: 24620950.

[26] Hayashi M, Kiumi F, Mitsuya K. Changes in platelet ATP secretion and aggregation during pregnancy and in preeclampsia. The American journal of the medical sciences. 1999 Aug;318(2):115-21. PubMed PMID: 10452571.

[27] Shanley DK, Kiely PA, Golla K, Allen S, Martin K, O'Riordan RT, et al. Pregnancy-specific glycoproteins bind integrin alphaIIbbeta3 and inhibit the platelet-fibrinogen interaction. PloS one. 2013;8(2):e57491. PubMed PMID: 23469002. Pubmed Central PMCID: 3585349.

[28] Moran N, Kiernan A, Dunne E, Edwards RJ, Shields DC, Kenny D. Monitoring modulators of platelet aggregation in a microtiter plate assay. Analytical biochemistry. 2006 Oct 1;357(1):77-84. PubMed PMID: 16920064.

[29] Edwards RJ, Moran N, Devocelle M, Kiernan A, Meade G, Signac W, et al. Bioinformatic discovery of novel bioactive peptides. Nature chemical biology. 2007 Feb;3(2): 108-12. PubMed PMID: 17220901.

[30] Mitrugno A, Williams D, Kerrigan SW, Moran N. A novel and essential role for FcgammaRIIa in cancer cell-induced platelet activation. Blood. 2014 Jan 9;123(2): 249-60. PubMed PMID: 24258815.

[31] Kim NS, Lee DH. Assessment of hemostatic function in pregnant women undergoing surgery using a Platelet Function Analyzer-100. Korean journal of anesthesiology. 2013 Feb;64(2):182-3. PubMed PMID: 23460935. Pubmed Central PMCID: 3581792.

[32] Karalis I, Nadar SK, Al Yemeni E, Blann AD, Lip GY. Platelet activation in pregnancy-induced hypertension. Thrombosis research. 2005;116(5):377-83. PubMed PMID: 16122550.

[33] Robb AO, Din JN, Mills NL, Smith IB, Blomberg A, Zikry MN, et al. The influence of the menstrual cycle, normal pregnancy and pre-eclampsia on platelet activation. Thrombosis and haemostasis. 2010 Feb;103(2):372-8. PubMed PMID: 20076841.

[34] Janes SL, Goodall AH. Flow cytometric detection of circulating activated platelets and platelet hyper-responsiveness in pre-eclampsia and pregnancy. Clinical science. 1994 Jun;86(6):731-9. PubMed PMID: 8062509.

[35] Battinelli EM, Markens BA, Italiano JE, Jr. Release of angiogenesis regulatory proteins from platelet alpha granules: modulation of physiologic and pathologic angiogenesis. Blood. 2011 Aug 4;118(5):1359-69. PubMed PMID: 21680800. Pubmed Central PMCID: 3152500. Epub 2011/06/18. eng.

[36] Ayhan A, Akkok E, Urman B, Yarali H, Dundar S, Kirazli S. Beta-thromboglobulin and platelet factor 4 levels in pregnancy and preeclampsia. Gynecologic and obstetric investigation. 1990;30(1):12-4. PubMed PMID: 2146196.

[37] Fitzgerald DJ, Mayo G, Catella F, Entman SS, FitzGerald GA. Increased thromboxane biosynthesis in normal pregnancy is mainly derived from platelets. American journal of obstetrics and gynecology. 1987 Aug;157(2):325-30. PubMed PMID: 3618681.

[38] Davi G, Basili S, Vieri M, Cipollone F, Santarone S, Alessandri C, et al. Enhanced thromboxane biosynthesis in patients with chronic obstructive pulmonary disease. The Chronic Obstructive Bronchitis and Haemostasis Study Group. American journal of respiratory and critical care medicine. 1997 Dec;156(6):1794-9. PubMed PMID: 9412557.

[39] Gurney D, Lip GY, Blann AD. A reliable plasma marker of platelet activation: does it exist? American journal of hematology. 2002 Jun;70(2):139-44. PubMed PMID: 12111787.

[40] Wetzka B, Charnock-Jones DS, Viville B, Cooper JC, Nusing R, Zahradnik HP, et al. Expression of prostacyclin and thromboxane synthases in placenta and placental bed

after pre-eclamptic pregnancies. Placenta. 1996 Nov;17(8):573-81. PubMed PMID: 8916205.

[41] Konijnenberg A, van der Post JA, Mol BW, Schaap MC, Lazarov R, Bleker OP, et al. Can flow cytometric detection of platelet activation early in pregnancy predict the occurrence of preeclampsia? A prospective study. American journal of obstetrics and gynecology. 1997 Aug;177(2):434-42. PubMed PMID: 9290465.

[42] Erez O, Romero R, Hoppensteadt D, Fareed J, Chaiworapongsa T, Kusanovic JP, et al. Premature labor: a state of platelet activation? Journal of perinatal medicine. 2008;36(5):377-87. PubMed PMID: 18958919. Pubmed Central PMCID: 3163447.

[43] Dean WL, Lee MJ, Cummins TD, Schultz DJ, Powell DW. Proteomic and functional characterisation of platelet microparticle size classes. Thrombosis and haemostasis. 2009 Oct;102(4):711-8. PubMed PMID: 19806257. Pubmed Central PMCID: 2861410.

[44] Marques FK, Campos FM, Filho OA, Carvalho AT, Dusse LM, Gomes KB. Circulating microparticles in severe preeclampsia. Clinica chimica acta; international journal of clinical chemistry. 2012 Dec 24;414:253-8. PubMed PMID: 23041217.

[45] Davies JR, Fernando R, Hallworth SP. Hemostatic function in healthy pregnant and preeclamptic women: an assessment using the platelet function analyzer (PFA-100) and thromboelastograph. Anesth Analg. 2007 Feb;104(2):416-20. PubMed PMID: 17242101.

[46] Yoneyama Y, Suzuki S, Sawa R, Otsubo Y, Power GG, Araki T. Plasma adenosine levels increase in women with normal pregnancies. American journal of obstetrics and gynecology. 2000 May;182(5):1200-3. PubMed PMID: 10819858.

[47] Sheu JR, Hsiao G, Lin WY, Chen TF, Chien YY, Lin CH, et al. Mechanisms involved in agonist-induced hyperaggregability of platelets from normal pregnancy. Journal of biomedical science. 2002 Jan-Feb;9(1):17-25. PubMed PMID: 11810021.

[48] Mellembakken JR, Solum NO, Ueland T, Videm V, Aukrust P. Increased concentrations of soluble CD40 ligand, RANTES and GRO-alpha in preeclampsia--possible role of platelet activation. Thrombosis and haemostasis. 2001 Nov;86(5):1272-6. PubMed PMID: 11816717.

[49] Sahin S, Ozakpinar OB, Eroglu M, Tulunay A, Ciraci E, Uras F, et al. The impact of platelet functions and inflammatory status on the severity of preeclampsia. The journal of maternal-fetal & neonatal medicine : the official journal of the European Association of Perinatal Medicine, the Federation of Asia and Oceania Perinatal Societies, the International Society of Perinatal Obstet. 2014 Jun 20:1-6. PubMed PMID: 24853491.

[50] Vincelot A, Nathan N, Collet D, Mehaddi Y, Grandchamp P, Julia A. Platelet function during pregnancy: an evaluation using the PFA-100 analyser. Br J Anaesth. 2001 Dec; 87(6):890-3. PubMed PMID: 11878692.

[51] Sheu JR, Hsiao G, Shen MY, Lin WY, Tzeng CR. The hyperaggregability of platelets from normal pregnancy is mediated through thromboxane A2 and cyclic AMP pathways. Clinical and laboratory haematology. 2002 Apr;24(2):121-9. PubMed PMID: 11985559.

[52] Lynch CM, O'Kelly R, Stuart B, Treumann A, Conroy R, Regan CL. The role of thromboxane A(2) in the pathogenesis of intrauterine growth restriction associated with maternal smoking in pregnancy. Prostaglandins & other lipid mediators. 2011 Aug;95(1-4):63-7. PubMed PMID: 21723954.

[53] Walsh SW. Eicosanoids in preeclampsia. Prostaglandins, leukotrienes, and essential fatty acids. 2004 Feb;70(2):223-32. PubMed PMID: 14683695.

[54] Fitzgerald DJ, Rocki W, Murray R, Mayo G, FitzGerald GA. Thromboxane A2 synthesis in pregnancy-induced hypertension. Lancet. 1990 Mar 31;335(8692):751-4. PubMed PMID: 1969511.

[55] Mills JL, DerSimonian R, Raymond E, Morrow JD, Roberts LJ, 2nd, Clemens JD, et al. Prostacyclin and thromboxane changes predating clinical onset of preeclampsia: a multicenter prospective study. JAMA. 1999 Jul 28;282(4):356-62. PubMed PMID: 10432033.

[56] Lewis DF, Canzoneri BJ, Gu Y, Zhao S, Wang Y. Maternal levels of prostacyclin, thromboxane, ICAM, and VCAM in normal and preeclamptic pregnancies. Am J Reprod Immunol. 2010 Dec;64(6):376-83. PubMed PMID: 20482519. Pubmed Central PMCID: 3062267.

[57] Tesse A, Meziani F, David E, Carusio N, Kremer H, Schneider F, et al. Microparticles from preeclamptic women induce vascular hyporeactivity in vessels from pregnant mice through an overproduction of NO. American journal of physiology Heart and circulatory physiology. 2007 Jul;293(1):H520-5. PubMed PMID: 17369461.

[58] Wong AE, Kwaan HC, Grobman WA, Weiss I, Wong CA. Microparticle source and tissue factor expression in pregnancy. Annals of hematology. 2015 Apr 1. PubMed PMID: 25823853.

[59] Sato Y, Fujiwara H, Zeng BX, Higuchi T, Yoshioka S, Fujii S. Platelet-derived soluble factors induce human extravillous trophoblast migration and differentiation: platelets are a possible regulator of trophoblast infiltration into maternal spiral arteries. Blood. 2005 Jul 15;106(2):428-35. PubMed PMID: 15797992.

[60] Krupp J, Boeldt DS, Yi FX, Grummer MA, Bankowski Anaya HA, Shah DM, et al. The loss of sustained Ca(2+) signaling underlies suppressed endothelial nitric oxide production in preeclamptic pregnancies: implications for new therapy. American

journal of physiology Heart and circulatory physiology. 2013 Oct 1;305(7):H969-79. PubMed PMID: 23893163. Pubmed Central PMCID: 3798749.

[61] Feuring M, Christ M, Roell A, Schueller P, Losel R, Dempfle CE, et al. Alterations in platelet function during the ovarian cycle. Blood coagulation & fibrinolysis : an international journal in haemostasis and thrombosis. 2002 Jul;13(5):443-7. PubMed PMID: 12138372.

[62] Sood R, Sholl L, Isermann B, Zogg M, Coughlin SR, Weiler H. Maternal Par4 and platelets contribute to defective placenta formation in mouse embryos lacking thrombomodulin. Blood. 2008 Aug 1;112(3):585-91. PubMed PMID: 18490515. Pubmed Central PMCID: 2481555.

[63] Zufferey A, Schvartz D, Nolli S, Reny JL, Sanchez JC, Fontana P. Characterization of the platelet granule proteome: evidence of the presence of MHC1 in alpha-granules. J Proteomics. 2014 Apr 14;101:130-40. PubMed PMID: 24549006.

[64] Sood R, Zogg M, Westrick RJ, Guo YH, Kerschen EJ, Girardi G, et al. Fetal gene defects precipitate platelet-mediated pregnancy failure in factor V Leiden mothers. J Exp Med. 2007 May 14;204(5):1049-56. PubMed PMID: 17438064. Pubmed Central PMCID: 2118565.

[65] Meziani F, Tesse A, Andriantsitohaina R. Microparticles are vectors of paradoxical information in vascular cells including the endothelium: role in health and diseases. Pharmacol Rep. 2008 Jan-Feb;60(1):75-84. PubMed PMID: 18276988.

[66] Moore T, Dveksler GS. Pregnancy-specific glycoproteins: complex gene families regulating maternal-fetal interactions. The International journal of developmental biology. 2014;58(2-4):273-80. PubMed PMID: 25023693.

[67] Ballesteros A, Mentink-Kane MM, Warren J, Kaplan GG, Dveksler GS. Induction and activation of latent transforming growth factor-beta1 are carried out by two distinct domains of pregnancy-specific glycoprotein 1 (PSG1). The Journal of biological chemistry. 2015 Feb 13;290(7):4422-31. PubMed PMID: 25548275. Pubmed Central PMCID: 4326847.

[68] Blois SM, Tirado-Gonzalez I, Wu J, Barrientos G, Johnson B, Warren J, et al. Early expression of pregnancy-specific glycoprotein 22 (PSG22) by trophoblast cells modulates angiogenesis in mice. Biology of reproduction. 2012 Jun;86(6):191. PubMed PMID: 22423048. Pubmed Central PMCID: 3386151.

[69] Labelle M, Begum S, Hynes RO. Direct signaling between platelets and cancer cells induces an epithelial-mesenchymal-like transition and promotes metastasis. Cancer Cell. 2011 Nov 15;20(5):576-90. PubMed PMID: 22094253. Epub 2011/11/19. eng.

[70] Peracoli MT, Menegon FT, Borges VT, de Araujo Costa RA, Thomazini-Santos IA, Peracoli JC. Platelet aggregation and TGF-beta(1) plasma levels in pregnant women

with preeclampsia. J Reprod Immunol. 2008 Oct;79(1):79-84. PubMed PMID: 18805591.

[71] Pfeiler S, Massberg S, Engelmann B. Biological basis and pathological relevance of microvascular thrombosis. Thrombosis research. 2014 May;133 Suppl 1:S35-7. PubMed PMID: 24759139.

[72] Uyama O, Shimizu S, Nakanishi T, Nakahama H, Takiguchi A, Hayashi Y, et al. Urinary 11-dehydro-thromboxane B2: a quantitative index of platelet activation in cerebral infarction. Internal medicine. 1992 Jun;31(6):735-9. PubMed PMID: 1392173.

[73] Lopez LR, Guyer KE, Torre IG, Pitts KR, Matsuura E, Ames PR. Platelet thromboxane (11-dehydro-Thromboxane B2) and aspirin response in patients with diabetes and coronary artery disease. World journal of diabetes. 2014 Apr 15;5(2):115-27. PubMed PMID: 24748925. Pubmed Central PMCID: 3990310.

[74] Suzuki K, Nishioka J, Hayashi T, Kosaka Y. Functionally active thrombomodulin is present in human platelets. J Biochem. 1988 Oct;104(4):628-32. PubMed PMID: 2853710.

Chapter 9

# Mechanisms Involved in Diabetes-Associated Platelet Hyperactivation

Voahanginirina Randriamboavonjy

Additional information is available at the end of the chapter

http://dx.doi.org/10.5772/60539

## 1. Introduction

Diabetes mellitus is a multi-factorial disease caused by a combination of genetic and environmental factors. Although insulin resistance and dysregulation of glucose and lipid homeostasis are the primary hallmarks of the disease, it is now well accepted that the morbidity and mortality associated with diabetes mostly result from micro- and macro-vascular complications [1]. An early step in the pathogenesis of the vascular complications of diabetes is the development of endothelial dysfunction which is characterised by a decrease in nitric oxide (NO) bioavailability, prostacyclin production and a general reduction in the anti-thrombogenic properties of vascular wall [2]. Diabetes is also characterised by an alteration of platelet function. Indeed, platelets from patients with type 1 or type 2 diabetes are hyperreactive and demonstrate increased adhesiveness as well as exaggerated aggregation and thrombus formation. Several mechanisms have been reported to mediate the hyperreactivity of platelets from diabetic patients including morphological changes such as increased mean platelet volume and accelerated platelet turnover, biochemical changes such as increased reactive oxygen species (ROS) production, increased synthesis of thromboxane A2 (TXA2) and thrombin and a dysregulated $Ca^{2+}$ homeostasis. Platelets from diabetic patients also demonstrate increased surface expression of adhesion proteins such as P-selectin and the $\alpha IIb\beta 3$ integrin and reduced membrane fluidity. These changes characteristic of the "diabetic platelet" have been mostly attributed to the metabolic dysregulation associated to the insulin resistance and dyslipidemia. However, given that platelet hyperreactivity has also been found in patients with type 1 diabetes mellitus it is suggested that hyperglycemia alone can account for at least part of the altered platelet response in patients with diabetes mellitus. Oxidative stress which characterizes both types of diabetes has also been shown to be an important factor mediating the phenotypic changes of diabetic platelets. In this chapter I will first give an overview of the physiological platelet activation, and then discuss the role of factors such as insulin resistance, hyperglycemia, dyslipidemia on platelet function. Next, I will describe the intracellular mechanisms underlying platelet hyperreactivity in diabetes. Finally, the impact of diabetes on the responsiveness to anti-platelet therapy will be discussed.

## 2. Physiological platelet activation

Platelets are anucleated cells generated from megakaryocytes, and after their release into the blood, circulate for approximately 10 days. The main role of platelets is to maintain hemostasis. Under normal conditions, platelet adhesion to the vascular wall is inhibited due to the anti-thrombotic nature of the endothelial cell surface and the permanent release of anti-platelet factors by the endothelium [3]. Following vascular injury, especially under the influence of high shear stress, platelets tether and adhere to the exposed subendothelial collagen via the von Willebrand factor (vWF)-mediated binding to platelet glycoprotein Ib/V/IX complex. The initial interaction is subsequently strengthened by the interaction of collagen to its receptor glycoprotein VI (GPVI) and the integrin $\alpha 2\beta 1$. The ligation of these receptors activates Src family tyrosine kinases (SFKs) which lead to the phosphorylation and activation of the phospholipase C$\gamma$2 (PLC $\gamma$2). The latter hydrolyses membrane Phosphatidylinositol-4, 5-bisphosphate (PIP2) into diacylglycerol (DAG) and inositol 1, 4, 5-triphosphate (IP3) which respectively activates the protein kinase C (PKC) and stimulates the release of $Ca^{2+}$ from the intracellular stores. PKC binds to and phosphorylates the cytoplasmic tail of the $\beta 3$ subunit of the $\alpha IIb\beta 3$ integrin complex, which then recruits talin and kindlin-3. This in turns causes a conformational change in the extracellular domain of the integrin and enables the binding of circulating fibrinogen (inside-out signalling). Fibrinogen links activated $\alpha IIb\beta 3$ integrins of neighbouring platelets and initiates platelet aggregation. After its binding, fibrinogen initiates the so-called "outside-in" signalling of the integrin. This step includes the activation of SFKs which promotes the tyrosine phosphorylation of $\beta 3$ integrin and the binding of cytoskeletal proteins leading to the activation of the phosphatidylinositide 3-kinases (PI3K) and platelet adhesion. $Ca^{2+}$ and DAG also act together to activate the calcium- and diacylglycerol-regulated guanosine exchange factor (CalDAGGEF), a guanosine exchange factor important for the activation of the small GTPase Rap1. The latter activates mitogen-activated protein kinases (MAPKs) which are known to be upstream of the phospholipase A2 (PLA2)/cyclooxygenase (COX) signalling cascade resulting into the production of thromboxane A2. PKC and MAPK act in concert to stimulate the release of different second mediators from platelet granules. These agonists; including adenosine diphosphate (ADP), serotonin and the formed thromboxane A2 bind to their respective G protein–coupled receptors (GPCRs). Through the activation of G protein-mediated signalling pathways, they can further increase their own formation and/or release, thus acting as positive-feedback amplifying platelet responses by recruiting additional platelets and promoting aggregation. (for review see references [4, 5]) (figure 1). In addition to stimulating degranulation, the increase in platelet $[Ca^{2+}]_i$ also leads to the activation of calpains, a family of $Ca^{2+}$-dependent neutral cysteine proteases. While some calpains are expressed only in specific tissues, platelets are known to express at least two

http://dx.doi.org/10.5772/60539

isoforms of this enzyme i.e μ-calpain (calpain 1) and m-calpain (calpain 2). The μ- and m-calpain were initially named for the $Ca^{2+}$ concentration (micromolar versus millimolar) required for their activation in vitro [6]. However it is now clear that additional mechanisms such as phosphorylation also regulate their proteolytic activity [7]. Several reports have highlighted the importance of μ- and m-calpain in platelet activation. Indeed, once activated, calpains induce the limited proteolysis of a number of proteins implicated in cytoskeletal rearrangement, degranulation and aggregation. Proteins identified to-date that are targeted by calpain include spectrin, adducin and talin as well as platelet-endothelial cell adhesion molecule-1 (PECAM-1), the myosin light chain kinase and N-ethylmaleimide-sensitive-factor attachment receptor proteins such as N-ethylmaleimide sensitive factor attachment protein-23 and vesicle-associated membrane protein-3. Furthermore, μ-calpain modulates $\alpha IIb\beta 3$ integrin-mediated outside-in signaling and platelet spreading by cleaving the $\beta 3$ subunit of the $\alpha IIb\beta 3$ integrin [8]. In the final stages of platelet activation, phosphatidylserine, which is normally sequestered in the inner leaflet of the plasma membrane, is relocated to the outer leaflet leading to the shedding of microparticles and giving platelets a procoagulant surface. After stimulation, $Ca^{2+}$ is removed from the cytosol and sequestred into the intracellular stores and/or extruded into the extracellular space by the action of the sarco-endoplasmic reticulum $Ca^{2+}$-ATPase (SERCA) and the plasma membrane $Ca^{2+}$-ATPase (PMCA), respectively. Formation of platelet plug or primary hemostasis is associated with the activation of the coagulation cascade which results into fibrin deposition and linking (secondary hemostasis) and the formation of a red clot. After the clot has been formed, platelets rearrange and contract their intracellular actin/myosin cytoskeleton. Given that the intracellular actin network is connected to the internal part of the integrin $\alpha IIb\beta 3$, platelet contractile force on the fibrin network will lead to "clot retraction". Finally, the fibrin is slowly dissolved by the fibrinolytic enzyme, plasmin, and the platelets are cleared by phagocytosis and wound healing will take place.

Platelets store quite high concentrations of chemokines, cytokines, growth factors and vasoactive substances. The latter are sequestered into 2 major types of granules; $\alpha$-granules and dense granules. On the one hand, alpha-granules are known to contain growth factors including vascular endothelial growth factor, platelet-derived growth factor, endostatin, transforming growth factor-β; chemokines such as platelet factor 4 (CXCL4) and CCL5 and adhesion molecules such as P-selectin. Dense granules, on the other hand, store mainly small molecules (e.g ADP and serotonin) and ions (such as $Ca^{2+}$ and $Mg^{2+}$). Upon activation, platelets release soluble proteins contained in their granules and redistribute some $\alpha$-granules contents to the membrane (e.g P-selectin, CD40 ligand). Given the variety of proteins released upon platelet activation, it is clear that platelets may affect the vascular wall in different ways. Indeed, beyond their role in hemostasis, platelets are involved in angiogenesis as well as in vascular inflammation.

## 3. Effect of insulin resistance on platelet function

Insulin exerts an inhibitory effect on platelets but the intracellular mechanisms remain not fully characterized and whether the effects are mediated by the insulin receptor is unclear.

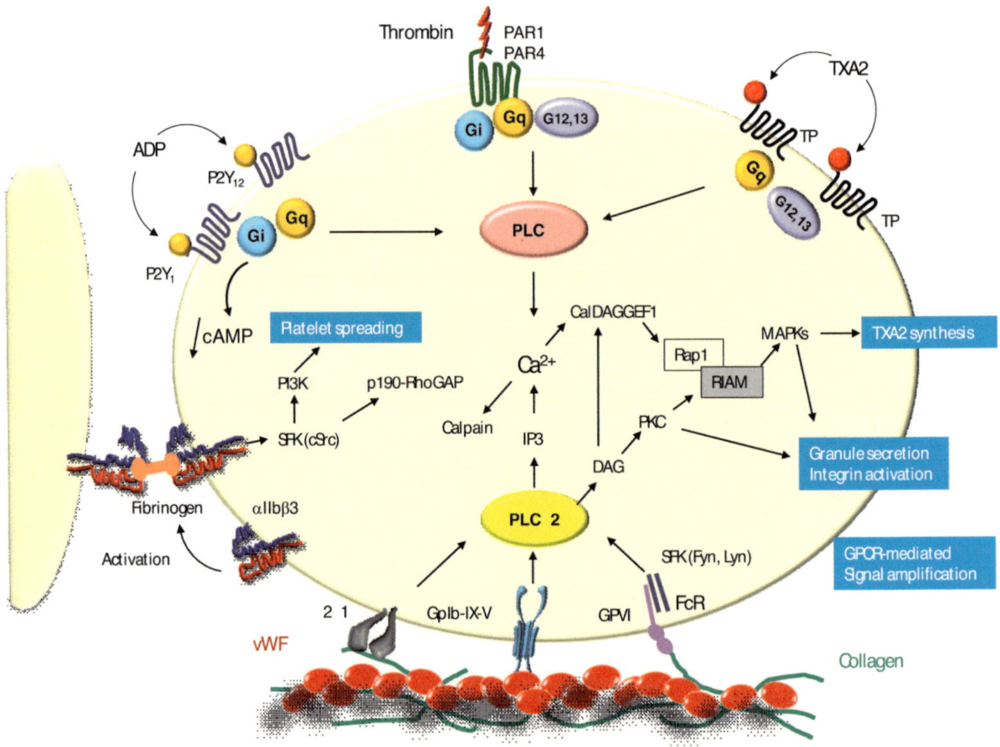


**Figure 1. Platelet major signalling pathways.** Collagen binding either to GPVI or $\alpha2\beta1$ integrin or vWF binding to Gp1b-IX-V leads to the activation of Src family kinases and tyrosine phosphorylation of the phospholipase $C\gamma2$. $PLC\gamma2$ cleaves phosphatidylinositol (4, 5)-bisphosphate PIP2 to generate inositol (1, 4, 5)-trisphosphate (IP3) and diacylglycerol (DAG). IP3 and DAG are responsible for the mobilization of calcium from intracellular stores leading to calpain activation and the activation of isoforms of protein kinase C (PKC), respectively. $Ca^{2+}$ and DAG activate the $Ca^{2+}$ and DAG-regulated guanosine exchange factor (CalDAGGEF) which in turn activate the small GTPase Rap1. The latter activates the mitogen-activated kinase (MAPK) which leads to thromboxane A2 generation, granule secretion and integrin activation. The released factors potentiate platelet signaling via the activation of G protein-coupled receptors/ phospholipase $C\beta$ pathway. The binding of fibrinogen to activated integrin initiates platelet spreading by activating the Phosphoinositide 3-kinase (PI3K) pathway.

Indeed, there is no evidence of the expression of insulin receptor on platelets [9] and it is speculated that the effects are rather mediated by the activation of insulin-like growth factor (IGF) receptor [10, 11]. Insulin decreases thrombin-induced increase in $Ca^{2+}$ and attenuates agonist-induced platelet aggregation [12]. One of the mechanisms described to mediate the anti-platelet effect of insulin is the activation of the AMP-activated protein kinase (AMPK) and Akt by the PI3K [13]. Insulin can also inhibit $Ca^{2+}$ mobilization by activating the inhibitory G-protein Gi [14]. However, given that insulin can also stimulate the release of ADP [15], it is assumed that whether insulin activates or inhibits platelets may depend on its concentration. Although the insulin effect in platelets has been initially believed to involve the activation of nitric oxide synthase (NOS), there are contradictory reports on the expression and function of NOS in human platelets [13, 16]. Insulin resistance refers to the loss of response to insulin stimulation. The molecular mechanisms of insulin resistance are complex but it has been

http://dx.doi.org/10.5772/60539

shown that the faculty of insulin to inhibit platelet activation is lost in diabetic patients [17] and the inhibitory effect of insulin on the interaction of platelet with collagen and other agonists is blunted by insulin resistance in obese subjects [18]. Moreover, in non diabetic, obese women, there is a direct correlation between platelet reactivity assessed by thromboxane A2 generation and insulin resistance [19].

## 4. Effect of hyperglycemia and AGEs

Despite the fact that diabetes is characterized by chronic hyperglycemia, there is evidence that acute hyperglycemia can directly affect platelet reactivity. Indeed, a prospective randomised double blind controlled study has shown that 24h euglycaemic treatment significantly increased the plasma levels of the platelet and endothelial activation markers soluble P-selectin and vWF [20]. Moreover, it has been shown that challenging healthy non-diabetic subjects with 24h hyperglycemia-hyperinsulinemia altered the insulin signaling pathway [21]. Indeed, the glycogen synthase kinase 3β (GSKβ3) and the tyrosine phosphatase SHP2 as well as tissue factor were upregulated on mRNA and protein levels while mRNA for the syntaxin 4-binding protein was downregulated. High glucose can also increase calcium influx in platelets by enhancing a PI3K-dependent transient receptor potential channel canonical type 6 [22]. The latter is known to be significantly highly expressed in diabetic platelets. Hyperglycemia is able to increase the expression and/or activity of PKC [23, 24], a central kinase in the regulation of platelet activity. Another consequence of hyperglycemia in platelets is the induction of mitochondrial dysfunction. One of the recent mechanisms linking hyperglycemia and mitochondrial dysfunction is the activation of aldose reductase and subsequent ROS production which result to p53 phosphorylation [25] or the stimulation of the PLCγ2/PKC/p38α MAPK pathway and the increase in TXA2 production [26]. More recent findings showed that the hyperglycemia-induced platelet activation could be attributed to the downregulation of different micro-RNA (miR) such as miR-223 and miR-146a. Indeed, low platelet and plasma miR-223 and miR-146a expression has been associated with an increased risk for ischemic stroke in patients with diabetes mellitus [27]. Many of the deleterious effects of glucose have been attributed to its metabolite methylgyloxal (MG), a highly reactive dicarbonyl metabolite that is generated endogenously by the nonenzymatic degradation of the glycolytic intermediates, dihydroxyacetone phosphate and glyceraldehyde-3-phosphate [28]. It is known that plasma levels of MG in diabetic individuals are enhanced. Study investigating the effect of MG on platelets showed that acute application of MG to platelets increases intracellular $Ca^{2+}$ levels and activates classical PKCs at the same time as inhibiting PI3K/Akt and the β3-integrin outside-in signalling. Moreover, *in vivo*, MG increases thrombus size but reduces its stability in mice [29]. Although most of the effects of MG have been attributed to the formation of advanced glycation end-products (AGEs) and the subsequent activation of the AGE receptor; RAGE, this study has highlighted a direct effect of MG on platelets which may contribute to the diabetes-associated platelet hyperaggregability. Several studies have shown that AGEs can activate platelets and that platelets express RAGE. The expression of surface markers such as P-selectin (CD62) and CD63 (a lysosomal glycoprotein) has been shown to be significantly increased by AGE stimulation [30] suggesting AGE-induced platelet degranulation. However, this study failed to report the detailed intracellular mechanism involved. Studies performed in mice could show that AGEs induce a prothrombotic phenotype via interaction with platelet glycoprotein IV (CD36) [31]. The serum- and glucocorticoid-inducible kinase 1 (SGK1) has been also suggested to mediate AGE-induced platelet hyperactivation [32]. Indeed, SGK1 expression is known to be regulated by hyperglycaemia and AGEs. In platelets, SGK1 increases store-operated calcium entry (SOCE) and thereby regulates several $Ca^{2+}$-dependent platelet functions such as degranulation, integrin $\alpha_{IIb}\beta_3$ activation, phosphatidylserine exposure, aggregation and thrombus formation.

## 5. Effect of dyslipidemia

The fact that glycemic control alone has proven insufficient to reduce thrombotic complications in diabetic patients suggests that other factors may contribute to platelet hyperreactivity in diabetes [33]. One feature of diabetes is the presence of dyslipidemia which is characterized by high plasma triglyceride concentration, reduced high density lipoprotein (HDL) concentration, and increased concentration of low density lipoprotein (LDL)[34]. There is evidence that dyslipidemia contributes to the diabetes-associated platelet hyperactivation. By binding to a pertussis sensitive G-protein coupled receptor on platelets, LDL induces an increase in cytosolic $[Ca^{2+}]_i$, IP3 formation and activation of PKC [35]. However, the pro-thrombotic properties of LDL seem to be rather associated to its oxidation. Indeed, oxidized-LDL can directly interact with platelets specific receptors such as the lectin-like oxidized LDL receptor-1 [36] or the CD36 [37, 38]. The latter involves the activation of the MAPK c-Jun N-terminal kinase (JNK)2 and its upstream activator MKK4. Not only are platelets activated by ox-LDL but activated platelets are also known to be able to form ox-LDL via platelet gp91phox (NOX2)-dependent ROS generation [39] suggesting the contribution of platelets to circulating ox-LDL. The formed ox-LDL has been demonstrated to be either uptaken by monocytes [39] or amplify platelet activation [40]. On the molecular levels, LDL activates the platelet arachidonic acid signalling cascade, i.e phosphorylation of p38 MAPK and cytosolic phospholipase A2, leading to increased TXA2 formation [41]. Interestingly, there is less information on the direct effects of triglycerides on platelets. However, the link between hyperlipidemia and platelet hyperactivation is supported by the fact that lipid-lowering agents possess anti-thrombotic properties [42, 43].

## 6. Dysregulation of calcium signalling

One of the characteristics of platelets from patients with type 2 diabetes is the alteration of the intracellular $Ca^{2+}$ homeostasis. Different mechanisms have been reported to be responsible for this abnormality. One of the mechanisms leading to the latter phenomenon is the reduction in platelet $Ca^{2+}$-ATPase activity in diabetic subjects [44, 45]. Moreover, the function of the $Na^+/Ca^{2+}$ exchanger is known to be significantly altered in platelets from diabetic patients [46]. Another mechanism contributing to the enhanced resting cytosolic calcium in platelets from diabetic patients is the increased passive $Ca^{2+}$ leakage rate from the intracellular stores [47]. Given that most of the intracellular signalling in platelets is regulated by calcium, it is more than expected that a dysregulation in calcium homeostasis would affect platelet function in many ways. One of the consequences of the increased $[Ca^{2+}]_i$ in platelet is the activation of calpains. Although calpain-mediated proteolysis is involved in physiological platelet activation, type 2 diabetes has been shown to be associated with the overactivation of calpain in platelets [45] leading to marked changes in the platelet proteome [48]. In platelets from diabetic patients, the integrin-linked kinase and septin-5 were found to be new calpain substrates and their cleavage was shown to be involved in the enhanced platelet adhesion and spreading as well as enhanced $\alpha$-granule secretion, respectively. Moreover, calpain was able to cleave the chemokine RANTES into a variant with an enhanced chemotactic activity. The *in vivo* relevance of calpain in inducing the hyperreactivity of platelets from diabetic patients was supported by the finding that treatment of diabetic mice with calpain inhibitor preserved the platelet proteome, and reversed the diabetes-associated platelet hyperactivation [48].

## 7. Increased apoptosis

Although being anucleated, there is evidence demonstrating that platelets possess the necessary machinery to undergo apoptosis [49]. Among other mechanisms, calpain seems to play an important role in platelet apoptosis [50, 51]. Indeed, although caspase is activated during platelet apoptosis, this seems to be downstream of calpain activation. The increased calpain activation in platelets from diabetic patients described above suggests that diabetic platelets may be more prone to apoptosis. Several factors have been reported to induce platelet apoptosis including the diabetes-associated oxidative stress which is an important stimulus for inducing mitochondrial damage [52]. Mitochondria not only are the target of oxidative stress but are also able to generate ROS therefore amplifying the reaction to oxidative stress [52, 53]. Platelets from patients with type 2 diabetes demonstrate an increased ATP content but decreased mitochondrial membrane potential [54] supporting the alteration of mitochondrial function. Another mechanism involved in platelet apoptosis is the development of endoplasmic reticulum (ER) stress. It has been shown that diabetes mellitus was associated with the production of hyperreactive platelets expressing an altered protein disulfide isomerase and 78-kDa glucose-regulated protein [55]. Moreover, homocysteine, which levels are known to be significantly increased in diabetic patients, has been shown to stimulate ER stress-mediated platelet apoptosis by activating the caspase pathway [56]. One of the consequences of platelet activation and apoptosis is the generation of intact membrane vesicles known as microparticles. The formation of platelet-derived microparticles (PMPs) is known to be $Ca^{2+}$- and calpain-dependent. Although PMPs are involved in hemostasis due to their procoagulant properties, elevated levels of PMPs in blood from diabetic patients has been suggested to participate in the increased vascular complications in diabetes [57, 58].

## 8. Increased mean platelet volume

Platelet reactivity and size have been shown to directly correlate. Indeed, young and large platelets exhibit higher activity than old and small ones. The mean platelet volume (MPV) is an indicator of the average size of platelets which has been largely used to investigate the relationship between platelet size and activity. There is evidence that MPV is significantly increased in diabetic patients and that it directly correlates with glycemic control [59-61].

## 9. Hyporesponsiveness to anti-platelet therapy

One feature of platelets from diabetic patients is their hyporesponsiveness to anti-platelet therapy. Indeed, there is evidence that anti-platelet therapy is less effective in diabetic patients when compared with patients without diabetes [62]. One example is the so-called "aspirin resistance" in which diabetic patients are refractory to the anti-platelet effect of aspirin [63]. Aspirin or salicylic acid acetylates and irreversibly inhibits cyclooxygenase thereby inhibiting the TXA2 formation. Aspirin has been also shown to activate the NO/cGMP pathway. Although aspirin resistance is seen in the majority of diabetic patients, the exact molecular mechanism is still unclear. One of the mechanisms proposed to mediate aspirin-resistance is the increased glycation of platelet proteins which may alter the acetylation process [64]. Some *in vitro* studies have also shown a direct link between hyperglycemia and aspirin resistance. Certainly, high glucose can acutely reduce the antiaggregating effect of aspirin by inhibiting the aspirin-induced activation of the NO/cGMP/PKG pathway without affecting the aspirin-induced inhibition of TXA2 synthesis [65]. Given that acute stimulation of platelets with other monosaccharides such as fructose and galactose was shown to lead to a similar alteration of the aspirin effect on platelets and that lactic acid also impaired the inhibition of platelet aggregation with aspirin, it has been suggested that lactic acid might be the mediator of the glucose-induced inhibition of the aspirin effect in platelets [66]. Interestingly, the platelet resistance seems to be specific to aspirin since hyperglycemia-induced platelet hyperactivation in type 2 diabetes could be reversed by a nitric oxide-donating agent [67]. More recently, non-HDL cholesterol has been reported to be an independent risk factor for aspirin resistance in patients with type 2 diabetes [68].

Diabetes is also known to be associated to a reduced responsiveness of platelets to the P2Y12 ADP receptor antagonist clopidogrel [69, 70]. Although not directly investigated in diabetic patients, upregulation of ADP receptor levels, increase in ADP exposure or accelerated platelet turnover may contribute to clopidogrel resistance.

## 10. Conclusions

The fact that the diabetic milieu can affect platelet function in several ways explains the failure of glycemic control alone to reduce the risk of atherothrombotic events in diabetic patients.

http://dx.doi.org/10.5772/60539

Indeed, the increased platelet hyperreactivity is the result of complicated inter-regulated mechanisms. Moreover, given that diabetic platelets are resistant to most anti-platelet therapy, there is a need of new therapeutical strategies to improve platelet function in diabetes. Certainly, management of both glycemia and dyslipidemia would improve the effects of anti-platelet therapy. Moreover, the facts that calpain plays a key role in platelet activation and that calpain activity is elevated in diabetic platelets, makes it tempting to suggest the $Ca^{2+}$-activated proteases as a promising therapeutic target to prevent thrombotic complications in diabetic patients.

## Author details

Voahanginirina Randriamboavonjy*

Address all correspondence to: voahangy@vrc.uni-frankfurt.de

Institute for Vascular Signalling, Centre for Molecular Medicine, Goethe University, Frankfurt am Main, Germany

## References

[1] Beckman JA, Creager MA, Libby P. Diabetes and atherosclerosis: epidemiology, pathophysiology, and management. JAMA 2002;287:2570-81.

[2] Schafer A, Bauersachs J. Endothelial dysfunction, impaired endogenous platelet inhibition and platelet activation in diabetes and atherosclerosis. Curr Vasc Pharmacol 2008;6:52-60.

[3] Bunting S, Moncada S, Vane JR. Antithrombotic properties of vascular endothelium. Lancet 1977;2:1075-6.

[4] Gibbins JM. Platelet adhesion signalling and the regulation of thrombus formation. J Cell Sci 2004;117:3415-25.

[5] Li Z, Delaney MK, O'Brien KA, et al. Signaling during platelet adhesion and activation. Arterioscler Thromb Vasc Biol 2010;30:2341-9.

[6] Suzuki K, Hata S, Kawabata Y, et al. Structure, activation, and biology of calpain. Diabetes 2004;53 Suppl 1:S12-S18.

[7] Goll DE, Thompson VF, Li H, et al. The calpain system. Physiol Rev 2003;83:731-801.

[8] Kuchay SM, Chishti AH. Calpain-mediated regulation of platelet signaling pathways. Curr Opin Hematol 2007;14:249-54.

[9] Rauchfuss S, Geiger J, Walter U, et al. Insulin inhibition of platelet-endothelial interaction is mediated by insulin effects on endothelial cells without direct effects on platelets. J Thromb Haemost 2008;6:856-64.

[10] Blair TA, Moore SF, Williams CM, et al. Phosphoinositide 3-kinases p110alpha and p110beta have differential roles in insulin-like growth factor-1-mediated Akt phosphorylation and platelet priming. Arterioscler Thromb Vasc Biol 2014;34:1681-8.

[11] Hers I. Insulin-like growth factor-1 potentiates platelet activation via the IRS/PI3Kalpha pathway. Blood 2007;110:4243-52.

[12] Ishida M, Ishida T, Ono N, et al. Effects of insulin on calcium metabolism and platelet aggregation. Hypertension 1996;28:209-12.

[13] Fleming I, Schulz C, Fichtlscherer B, et al. AMP-activated protein kinase (AMPK) regulates the insulin-induced activation of the nitric oxide synthase in human platelets. Thromb Haemost 2003;90:863-71.

[14] Ferreira IA, Eybrechts KL, Mocking AI, et al. IRS-1 mediates inhibition of Ca2+ mobilization by insulin via the inhibitory G-protein Gi. J Biol Chem 2004;279:3254-64.

[15] Randriamboavonjy V, Schrader J, Busse R, et al. Insulin induces the release of vasodilator compounds from platelets by a nitric oxide-G kinase-VAMP-3-dependent pathway. J Exp Med 2004;199:347-56.

[16] Bohmer A, Gambaryan S, Tsikas D. Human blood platelets lack nitric oxide synthase activity. Platelets 2014;1-6.

[17] Ferreira IA, Mocking AI, Feijge MA, et al. Platelet inhibition by insulin is absent in type 2 diabetes mellitus. Arterioscler Thromb Vasc Biol 2006;26:417-22.

[18] Westerbacka J, Yki-Jarvinen H, Turpeinen A, et al. Inhibition of platelet-collagen interaction: an in vivo action of insulin abolished by insulin resistance in obesity. Arterioscler Thromb Vasc Biol 2002;22:167-72.

[19] Basili S, Pacini G, Guagnano MT, et al. Insulin resistance as a determinant of platelet activation in obese women. J Am Coll Cardiol 2006;48:2531-8.

[20] Kotzailias N, Graninger M, Knechtelsdorfer M, et al. Acute effects of hyperglycaemia on plasma concentration of soluble P-selectin and von Willebrand factor in healthy volunteers -a prospective randomised double blind controlled study. Thromb Res 2009;123:452-9.

[21] Rao AK, Freishtat RJ, Jalagadugula G, et al. Alterations in insulin-signaling and coagulation pathways in platelets during hyperglycemia-hyperinsulinemia in healthy non-diabetic subject. Thromb Res 2014;134:704-10.

[22] Liu D, Maier A, Scholze A, et al. High glucose enhances transient receptor potential channel canonical type 6-dependent calcium influx in human platelets via phosphati-

dylinositol 3-kinase-dependent pathway. Arterioscler Thromb Vasc Biol 2008;28:746-51.

[23] Assert R, Scherk G, Bumbure A, et al. Regulation of protein kinase C by short term hyperglycaemia in human platelets in vivo and in vitro. Diabetologia 2001;44:188-95.

[24] Kimura M, Ishizawa M, Miura A, et al. Platelet protein kinase C isoform content in type 2 diabetes complicated with retinopathy and nephropathy. Platelets 2001;12:138-43.

[25] Tang WH, Stitham J, Jin Y, et al. Aldose reductase-mediated phosphorylation of p53 leads to mitochondrial dysfunction and damage in diabetic platelets. Circulation 2014;129:1598-609.

[26] Tang WH, Stitham J, Gleim S, et al. Glucose and collagen regulate human platelet activity through aldose reductase induction of thromboxane. J Clin Invest 2011;121:4462-76.

[27] Duan X, Zhan Q, Song B, et al. Detection of platelet microRNA expression in patients with diabetes mellitus with or without ischemic stroke. J Diabetes Complications 2014;28:705-10.

[28] Thornalley PJ. The glyoxalase system in health and disease. Mol Aspects Med 1993;14:287-371.

[29] Hadas K, Randriamboavonjy V, Elgheznawy A, et al. Methylglyoxal induces platelet hyperaggregation and reduces thrombus stability by activating PKC and inhibiting PI3K/Akt pathway. PLoS One 2013;8:e74401.

[30] Gawlowski T, Stratmann B, Ruetter R, et al. Advanced glycation end products strongly activate platelets. Eur J Nutr 2009;48:475-81.

[31] Zhu W, Li W, Silverstein RL. Advanced glycation end products induce a prothrombotic phenotype in mice via interaction with platelet CD36. Blood 2012;119:6136-44.

[32] Lang F, Gawaz M, Borst O. The serum- & glucocorticoid-inducible kinase in the regulation of platelet function. Acta Physiol (Oxf) 2014.

[33] Stolar M. Glycemic control and complications in type 2 diabetes mellitus. Am J Med 2010;123:S3-11.

[34] Chehade JM, Gladysz M, Mooradian AD. Dyslipidemia in type 2 diabetes: prevalence, pathophysiology, and management. Drugs 2013;73:327-39.

[35] Pedreno J, Hurt-Camejo E, Wiklund O, et al. Low-density lipoprotein (LDL) binds to a G-protein coupled receptor in human platelets. Evidence that the proaggregatory effect induced by LDL is modulated by down-regulation of binding sites and desensitization of its mediated signaling. Atherosclerosis 2001;155:99-112.

[36] Chen M, Kakutani M, Naruko T, et al. Activation-dependent surface expression of LOX-1 in human platelets. Biochem Biophys Res Commun 2001;282:153-8.

[37] Chen K, Febbraio M, Li W, et al. A specific CD36-dependent signaling pathway is required for platelet activation by oxidized low-density lipoprotein. Circ Res 2008;102:1512-9.

[38] Podrez EA, Byzova TV, Febbraio M, et al. Platelet CD36 links hyperlipidemia, oxidant stress and a prothrombotic phenotype. Nat Med 2007;13:1086-95.

[39] Carnevale R, Pignatelli P, Lenti L, et al. LDL are oxidatively modified by platelets via GP91(phox) and accumulate in human monocytes. FASEB J 2007;21:927-34.

[40] Carnevale R, Bartimoccia S, Nocella C, et al. LDL oxidation by platelets propagates platelet activation via an oxidative stress-mediated mechanism. Atherosclerosis 2014;237:108-16.

[41] Colas R, Sassolas A, Guichardant M, et al. LDL from obese patients with the metabolic syndrome show increased lipid peroxidation and activate platelets. Diabetologia 2011;54:2931-40.

[42] Tehrani S, Mobarrez F, Antovic A, et al. Atorvastatin has antithrombotic effects in patients with type 1 diabetes and dyslipidemia. Thromb Res 2010;126:e225-e231.

[43] Tsai NW, Lin TK, Chang WN, et al. Statin pre-treatment is associated with lower platelet activity and favorable outcome in patients with acute non-cardio-embolic ischemic stroke. Crit Care 2011;15:R163.

[44] Rosado JA, Saavedra FR, Redondo PC, et al. Reduced plasma membrane Ca2+-ATPase function in platelets from patients with non-insulin-dependent diabetes mellitus. Haematologica 2004;89:1142-4.

[45] Randriamboavonjy V, Pistrosch F, Bolck B, et al. Platelet sarcoplasmic endoplasmic reticulum Ca2+-ATPase and mu-calpain activity are altered in type 2 diabetes mellitus and restored by rosiglitazone. Circulation 2008;117:52-60.

[46] Li Y, Woo V, Bose R. Platelet hyperactivity and abnormal $Ca^{2+}$ homeostasis in diabetes mellitus. Am J Physiol Heart Circ Physiol 2001;280:H1480-H1489.

[47] Zbidi H, Jardin I, Bartegi A, et al. Ca2+ leakage rate from agonist-sensitive intracellular pools is altered in platelets from patients with type 2 diabetes. Platelets 2011;22:284-93.

[48] Randriamboavonjy V, Isaak J, Elgheznawy A, et al. Calpain inhibition stabilizes the platelet proteome and reactivity in diabetes. Blood 2012;120(2):415-23.

[49] Leytin V. Apoptosis in the anucleate platelet. Blood Rev 2012;26:51-63.

[50] Wolf BB, Goldstein JC, Stennicke HR, et al. Calpain functions in a caspase-independent manner to promote apoptosis-like events during platelet activation. Blood 1999;94:1683-92.

[51] Zhang W, Liu J, Sun R, et al. Calpain activator dibucaine induces platelet apoptosis. Int J Mol Sci 2011;12:2125-37.

[52] Garcia-Souza LF, Oliveira MF. Mitochondria: Biological roles in platelet physiology and pathology. Int J Biochem Cell Biol 2014;50:156-60.

[53] Pietraforte D, Vona R, Marchesi A, et al. Redox control of platelet functions in physiology and pathophysiology. Antioxid Redox Signal 2014;21:177-93.

[54] Guo X, Wu J, Du J, et al. Platelets of type 2 diabetic patients are characterized by high ATP content and low mitochondrial membrane potential. Platelets 2009;20:588-93.

[55] Hernandez VR, Vilahur G, Ferrer-Lorente R, et al. Platelets derived from the bone marrow of diabetic animals show dysregulated endoplasmic reticulum stress proteins that contribute to increased thrombosis. Arterioscler Thromb Vasc Biol 2012;32:2141-8.

[56] Zbidi H, Redondo PC, Lopez JJ, et al. Homocysteine induces caspase activation by endoplasmic reticulum stress in platelets from type 2 diabetics and healthy donors. Thromb Haemost 2010;103:1022-32.

[57] Nomura S, Miyazaki Y, Miyake T, et al. Detection of platelet-derived microparticles in patients with diabetes. Am J Hematol 1993;44:213.

[58] Nomura S, Suzuki M, Katsura K, et al. Platelet-derived microparticles may influence the development of atherosclerosis in diabetes mellitus. Atherosclerosis 1995;116:235-40.

[59] Hekimsoy Z, Payzin B, Ornek T, et al. Mean platelet volume in Type 2 diabetic patients. J Diabetes Complications 2004;18:173-6.

[60] Kodiatte TA, Manikyam UK, Rao SB, et al. Mean platelet volume in Type 2 diabetes mellitus. J Lab Physicians 2012;4:5-9.

[61] Papanas N, Symeonidis G, Maltezos E, et al. Mean platelet volume in patients with type 2 diabetes mellitus. Platelets 2004;15:475-8.

[62] Angiolillo DJ. Antiplatelet therapy in diabetes: efficacy and limitations of current treatment strategies and future directions. Diabetes Care 2009;32:531-40.

[63] Ajjan R, Storey RF, Grant PJ. Aspirin resistance and diabetes mellitus. Diabetologia 2008;51:385-90.

[64] Watala C, Pluta J, Golanski J, et al. Increased protein glycation in diabetes mellitus is associated with decreased aspirin-mediated protein acetylation and reduced sensitivity of blood platelets to aspirin. J Mol Med (Berl) 2005;83:148-58.

[65] Russo I, Viretto M, Barale C, et al. High glucose inhibits the aspirin-induced activation of the nitric oxide/cGMP/cGMP-dependent protein kinase pathway and does not affect the aspirin-induced inhibition of thromboxane synthesis in human platelets. Diabetes 2012;61:2913-21.

[66] Kobzar G, Mardla V, Samel N. Short-term exposure of platelets to glucose impairs inhibition of platelet aggregation by cyclooxygenase inhibitors. Platelets 2011;22:338-44.

[67] Gresele P, Marzotti S, Guglielmini G, et al. Hyperglycemia-induced platelet activation in type 2 diabetes is resistant to aspirin but not to a nitric oxide-donating agent. Diabetes Care 2010;33:1262-8.

[68] Kim JD, Park CY, Ahn KJ, et al. Non-HDL cholesterol is an independent risk factor for aspirin resistance in obese patients with type 2 diabetes. Atherosclerosis 2014;234:146-51.

[69] Angiolillo DJ, Fernandez-Ortiz A, Bernardo E, et al. Platelet function profiles in patients with type 2 diabetes and coronary artery disease on combined aspirin and clopidogrel treatment. Diabetes 2005;54:2430-5.

[70] Geisler T, Anders N, Paterok M, et al. Platelet response to clopidogrel is attenuated in diabetic patients undergoing coronary stent implantation. Diabetes Care 2007;30:372-4.

Chapter 10

# Platelets in Alzheimer's Disease

Barbara Plagg and Christian Humpel

Additional information is available at the end of the chapter

http://dx.doi.org/10.5772/60535

## 1. Introduction

Alzheimer's disease (AD) is a progressive neurodegenerative disorder that gradually leads to severe cognitive impairment. The neuropathological hallmarks of AD include beta-amyloid plaques, tau neurofibrillary tangles, inflammation and glial responses, vascular dysfunction, synapse loss and cholinergic neurodegeneration. Currently, the diagnosis of possible or probable AD is based on a time consuming combination of clinical and psychological testing, imaging, and the analysis of three well-established biomarkers (beta-amyloid(42), total tau and phospho-tau-181) in cerebrospinal fluid. The search for biomarkers in blood is of high importance to avoid invasive lumbar puncture and to allow fast and easy analysis of a high number of patients. Biomarkers have been screened in blood of AD patients in plasma/serum, peripheral blood mononuclear cells (PBMCs), monocytes or also in platelets.

Platelets are interesting targets to study AD because they share some properties with neurons: they contain the neurotransmitter serotonin and the amyloid-precursor protein (APP), which produces the beta-amyloid, which aggregates in the brain of AD patients. Moreover, platelets are an easily accessible source of human cells. This review focuses on changes in the platelets of AD patients and will summarize (1) platelet activation including mean platelet volume, membrane fluidity and coated platelets, (2) serotonin metabolism, (3) APP isoforms and processing enzymes, including secretases, (4) oxidative stress and radicals, including nitric oxide metabolism and mitochondrial pathologies, including cytochrome-c oxidase and monoamino-oxidase-B and (5) enzymatic activity, such as glycogen synthase kinase-3 or phospholipase A2. In spite of all efforts, the discrepant results so far have prevented the establishment of a valid platelet-derived AD biomarker. With this survey we provide a detailed review about the major current findings on the potential use of platelet markers in AD.

Alzheimer's disease (AD) is a progressive neurodegenerative disorder characterized by progressive deterioration in cognition leading to premature death. The neuropathological hallmarks of AD include beta-amyloid (Aβ) plaques, neurofibrillary tau tangles, inflammation and glial responses, synapse loss and cholinergic neurodegeneration among others. The worldwide prevalence of dementia was estimated as high as 24.2 million by 2005 and is expected to quadruplicate by 2050 [1, 2]. North America and Western Europe show the highest prevalence rate of dementia for persons >60 years [3]. Most dementia cases (70%) are attributed to AD, placing a considerable burden on society [2]. The increasing rate of AD cases not only stresses the establishment of efficient therapeutic intervention but also the identification of economic and reliable biomarkers. In both domains great efforts and smaller progress have been made in the last decades, while the desired breakthrough has yet to be awaited.

AD is classified into clinically indistinguishable early onset genetic AD (onset < 60 years) and late onset sporadic AD (> 60 years). Early onset AD accounts for approx. 1-5% of all cases and is associated with a more rapid progression of the neurodegenerative process and autosomal dominantly inherited mutations with a high penetrance. Sporadic AD accounts for >95% of all dementia cases and turned out to be a more heterogeneous disease. Currently, the diagnosis of possible or probable AD according to the NINCDS-ADRDA criteria is based on a time consuming combination of psychological testing, imaging, and the analysis of three well-established biomarkers (beta-amyloid(42), total tau and phospho-tau-181) in cerebrospinal fluid (CSF).

Biochemical markers mirror the physiological changes and can be objectively measured and evaluated as an indicator of pathological changes. A good biomarker must be sufficiently sensitive to detect early changes and specific to differentiate AD from clinically similar conditions. Besides high diagnostic and prognostic accuracy, biomarkers should allow global reproducibility with non-invasive and easy-to-perform tests. Within the search for peripheral AD-specific biomarkers, anucleated blood platelets have shown to be a promising target, since they represent the principal component of human blood affected by (early) biochemical alterations during AD. Moreover, platelets are an easily accessible source of human tissue and contain proteins found in neuronal cells.

In this chapter we aim to review changes in AD occurring in platelets to understand whether they may have a potential as putative biomarkers for diagnosing AD. We will focus on (1) platelet activation including mean platelet volume, membrane fluidity and coated platelets, (2) serotonin metabolism, (3) APP isoforms and processing enzymes, including secretases, (4) oxidative stress and radicals, including nitric oxide metabolism and mitochondrial pathologies, including cytochrome-c oxidase and monoamino-oxidase-B activity and (5) enzymatic activity, such as glycogen synthase kinase-3 or phospholipase A2. In spite of all efforts made, the discrepant results so far have prevented the establishment of a valid platelet-derived AD biomarker. With this survey we provide a detailed review about the major current findings on the potential use of platelet markers in AD.

## 2. Platelet activation

Vascular risk factors were traditionally considered to distinguish between vascular dementia and AD. However, in the last decade a series of studies revealed that vascular events are

http://dx.doi.org/10.5772/60535

involved in the development of AD and the arbitrary classification into vascular dementia and AD is very much outdated [4-7]. Several studies reported vascular alterations such as an increased number of fragmented vessels, atrophic string vessels, changed vessel diameters, altered capillary membrane and collagen accumulation in the basement membrane of AD patients [8, 9]. Besides, deposits of Aβ in cerebral vessels (cerebral amyloid angiopathy (CAA)) induce severe damage of the vessel wall and alter the cerebral blood flow promoting the progression of AD [10]. Moreover, it became clear that AD associated alterations are not solely limited to the brain and occur in vessels and blood cells of the peripheral system [11].

Activation and aggregation of platelets are important steps for haemostasis at sites of vascular injury, while uncontrolled activation can trigger thrombotic vessel occlusion at sides of atherosclerotic plaque rupture [12] and lead to chronic inflammatory reactions. In AD, activated platelets are strongly linked to vascular processes and are proposed to be the missing link for the association between atherosclerotic events and AD [13]. Adhesion and activation of platelets on the vascular wall progressively lead to vascular inflammation and atherosclerosis, thus playing a key role in the development of AD-associated conditions. Increased platelet activation has been identified in the late 90s, due to damaged cerebral endothelial cells or membrane abnormalities in the AD brain [14].

Moreover, increased platelet activation, measured by GPIIb-IIIa complex activation or P-selectin expression is significantly higher in AD patients with fast cognitive decline compared to slow cognitive decline [13]. Furthermore it is known, that peripheral Aβ peptides contribute to platelet adhesion and activation in the initiation of thrombus formation [15, 16]. Recently it has been shown that activated platelets aggregate at sites of vascular Aβ promoting CAA by inducing platelet thrombus formation leading to vessel occlusion at vascular Aβ plaques [17, 18]. Because platelets are major players in blood flow alterations and vascular diseases, it was suggested that they do not only mirror AD related changes, but promote actively the progression of AD. In light of these findings it is conceivable that increased platelet activity could induce the progression of AD by contributing to peripheral vascular damage and endothelial senescence. Uncontrolled activation of platelets in AD-subjects may result in chronic inflammation mediating endothelial cell stress, which, in turn, may trigger platelet activation [19]. Alternatively, systemic inflammation in AD patients may result in platelet activation creating a vicious, self-amplifying circle [20]. Thus, it is conceivable that activated platelets contribute at different sites to the progression of AD.

| References | Effect on platelet activation |
|---|---|
| Sevush et al., 1998 | ↑ in AD |
| Stellos et al., 2010, 2014 | ↑ in AD with faster cognitive decline compared to AD with slow decline<br>↑ in coronary artery disease with cognitive impairment |

**Table 1.** Platelet activation in AD

### 2.1. Effects on platelet volume

The platelet volume is a marker of platelet activation and thus involved in the pathophysiology of multiple pro-inflammatory diseases. Along with platelet activation, platelet volume values are considered indicators for vascular events linked to cerebral vascular dementia. In AD, both increased [21, 22] and decreased [23, 24] mean platelet volume has been reported. These heterogeneous results point out the importance of establishing methodological consensus in the isolation and processing of platelets, since they are very sensitive to cellular damage.

| References | Effect on platelet volume |
|---|---|
| Yagi et al., 1984 | ↑ in vascular dementia compared to AD |
| Yesil et al., 2012 | ↑ in AD |
| Wang et al., 2013 | ↓ in AD and MCI; associated with MMSE |
| Liang et al., 2013 | ↓ in vascular dementia and AD |

**Table 2.** Platelet volume in AD

### 2.2. Effects on membrane fluidity

Discrepant results have been published concerning platelet membrane fluidity: while decreased fluidity of cell membranes from platelets is associated with normal ageing, increased internal membrane fluidity is one of the first alterations to be reported in platelets [25, 26]. Increased platelet membrane fluidity becomes apparent by a decrease in the fluorescence anisotropy of 1,6-diphenyl-1,3,5-hexatriene (DPH) in labelled membranes. It was proposed, that this apparent abnormality of membranes in AD patients is due to an increase in internal membranes [26]. However, no significant differences in either cholesterol or phospholipid compared to healthy subjects has been observed [26], while an increase of intracellular platelet membranes in AD patients has been reported [27]. Other findings suggest furthermore that demented patients with increased platelet membrane fluidity display an earlier onset and a more rapid deterioration of cognitive symptoms compared to other demented subjects [25]. In light of these findings, platelet membrane fluidity was proposed as a biological risk factor for AD, since it is associated with significant contributions to the risk of developing AD [28, 29]. However, others failed to demonstrate differences in platelet membrane fluidity between AD patients and healthy controls, concluding that platelet membrane fluidity cannot be considered as antemortem biomarker for AD [30-32]. An increase in DPH fluorescence anisotropy has been reported [33-36] and as anisotropy is inversely related to membrane fluidity, these results indicate in contrast to the previously mentioned studies a decrease of the external and internal membrane fluidity in AD [33]. It was suggested that the short life span of platelets makes them less susceptible for long-term modifications. And finally, a reduced fluidity in the platelet inner mitochondrial membrane has been reported, which was associated with oxidative damage [37], while others correlated membrane fluidity with alterations of APP fragments [38].

http://dx.doi.org/10.5772/60535

| References | Effects on membrane fluidity |
|---|---|
| Zubenko et al., 1987, 1990 | ↑ in familial AD by fluorescence anisotropy |
| Kozubski et al., 1999, 2002 | ↑ in AD with 2 spin-labelled markers |
| Cohen et al., 1987: Piletz et al.,1991 | ↑ by fluorescence anisotropy, ↓ ratio of cholesterol to phospholipid |
| Kaakkola et al., 1991 | ↑ in AD and multi-infarct dementia compared to controls |
| Ortiz et al., 2008 | ↓ fluidity of platelet inner mitochondrial membrane |
| Fernandes et al., 1999 | unchanged in AD by fluorescence anisotropy |
| Kukull et al., 1992 | unchanged |
| Kálmàn et al., 1994 | ↑ in AD by fluorescence anisotropy |
| Cardoso et al., 2004 | unchanged in AD compared to controls |
| Zainaghi et al., 2007 | membrane fluidity correlated with alteration of APP fragments |
| Vignini et al., 2013 | ↓ in AD by fluorescence anisotropy, worse profile for male patients |
| Hajimohammadreza et al., 1990 | ↑ in AD by fluorescence anisotropy |

**Table 3.** Platelet membrane fluidity in AD

### 2.3. Coated platelets

Coated-platelets (PLTs) are a subset of platelets produced upon dual-agonist stimulation with collagen und thrombin retaining several procoagulant $\alpha$-granule proteins on their surface [39]. PLTs are important for the coagulation cascade because of their ability to generate thrombin at sites of vascular damage. Effectively, it was suggested that increased levels of PLTs may be related to prothrombotic conditions [40], while decreased levels of PLTs were linked to an increased risk for haemorrhage [41]. It was also demonstrated that coated-platelet levels are elevated in amnestic mild cognitive impairment (MCI) and correlate with the progression of AD [40, 42-45]. Additionally, the same group showed that MCIs with elevated coated-platelet levels are more likely to develop AD, while they found no significant alterations in patients with frontotemporal lobe dementia [44, 45]. So far, coated platelets seem to be an interesting target, which needs to be reproduced internationally by other research groups.

## 3. Serotonin

Several studies report abnormalities in serotonin (5-HT) concentration as well as alterations in its uptake during AD, possibly linked to psychobehavioral problems such as e.g. depression [46-48]. Platelets accumulate high levels of serotonin in dense granules and release it upon activation [49]. Early studies failed to demonstrate altered serotonin processing in platelets [50,

51], while in the early 90s heterogeneous results regarding 5-HT Km (Michaelis-Menten constant) and maximal velocity (Vmax) binding affinity were published [52, 53, 54]. Compared to controls, patients with AD demonstrated in different studies significantly lower platelet serotonin concentrations [55-58]. However, an increased 5-HT concentration in low-density platelet populations was recently reported [59]. Likewise, heterogeneous results have been reported for serotonin uptake: both increased and decreased serotonin uptake was found in AD platelets [52, 60]. In light of these data and despite great efforts, so far platelet-derived serotonin has not been established as a reliable biomarker for AD.

| References | Effects on serotonin |
|---|---|
| Tukiainen et al., 1981 | unchanged 5-HT uptake in |
| Andersson et al., 1991 | unchanged maximum number of binding sites (Bmax) and binding affinity |
| Inestrosa et al., 1993 | ↓ ability to accumulate 5-HT<br>↓ Km and Vmax |
| Kumar et al., 1995a | ↓ 5-HT concentration |
| Kumar et al., 1995b | ↑ affinity of binding of 5-HT to the platelet membrane in AD (only females tested) |
| Arora et al., 1991 | ↑ Vmax 5-HT-uptake in mild and moderate AD<br>Trend ↓ Vmax 5-HT-uptake in severe AD |
| Koren et al., 1993 | ↓ [3H]-5-HT uptake |
| Mimica et al., 2008 | ↓ 5-HT concentrations in non-psychotic female and psychotic male AD patients compared to controls |
| Muck-Seler et al., 2009 | ↓ 5-HT concentrations in the late phase of AD compared to other phases and controls |
| Milovanovic et al., 2014 | ↑ in low-density platelet populations |
| Prokselj et al., 2014 | ↓ 5-HT concentrations in AD compared to AD controls |

Vmax = maximum number of 5-HT uptake sites; Km = Michaelis-Menten constant; EOAD = Early Onset AD

**Table 4.** Platelet 5-HT in AD

# 4. Amyloid Precursor protein (APP) and secretases

## 4.1. APP isoforms and ratios

APP is an integral membrane protein with a large extracellular domain and a shorter, intracellular C-terminal tail. Three major APP isoforms (770, 751 and 695 kDa) have been described.

APP 751 und APP 770 contain a Kunitz-type serine protease inhibitor domain (APP KPI), while APP 695 lacks this domain. The APP isoforms are cut by different enzymes (secretases) into smaller peptides, whereas sequential cleavage by β-secretase (BACE1) and γ-secretase (ADAM-10) generates the neurotoxic Aβ fragments. Conversely, cleavage by α-secretase precludes the formation of amyloid fragments by processing APP within the Aβ domain.

Platelets are of particular interest in AD research, because they contain high levels of APP [61-63]. In contrast to neuronal tissues where isoform 695 lacking the KPI domain is the most abundant one, platelets express mainly APP770 whereas APP695 is marginally present [64]. Platelets contain α-, β-, γ- secretase activities and generate different APP fragments: sAPPα, sAPPβ, the amyloidogenic fragment (C99) and Aβ peptides [65, 66]. Platelet APP is mainly processes by the α-secretase pathway releasing soluble APP (sAPP) [66] and predominantly Aβ(40). Both APP and Aβ are stored in α-granules of platelets and become released upon activation by agents like the physiological agonists thrombin and collagen. A recent study reports significant up-regulation of platelet APP isoforms compared to controls, and a correlation between APP mRNA levels and cognitive impairment [67]. The same group found significant up-regulation of platelet mRNA expression level of total APP and APP containing a KPI domain in patients with AD and frontotemporal lobe dementia compared to controls [68]. We have recently shown that platelet-secreted APPβ in MCI and AD is significantly increased when measured with ELISA compared to control subjects, while no changes in sAPPα are seen [69].

| References | APP expression and release |
|---|---|
| Vignini et al., 2013 | ↑ mRNA of total APP and APP containing KPI domain in AD and FTLD<br>↑ APP isoforms compared to controls |
| Marksteiner and Humpel, 2013 | ↑ sAPP–β in MCI and AD compared to controls<br>unchanged sAPP-α in MCI and AD compared to controls |

**Table 5.** Platelet APP expression in AD

Several studies showed that the platelet APP ratio (defined as the ratio between the upper 130kDa and the lower 106-110kDa isoforms) is significantly lower in AD patients compared to controls and patients with other forms of dementia [70-77]. It seems that the alteration of platelet APP isoforms is an early event in AD and the ratio shows to be a consistent predictor for the conversion from MCI to AD. In fact, MCI subjects converting to AD showed significantly decreased APP ratios at baseline compared to other dementia forms and stable MCI subjects [78-80]. Furthermore, the APP ratio positively correlates with cognitive decline, i.e. the lower the ratio, the more severe the disease [38, 73]. Furthermore, it has been shown that carriers of the APOE4 allele are associated with a larger reduction in the APP ratio [81]. Moreover, administration of acetylcholine esterase inhibitors [82, 83] increases the ratio of APP forms in AD suggesting a possible effect of these drugs on APP trafficking in platelets. The proposed cut-off scores are around 0.56 with a sensitivity of 88% and specificity of 89% [80, 84]. Thus, the APP ratio has been proposed as a potential biomarker in prodromal AD-stages and a reliable indicator for the disease progress. Despite the promising homogeneous findings the validity of APP ratio as a useful supportive biomarker for AD diagnosis is not yet internationally established. Methodological problems including lack of sensitivity and diversity of the used antibodies and different isolation procedures of platelets may account for this problem.

| References | Effects on APP ratio |
|---|---|
| Di Luca et al., 1996, 1998 | ↓ in AD and elderly patients with Down Syndrom; ratio correlated with the severity of the disease |
| Rosenberg et al., 1997 | ↓ in AD compared to controls |
| Baskin et al., 2000, 2001 | ↓ specific in AD compared to PD and HS (Hemorrhagic Stroke);<br>unchanged in cognitively normal young adults carrying PS-1 mutations |
| Padovani et al., 2001, 2002 | ↓ in MCI and mild and very mild AD |
| Borroni et al., 2002, 2003, 2004 | ↓ in MCIs converting to AD and early stages of probable AD |
| Liu et al., 2005 | ↓ in AD; increases with galantamine treatment for 12 weeks |
| Tang et al., 2006 | ↓ in AD |
| Zainaghi et al., 2007, 2012 | ↓ in MCI converting to dementia upon follow-up |
| Srisawat et al., 2013 | ↓ in Thai patients with AD |

**Table 6.** Platelet APP ratio in AD

### 4.2. Enzymatic activity: BACE1 and ADAM-10

APP is cleaved into secreted (soluble) APP (sAPP), smaller intracellular fragments and the A$\beta$ peptides (40, 42 or 43 amino acids) by three secretases ($\alpha$, $\beta$, $\gamma$). The $\alpha$-secretase leads to the non-amyloidogenic pathway, while cleavage of APP by $\beta$ -secretase (BACE1) and $\gamma$-secretase (ADAM-10) generates the toxic A$\beta$ fragments. So far, several authors report increased BACE1 in AD by Western blotting or ELISA analysis [69, 73, 85, 86]. However, using a novel ELISA system a significant decrease of BACE1 N-terminal and C-terminal fragments has been reported in AD [87]. ADAM-10 is the major constitutive $\alpha$-secretase for APP processing [88, 89]. To date, platelet ADAM10 (a disintegrin and metalloprotease) has been reported to be significantly reduced in platelets in AD [85, 90, 91] while others failed to detect changes in alpha- and beta-secretase activities in AD [92]. Moreover, reduction in ADAM-10 levels correlates with the progression and seems to be stage-dependent [91].

http://dx.doi.org/10.5772/60535

| References | Effects on secretases |
|---|---|
| Johnston et al., 2008 | ↑ platelet membrane ß-secretase activity in AD compared to controls; |
| Colciaghi et al., 2002, 2004 | ↓ ADAM10 in AD compared to controls<br>↓ level of alpha APPs<br>↑ BACE1 in AD |
| Tang et al., 2006 | ↑ BACE1 in AD<br>↓ ADAM10 in AD |
| Gorham et al., 2010 | unchanged alpha- and beta-secretase activities and -ratio in AD and MCI |
| Decourt et al., 2013 | ↓ BACE1 in AD (newly developed ELISA) |
| Manzine et al., 2013 | ↓ ADAM10 in AD |

**Table 7.** Platelet secretase activity in AD

### 4.3. Activation of platelets by beta-amyloid

It is well known that different heterogeneous amyloidogenic peptides (Aβ(1-40), Aβ(1-42), Aβ(25-36)) as well as aggregated Aβ can induce platelet aggregation [15, 16]. Platelets store and release preferentially the 40 amino acid Aβ fragment in their granules upon stimulation with physiological agonists like thrombin, collagen or calcium ionophores [93, 61, 94, 95]. Once released, Aβ peptides trigger platelet activation, initiating a vicious feedback loop of platelet activation and Aβ release. Further, apoptotic stimuli significantly increase platelet Aβ(40) but not Aβ(42) suggesting that this pathway determines altered APP processing [96, 97]. Recently it was shown that Aβ induces platelet activation independent of known physiological agonists [16]. It was furthermore suggested that platelets modulate aggregation of soluble Aβ into fibrillar Aβ and facilitate platelet adhesion at vascular Aβ accumulations, contributing to the full occlusion of the affected vessel [18]. At this point it seems therefore likely that platelets and platelet-derived Aβ may contribute to a significant degree to the amyloid burden in the vascular walls promoting CAA in AD patients [96].

## 5. Oxidative stress, radicals and mitochondrial pathologies

Excessive chronic oxidative stress and production of radicals in the AD brain has been considered to promote cellular degeneration. Especially, nitric oxide (NO) and peroxynitrite (ONOO) are very reactive toxic radicals (ROS). It becomes more and more clear that a dysregulation of mitochondria and the involvement of cytochrome C-oxidase may play a role in this process. Vascular damage and endothelial dysfunction may play a role in AD and platelets serve as a source of oxidative stress. Mitochondria are the major sites responsible for more than 90 % of the ROS generation. In AD, mitochondrial DNA of cortical neurons was reported to induce excessive oxidative damage and increased DNA mutations [98-100]. Moreover, abnormal mitochondrial size and decreased mitochondrial number in AD and MCI are likely to increase ROS generation and oxidative damage [99, 101]. In platelets reduced Complex IV and Complex III activity has been repeatedly associated with AD [102-105, 32]. Subsequently, Aβ was shown to interact directly with mitochondria and inhibit platelet Complex IV activity inducing oxidative stress [106].

### 5.1. Nitric oxide and peroxynitrite

An increase in nitric oxide synthase (NOS) has been associated with normal aging and with AD [107, 108, 33]. Similarly to NO, peroxynitrite (ONOO) was found to be increased in AD patients and both NO and ONOO are linked to reduced Na+/K+-ATPase activity in platelet membranes of AD patients [108]. Additionally, carriers of the epsilon 4 allele of apolipoprotein E (APOE) show higher NOS compared to non-carriers [109]. In contrast, others found significantly lower NO concentrations in platelets of AD patients and a generally higher platelet aggregation rate. Since NO is known to inhibit platelet aggregation, NO might be responsible for the aggregation of platelets in the observed AD cohort [110].

| References | Effects on nitric oxide |
|---|---|
| Kawamoto et al., 2005 | ↑ NO and peroxynitrite in AD |
| Vignini et al., 2007, 2013; | ↑ NO and ONOO(-) peroxynitrite in AD |
| Marcourakis et al., 2008 | ↑ NOS activity in APOE epsilon 4 carriers |
| Yu and Jia, 2009 | ↓ NO and eNOS (endothelial nitric oxide synthase) |

**Table 8.** Platelet nitric oxide and peroxynitrite concentrations in AD

### 5.2. Cytochrome c oxidase

Cytochrome C oxidase (COX) is an enzyme located in mitochondria and may play a role in the production of radicals. In most studies, reduced platelet COX activity has been found in AD [111-113, 102, 103, 32, 104] but also in cognitively normal individuals with a maternal history of AD [114]. However, another study did not find any differences in COX activity in AD [115]. Recently, reduced mitochondrial COX activity has been found, which correlates to decreased mitochondrial membrane potential, resulting in higher lipid peroxides, superoxide radicals and protein carbonyls [111]. It has been proposed, that reduced COX activity causes higher tissue vulnerability and reduced oxygen availability [104].

### 5.3. Monoamino-oxidase B

Monoamino-oxidase-B (MAO-B) is an important enzyme located in the mitochondria and plays a role in metabolic processes of serotonin. Studies on platelet MAO-B activity yielded inconsistent results up to date: increased MAO-B activity was reported by several groups [116-126], while few researchers could not find any abnormalities [127,128]. The decline of mini-mental state examination scores (MMSE) preceded the elevation of MAO-B activity

http://dx.doi.org/10.5772/60535

| References | Effects on COX activity |
|---|---|
| Silva et al., 2013 | ↓ COX, mitochondrial membrane potential , cytochrome c content |
| Burbaeva et al., 2012 | ↓ COX in AD and MCI |
| Mosconi et al., 2011 | ↓ COX activity in cognitively normal individuals with a history of maternal LOAD |
| Cardoso et al., 2004 | ↓ 15 % COX activity in AD despite COX subunits were present at normal levels |
| Bosetti et al., 2002 | ↓ COX in AD and MCI |
| Van Zuylen et al., 1992 | unchanged |
| Parker et al., 1990, 1991, 1994 | ↓ COX in AD |

**Table 9.** Platelet COX activity in AD

[116-119]. It has been suggested that MAO-B activity might be an indicator for severity and clinical progress in AD [57]. In another study, non-psychotic AD patients showed significantly higher platelet MAO-B activity, suggesting that MAO-B activity can differentiate between psychotic and non-psychotic subtypes of AD [56].

| References | Effects on MAO-B activity |
|---|---|
| Zellner et al., 2012 | ↑ MAO-B activity correlated with ↑ MAO-B protein expression in AD |
| Mimica et al., 2008 | ↑ in AD in non-psychotic patients |
| Soto et al., 1999 | ↑ 22% MAO-B activity in AD |
| Götz et al., 1998 | ↑ MAO-B activity in AD |
| Bongioanni et al., 1996 | ↑ MAO-B activity in AD |
| Ahlskop et al.,1996 | unchanged |
| Konings et al., 1995 | unchanged |
| Parnetti et al., 1992, 1994 | ↑ MAO-B activity in LOAD compared to controls and EOAD |
| Regland et al., 1991 | ↑ MAO-B activity in AD; after B12 therapy MAO-B activity was reduced to a normal level |
| Schneider et al., 1988 | ↑ MAO-B activity in female AD without agitation and delusions |
| Danielczyk et al., 1988 | ↑ MAO-B activity in AD (non-familial) |
| Alexopoulos et al., 1987 | ↑ MAO-B activity in demented patients with and without depression |
| Adolfsson et al., 1980 | ↑ MAO-B activity in AD |

**Table 10.** Platelet MAO-B activity in AD

## 6. Changes of other biological systems

### 6.1. GSK3β activity

Glycogen synthase kinase 3-beta (GSK3β) is involved in the regulation of glycogen synthesis by phosphorylating and inactivating the glycogen synthase and in the regulation of intracellular signalling pathways [129-131]. Moreover, in neural cell tissues GSK3β is the most important Tau kinase and has been linked to synaptic plasticity and neural injury [132, 133]. Therefore, deregulation of GSK3β has a significant impact on the formation of neurofibrillary tangles. GSK3β is also expressed in platelets and might be involved in platelet activation [134]. A substantial higher expression of GSK3β has been shown in AD and MCI platelets as compared to healthy controls, which also correlated with worse memory performance [135].

### 6.2. Phospholipase activity

It is known that AD is associated with chronic inflammatory responses and platelets express inflammatory mediators such as chemokines, interleukins, adhesive proteins and contain enzymes such as phospholipase-A2 (PLA2) [20]. Phospholipases are important platelet enzymes involved in the metabolism of membrane phospholipids and inflammatory synthesis. PLA2 and phospholipase C (PLC) are altered in peripheral blood cells and significantly decreased PLC activity in platelets of AD patients has been reported [136], suggesting aberrant phospholipase metabolism. Further, decreased PLA2 activity was found in human platelets [137, 138], which correlates with the degree of cognitive impairment and is modulated by cognitive training in healthy elders [139]. In contrast, an increased platelet PLA2 activity in individuals with AD has also been shown [140]. Thus, again the reports on these enzyme activities are very controversial and do not allow to establish a concluding interpretation.

| References | Effects on PLA2 and PLC activity |
|---|---|
| Krzystanek et al., 2007 | ↑ PLA2 in AD |
| Gattaz et al., 1995, 1996, 2004 | ↓ PLA2 in AD and MCI |
| Matushima et al., 1995, 1998 | ↓ PLC in AD |

**Table 11.** Platelet PLA2 and PLC activity in AD

### 6.3. Overview of other platelet components found to be altered in AD

Several other biological systems have been studied in platelets of AD patients, such as e.g. decreased plasma antioxidant power levels [107], decreased cathepsin D [141], increased platelet glutamine synthetase-like protein level in MCI [112], increased NA,K-ATPase activities in AD [107], unchanged Vitamin E and cholesterol content between AD and controls [32] or increased phenolsulphotransferase activity in demented patients [142] or decreased platelet peripheral-type benzodiazepine binding [143]. However, we do not claim to provide a complete overview of all markers. Anyhow, none of these markers has been found to be a suitable reproducible marker for AD.

## 7. Platelets as biomarkers

Biomarkers must objectively reflect physiological processes linked to AD and should be globally reproducible with easy-to-perform tests [144]. Moreover, besides being sensitive enough to differentiate AD from clinically similar diseases, a good biomarker should be able to detect early disease-associated changes. In AD, abnormal metabolism of APP, hyperphosphorylation of Tau, induction of oxidative stress and inflammatory cascades result in pathological changes in liquid fluids. Currently, the laboratory diagnosis of AD is based on the combination of three CSF biomarkers yielding a sensitivity of >95% and specificity of >85% [145, 146]. However, considering the invasiveness of lumbar puncture and the growing incidence rate of AD, the need for biomarkers in more accessible body fluids is necessary. Blood measurements are minimally invasive and less time-consuming compared to CSF. The establishment of new markers in plasma/serum has proven to be difficult because changes mirror a broad spectrum of physiological processes not necessarily related to AD [144]. Moreover, changes in plasma/serum are very small and heterogeneous, thus making the search for reliable and sensitive biomarkers challenging.

Within the search for peripheral biomarkers in AD, blood platelets have been of great interest during the last decades. These anuclear blood cells share several homeostatic functions with neurons such as accumulation and release of neurotransmitters like serotonin, and expression of receptors and enzymes [147]. Moreover, human platelets have shown to be the most important source of more than 90% of the circulating APP [148, 149]. On grounds of these findings, platelets can be considered a valid peripheral model for the analysis of metabolic pathways linked to AD. Despite great efforts, to date no specific platelet biomarker has been successfully established, while some platelet components have shown to be of greater validity than others.

Overall, the so far published studies underline the need to establish concurrent methods in order to yield comparable results and avoid methodological diversity among institutes. Platelets contain several types of surface receptors responding to external stimuli with activation or inhibitory actions [150]. In response to physiological and non-physiological stimuli, platelet granules and their contents are released, thus requiring careful handling during isolation and experimentation in order to avoid activation. Effectively, different platelet isolation and processing procedures may account to a significant extent for the observed inter-rater differences between institutes. Moreover, different phases of the disease, comorbidities or medications need to be taken into consideration when evaluating platelet status in AD patients. Additionally, further analysis and classification of platelets with respect to their different features (e.g. density fraction) might be helpful to generate more significant data. Besides a homogeneous patient group, the selection of healthy, age-matched controls is a known challenge in AD-research and might additionally explain varying data. Therefore, the so far obtained results need to be replicated in large and homogeneous cohorts according to the same methodological protocol by independent researchers. To date, the use of platelet biomarkers in the diagnostic routine of AD can yet not be recommended and is in urgent need of final evaluation.

## 8. Conclusions

In conclusion, the search for platelet biomarker so far has highlighted some candidates worth further investigation, while the breakthrough in identifying one satisfyingly specific and sensitive marker has yet to be awaited. Overall, among the studied platelet components and according to the available data, the platelet APP ratio and COX activity seem the most promising candidates for establishing new peripheral biomarkers for AD.

## Acknowledgements

This study has been supported by the Austrian Science Funds (P24734-B24).

## Author details

Barbara Plagg and Christian Humpel*

*Address all correspondence to: christian.humpel@i-med.ac.at

Laboratory of Psychiatry and Exp. Alzheimer's Research, Department of Psychiatry and Psychotherapy, Innsbruck Medical University, Austria

## References

[1] Ferri CP, Prince M, Brayne C, Brodaty H, Fratiglioni L, Ganguli M, Hall K, Hasegawa K, Hendrie H, Huang Y, Jorm A, Mathers C, Menezes PR, Rimmer E, Scazufca M; Alzheimer's Disease International. Global prevalence of dementia: a Delphi consensus study. Lancet. 2005; 366(9503) 2112-2117.

[2] Reitz C, Mayeux R. Alzheimer disease: epidemiology, diagnostic criteria, risk factors and biomarkers. Biochem Pharmacol. 2014; 88(4) 640-651.

[3] Mayeux R, Stern Y. Epidemiology of Alzheimer disease. Cold Spring Harb Perspect Med. 2012; 2(8).

[4] Schneider JA. High blood pressure and microinfarcts: a link between vascular risk factors, dementia, and clinical Alzheimer's disease. J Am Geriatr Soc. 2009; 57(11) 2146-2147.

[5] Breteler MM. Vascular involvement in cognitive decline and dementia. Epidemiologic evidence from the Rotterdam Study and the Rotterdam Scan Study. Ann N Y Acad Sci. 2000; 903 457-465.

[6] Purnell C, Gao S, Callahan CM, Hendrie HC. Cardiovascular risk factors and incident Alzheimer disease: a systematic review of the literature. Alzheimer Dis Assoc Disord. 2009; 23(1) 1-10.

[7] Zlokovic BV. Neurovascular mechanisms of Alzheimer's neurodegeneration. Trends Neurosci. 2005; 28(4) 202-208.

[8] Bailey TL, Rivara CB, Rocher AB, Hof PR. The nature and effects of cortical microvascular pathology in aging and Alzheimer's disease. Neurol Res. 2004; 26(5) 573-578.

[9] Farkas E, Luiten PG. Cerebral microvascular pathology in aging and Alzheimer's disease. Prog Neurobiol. 2001; 64(6) 575-611.

[10] Thal DR, Griffin WS, de Vos RA, Ghebremedhin E. Cerebral amyloid angiopathy and its relationship to Alzheimer's disease. Acta Neuropathol. 2008; 115(6) 599-609.

[11] Hardy J. Does Abeta 42 have a function related to blood homeostasis? Neurochem Res. 2007; 32(4-5) 833-835.

[12] Gawaz M, Langer H, May AE. Platelets in inflammation and atherogenesis. J Clin Invest. 2005; 115(12) 3378-3384.

[13] Stellos K, Panagiota V, Kögel A, Leyhe T, Gawaz M, Laske C. Predictive value of platelet activation for the rate of cognitive decline in Alzheimer's disease patients. J Cereb Blood Flow Metab. 2010; 30(11) 1817-1820.

[14] Sevush S, Jy W, Horstman LL, Mao WW, Kolodny L, Ahn YS. Platelet activation in Alzheimer disease. Arch Neurol. 1998; 55(4) 530-536.

[15] Canobbio I, Catricalà S, Di Pasqua LG, Guidetti G, Consonni A, Manganaro D, Torti M. Immobilized amyloid Aβ peptides support platelet adhesion and activation. FEBS Lett. 2013; 587(16) 2606-2611.

[16] Sonkar VK, Kulkarni PP, Dash D. Amyloid β peptide stimulates platelet activation through RhoA-dependent modulation of actomyosin organization. FASEB J. 2014; 28(4) 1819-1829.

[17] Roher AE, Esh CL, Kokjohn TA, Castaño EM, Van Vickle GD, Kalback WM, Patton RL, Luehrs DC, Daugs ID, Kuo YM, Emmerling MR, Soares H, Quinn JF, Kaye J, Connor DJ, Silverberg NB, Adler CH, Seward JD, Beach TG, Sabbagh MN. Amyloid

beta peptides in human plasma and tissues and their significance for Alzheimer's disease. Alzheimers Dement. 2009; 5(1) 18-29.

[18] Gowert NS, Donner L, Chatterjee M, Eisele YS, Towhid ST, Münzer P, Walker B, Ogorek I, Borst O, Grandoch M, Schaller M, Fischer JW, Gawaz M, Weggen S, Lang F, Jucker M, Elvers M. Blood platelets in the progression of Alzheimer's disease. PLoS One. 2014; 9(2).

[19] Catricala S, Torti M, Ricevuti G. Alzheimer disease and platelets: how's that relevant. Immun Ageing. 2012 Sep 17;9(1):20. Casoli T, Di Stefano G, Balietti M, Solazzi M, Giorgetti B, Fattoretti P. Peripheral inflammatory biomarkers of Alzheimer's disease: the role of platelets. Biogerontology. 2010; 11(5) 627-633.

[20] Casoli T, Di Stefano G, Balietti M, Solazzi M, Giorgetti B, Fattoretti P. Peripheral inflammatory biomarkers of Alzheimer's disease: the role of platelets. Biogerontology. 2010; 11(5) 627-633.

[21] Yagi T, Kohashi N, Katori R, Miyazaki M. [Mean platelet volume, platelet count and platelet retention rate in cerebral vascular disease and Alzheimer type dementia]. Nihon Ronen Igakkai Zasshi. 1984; 21(6) 545-549.

[22] Yesil Y, Kuyumcu ME, Cankurtaran M, Uz B, Kara A, Kilic MK, Halil M, Ulger Z, Yavuz BB, Haznedaroğlu IC, Ariogul S. Increased mean platelet volume (MPV) indicating the vascular risk in Alzheimer's disease (AD). Arch Gerontol Geriatr. 2012; 55(2) 257-260.

[23] Wang RT, Jin D, Li Y, Liang QC. Decreased mean platelet volume and platelet distribution width are associated with mild cognitive impairment and Alzheimer's disease. J Psychiatr Res. 2013; 47(5) 644-649.

[24] Liang QC, Jin D, Li Y, Wang RT. Mean platelet volume and platelet distribution width in vascular dementia and Alzheimer's disease. Platelets. 2013, 1-6.

[25] Zubenko GS, Cohen BM, Reynolds CF 3rd, Boller F, Teply I, Chojnacki B. Platelet membrane fluidity identifies a clinical subtype of Alzheimer's disease. Prog Neuropsychopharmacol Biol Psychiatry. 1987;11(6) 683-699.

[26] Cohen BM, Zubenko GS, Babb SM. Abnormal platelet membrane composition in Alzheimer's-type dementia. Life Sci. 1987; 40(25) 2445-2451.

[27] Piletz JE, Sarasua M, Whitehouse P, Chotani M. Intracellular membranes are more fluid in platelets of Alzheimer's disease patients. Neurobiol Aging. 1991; 12(5) 401-406.

[28] Zubenko GS, Kopp U, Seto T, Firestone LL. Platelet membrane fluidity individuals at risk for Alzheimer's disease: a comparison of results from fluorescence spectroscopy

and electron spin resonance spectroscopy. Psychopharmacology (Berl). 1999; 145(2) 175-180.

[29] Kozubski W, Swiderek M, Kloszewska I, Gwozdzinski K, Watala C. Blood platelet membrane fluidity and the exposition of membrane protein receptors in Alzheimer disease (AD) patients--preliminary Study. Alzheimer Dis Assoc Disord. 2002; 16(1) 52-54.

[30] Kukull WA, Hinds TR, Schellenberg GD, van Belle G, Larson EB. Increased platelet membrane fluidity as a diagnostic marker for Alzheimer's disease: a test in population-based cases and controls. Neurology. 1992; 42(3 Pt 1) 607-614.

[31] Fernandes MA, Proença MT, Nogueira AJ, Oliveira LM, Santiago B, Santana I, Oliveira CR. Effects of apolipoprotein E genotype on blood lipid composition and membrane platelet fluidity in Alzheimer's disease. Biochim Biophys Acta. 1999; 1454(1) 89-96.

[32] Cardoso SM, Proença MT, Santos S, Santana I, Oliveira CR. Cytochrome c oxidase is decreased in Alzheimer's disease platelets. Neurobiol Aging. 2004; 25(1) 105-110.

[33] Vignini A, Giusti L, Raffaelli F, Giulietti A, Salvolini E, Luzzi S, Provinciali L, Mazzanti L, Nanetti L. Impact of gender on platelet membrane functions of Alzheimer's disease patients. Exp Gerontol. 2013; 48(3) 319-325.

[34] Kaakkola S, Rosenberg PH, Alila A, Erkinjuntti T, Sulkava R, Palo J. Platelet membrane fluidity in Alzheimer's disease and multi-infarct dementia: a spin label study. Acta Neurol Scand. 1991; 84(1) 18-21.

[35] Kálmán J, Dey I, Ilona SV, Matkovics B, Brown D, Janka Z, Farkas T, Joó F. Platelet membrane fluidity and plasma malondialdehyde levels in Alzheimer's demented patients with and without family history of dementia. Biol Psychiatry. 1994; 35(3) 190-194.

[36] Hajimohammadreza I, Brammer MJ, Eagger S, Burns A, Levy R. Platelet and erythrocyte membrane changes in Alzheimer's disease. Biochim Biophys Acta. 1990; 1025(2) 208-214.

[37] Ortiz GG, Pacheco-Moisés F, El Hafidi M, Jiménez-Delgado A, Macías-Islas MA, Rosales Corral SA, de la Rosa AC, Sánchez-González VJ, Arias-Merino ED, Velázquez-Brizuela IE. Detection of membrane fluidity in submitochondrial particles of platelets and erythrocyte membranes from Mexican patients with Alzheimer disease by intramolecular excimer formation of 1,3 dipyrenylpropane. Dis Markers. 2008; 24(3) 151-156.

[38] Zainaghi IA, Forlenza OV, Gattaz WF. Abnormal APP processing in platelets of patients with Alzheimer's disease: correlations with membrane fluidity and cognitive decline. Psychopharmacology (Berl). 2007; 192(4) 547-553.

[39] Alberio L, Safa O, Clemetson KJ, Esmon CT, Dale GL. Surface expression and functional characterization of alpha-granule factor V in human platelets: effects of ionophore A23187, thrombin, collagen, and convulxin. Blood. 2000; 95(5) 1694-1702.

[40] Prodan CI, Joseph PM, Vincent AS, Dale GL. Coated-platelets in ischemic stroke: differences between lacunar and cortical stroke. J Thromb Haemost. 2008; 6(4) 609-614.

[41] Prodan CI, Vincent AS, Padmanabhan R, Dale GL. Coated-platelet levels are low in patients with spontaneous intracerebral hemorrhage. Stroke. 2009; 40(7) 2578-2580.

[42] Prodan CI, Szasz R, Vincent AS, Ross ED, Dale GL. Coated-platelets retain amyloid precursor protein on their surface. Platelets. 2006; 17(1) 56-60.

[43] Prodan CI, Ross ED, Vincent AS, Dale GL. Coated-platelets are higher in amnestic versus nonamnestic patients with mild cognitive impairment. Alzheimer Dis Assoc Disord. 2007; 21(3) 259-261.

[44] Prodan CI, Ross ED, Vincent AS, Dale GL. Differences in coated-platelet production between frontotemporal dementia and Alzheimer disease. Alzheimer Dis Assoc Disord. 2009; 23(3) 234-237.

[45] Prodan CI, Ross ED, Stoner JA, Cowan LD, Vincent AS, Dale GL. Coated-platelet levels and progression from mild cognitive impairment to Alzheimer disease. Neurology. 2011; 76(3) 247-52.

[46] Assal F, Alarcón M, Solomon EC, Masterman D, Geschwind DH, Cummings JL. Association of the serotonin transporter and receptor gene polymorphisms in neuropsychiatric symptoms in Alzheimer disease. Arch Neurol. 2004; 61(8) 1249-1253.

[47] Curcio CA, Kemper T. Nucleus raphe dorsalis in dementia of the Alzheimer type: neurofibrillary changes and neuronal packing density. J Neuropathol Exp Neurol. 1984; 43(4) 359-368.

[48] Zubenko GS, Moossy J, Martinez AJ, Rao G, Claassen D, Rosen J, Kopp U. Neuropathologic and neurochemical correlates of psychosis in primary dementia. Arch Neurol. 1991; 48(6) 619-624.

[49] De Clerck F, Xhonneux B, Leysen J, Janssen PA. Evidence for functional 5-HT2 receptor sites on human blood platelets. Biochem Pharmacol. 1984; 33(17) 2807-2811.

[50] Tukiainen E, Wikström J, Kilpeläinen H. Uptake of 5-hydroxytryptamine by blood platelets in Huntington's chorea and Alzheimer type of presenile dementia. Med Biol. 1981; 59(2) 116-120.

[51] Andersson A, Adolfsson R, Eriksson K, Marcusson J. Platelet [3H]paroxetine binding to 5-HT uptake sites in Alzheimer's disease. Neurobiol Aging. 1991; 12(5) 531-534.

[52] Arora RC, Emery OB, Meltzer HY. Serotonin uptake in the blood platelets of Alzheimer's disease patients. Neurology. 1991; 41(8) 1307-1309.

[53] Inestrosa NC, Alarcón R, Arriagada J, Donoso A, Alvarez J. Platelet of Alzheimer patients: increased counts and subnormal uptake and accumulation of [14C]5-hydroxytryptamine. Neurosci Lett. 1993; 163(1) 8-10.

[54] Kumar AM, Kumar M, Sevush S, Ruiz J, Eisdorfer C. Serotonin uptake and its kinetics in platelets of women with Alzheimer's disease. Psychiatry Res. 1995; 59(1-2) 145-150.

[55] Prokšelj T, Jerin A, Muck-Seler D, Kogoj A. Decreased platelet serotonin concentration in Alzheimer's disease with involuntary emotional expression disorder. Neurosci Lett. 2014; 578 71-74.

[56] Mimica N, Mück-Seler D, Pivac N, Mustapić M, Dezeljin M, Stipcević T, Presecki P, Radonić E, Folnegović-Smalc V. Platelet serotonin and monoamine oxidase in Alzheimer's disease with psychotic features. Coll Antropol. 2008; 32 Suppl 1 119-122.

[57] Muck-Seler D, Presecki P, Mimica N, Mustapic M, Pivac N, Babic A, Nedic G, Folnegovic-Smalc V. Platelet serotonin concentration and monoamine oxidase type B activity in female patients in early, middle and late phase of Alzheimer's disease. Prog Neuropsychopharmacol Biol Psychiatry. 2009; 33(7) 1226-1231.

[58] Kumar AM, Sevush S, Kumar M, Ruiz J, Eisdorfer C. Peripheral serotonin in Alzheimer's disease. Neuropsychobiology. 1995; 32(1) 9-12.

[59] Milovanovic M, Eriksson K, Winblad B, Nilsson S, Lindahl TL, Post C, Järemo P. Alzheimer and platelets: Low-density platelet populations reveal increased serotonin content in Alzheimer type dementia. Clin Biochem. 2014.

[60] Koren P, Diver-Haber A, Adunsky A, Rabinowitz M, Hershkowitz M. Uptake of serotonin into platelets of senile dementia of the Alzheimer type patients. J Gerontol. 1993; 48(3) B93-96.

[61] Bush AI, Martins RN, Rumble B, Moir R, Fuller S, Milward E, Currie J, Ames D, Weidemann A, Fischer P, et al. The amyloid precursor protein of Alzheimer's disease is released by human platelets. J Biol Chem. 1990; 265(26) 15977-15983.

[62] Gardella JE, Ghiso J, Gorgone GA, Marratta D, Kaplan AP, Frangione B, Gorevic PD. Intact Alzheimer amyloid precursor protein (APP) is present in platelet membranes and is encoded by platelet mRNA. Biochem Biophys Res Commun. 1990; 173(3) 1292-1298.

[63] Di Luca M, Colciaghi F, Pastorino L, Borroni B, Padovani A, Cattabeni F. Platelets as a peripheral district where to study pathogenetic mechanisms of alzheimer disease: the case of amyloid precursor protein. Eur J Pharmacol. 2000; 405(1-3) 277-283.

[64] Evin G, Li QX. Platelets and Alzheimer's disease: Potential of APP as a biomarker. World J Psychiatry. 2012; 2(6) 102-113.

[65] Li QX, Whyte S, Tanner JE, Evin G, Beyreuther K, Masters CL. Secretion of Alzheimer's disease Abeta amyloid peptide by activated human platelets. Lab Invest. 1998; 78(4) 461-469.

[66] Li QX, Cappai R, Evin G, Tanner JE, Gray CW, Beyreuther K, Masters CL. Products of the Alzheimer's disease amyloid precursor protein generated by b-secretase are present in human platelets, and secreted upon degranulation. Am J Alzheimers Dis. 1998; 13 236–244.

[67] Vignini A, Sartini D, Morganti S, Nanetti L, Luzzi S, Provinciali L, Mazzanti L, Emanuelli M. Platelet amyloid precursor protein isoform expression in Alzheimer's disease: evidence for peripheral marker. Int J Immunopathol Pharmacol. 2011; 24(2) 529-534.

[68] Vignini A, Morganti S, Salvolini E, Sartini D, Luzzi S, Fiorini R, Provinciali L, Di Primio R, Mazzanti L, Emanuelli M. Amyloid precursor protein expression is enhanced in human platelets from subjects with Alzheimer's disease and frontotemporal lobar degeneration: a real-time PCR study. Exp Gerontol. 2013; 48(12) 1505-1508.

[69] Marksteiner J, Humpel C. Platelet-derived secreted amyloid-precursor protein-β as a marker for diagnosing Alzheimer's disease. Curr Neurovasc Res. 2013; 10(4) 297-303.

[70] Di Luca M, Pastorino L, Cattabeni F, Zanardi R, Scarone S, Racagni G, Smeraldi E, Perez J. Abnormal pattern of platelet APP isoforms in Alzheimer disease and Down syndrome. Arch Neurol. 1996; 53(11) 1162-1166.

[71] Di Luca M, Pastorino L, Bianchetti A, Perez J, Vignolo LA, Lenzi GL, Trabucchi M, Cattabeni F, Padovani A. Differential level of platelet amyloid beta precursor protein isoforms: an early marker for Alzheimer disease. Arch Neurol. 1998; 55(9) 1195-1200.

[72] Borroni B, Colciaghi F, Archetti S, Marcello E, Caimi L, Di Luca M, Padovani A. Predicting cognitive decline in Alzheimer disease. Role of platelet amyloid precursor protein. Alzheimer Dis Assoc Disord. 2004; 18(1) 32-34.

[73] Tang K, Hynan LS, Baskin F, Rosenberg RN. Platelet amyloid precursor protein processing: a bio-marker for Alzheimer's disease. J Neurol Sci. 2006; 240(1-2) 53-58.

[74] Zainaghi IA, Talib LL, Diniz BS, Gattaz WF, Forlenza OV. Reduced platelet amyloid precursor protein ratio (APP ratio) predicts conversion from mild cognitive impairment to Alzheimer's disease. J Neural Transm. 2012; 119(7) 815-819.

[75] Baskin F, Rosenberg RN, Iyer L, Hynan L, Cullum CM. Platelet APP isoform ratios correlate with declining cognition in AD. Neurology. 2000; 54(10) 1907-9.

[76] Baskin F, Rosenberg RN, Iyer L, Schellenberg GD, Hynan L, Nee LE. Platelet APP isoform ratios in asymptomatic young adults expressing an AD-related presenilin-1 mutation. J Neurol Sci. 2001; 183(1) 85-88.

[77] Srisawat C, Junnu S, Peerapittayamongkol C, Futrakul A, Soi-ampornkul R, Senanarong V, Praditsuwan R, Assantachai P, Neungton N. The platelet amyloid precursor protein ratio as a diagnostic marker for Alzheimer's disease in Thai patients. J Clin Neurosci. 2013; 20(5) 644-8.

[78] Borroni B, Colciaghi F, Corsini P, Akkawi N, Rozzini L, Del Zotto E, Talarico G, Cattabeni F, Lenzi GL, Di Luca M, Padovani A. Early stages of probable Alzheimer disease are associated with changes in platelet amyloid precursor protein forms. Neurol Sci. 2002; 23(5) 207-210.

[79] Padovani A, Borroni B, Colciaghi F, Pettenati C, Cottini E, Agosti C, Lenzi GL, Caltagirone C, Trabucchi M, Cattabeni F, Di Luca M. Abnormalities in the pattern of platelet amyloid precursor protein forms in patients with mild cognitive impairment and Alzheimer disease. Arch Neurol. 2002; 59(1) 71-75.

[80] Borroni B, Colciaghi F, Caltagirone C, Rozzini L, Broglio L, Cattabeni F, Di Luca M, Padovani A. Platelet amyloid precursor protein abnormalities in mild cognitive impairment predict conversion to dementia of Alzheimer type: a 2-year follow-up study. Arch Neurol. 2003; 60(12) 1740-1744.

[81] Rosenberg RN, Baskin F, Fosmire JA, Risser R, Adams P, Svetlik D, Honig LS, Cullum CM, Weiner MF. Altered amyloid protein processing in platelets of patients with Alzheimer disease. Arch Neurol. 1997; 54(2) 139-144.

[82] Borroni B, Colciaghi F, Pastorino L, Pettenati C, Cottini E, Rozzini L, Monastero R, Lenzi GL, Cattabeni F, Di Luca M, Padovani A. Amyloid precursor protein in platelets of patients with Alzheimer disease: effect of acetylcholinesterase inhibitor treatment. Arch Neurol. 2001; 58(3) 442-446.

[83] Liu HC, Chi CW, Ko SY, Wang HC, Hong CJ, Lin KN, Wang PN, Liu TY. Cholinesterase inhibitor affects the amyloid precursor protein isoforms in patients with Alzheimer's disease. Dement Geriatr Cogn Disord. 2005; 19(5-6) 345-8.

[84] Padovani A, Pastorino L, Borroni B, Colciaghi F, Rozzini L, Monastero R, Perez J, Pettenati C, Mussi M, Parrinello G, Cottini E, Lenzi GL, Trabucchi M, Cattabeni F, Di Luca M. Amyloid precursor protein in platelets: a peripheral marker for the diagnosis of sporadic AD. Neurology. 2001; 57(12) 2243-8.

[85] Colciaghi F, Marcello E, Borroni B, Zimmermann M, Caltagirone C, Cattabeni F, Padovani A, Di Luca M. Platelet APP, ADAM 10 and BACE alterations in the early stages of Alzheimer disease. Neurology. 2004; 62(3) 498-501.

[86] Johnston JA, Liu WW, Coulson DT, Todd S, Murphy S, Brennan S, Foy CJ, Craig D, Irvine GB, Passmore AP. Platelet beta-secretase activity is increased in Alzheimer's disease. Neurobiol Aging. 2008; 29(5) 661-668.

[87] Decourt B, Walker A, Gonzales A, Malek-Ahmadi M, Liesback C, Davis KJ, Belden CM, Jacobson SA, Sabbagh MN. Can platelet BACE1 levels be used as a biomarker

for Alzheimer's disease? Proof-of-concept study. Platelets. 2013;24(3):235-8. Marksteiner J, Humpel C. Platelet-derived secreted amyloid-precursor protein-β as a marker for diagnosing Alzheimer's disease. Curr Neurovasc Res. 2013; 10(4) 297-303.

[88] Kuhn PH, Koroniak K, Hogl S, Colombo A, Zeitschel U, Willem M, Volbracht C, Schepers U, Imhof A, Hoffmeister A, Haass C, Roßner S, Bräse S, Lichtenthaler SF. Secretome protein enrichment identifies physiological BACE1 protease substrates in neurons. EMBO J. 2012; 31(14) 3157-68.

[89] Jorissen E, Prox J, Bernreuther C, Weber S, Schwanbeck R, Serneels L, Snellinx A, Craessaerts K, Thathiah A, Tesseur I, Bartsch U, Weskamp G, Blobel CP, Glatzel M, De Strooper B, Saftig P. The disintegrin/metalloproteinase ADAM10 is essential for the establishment of the brain cortex. J Neurosci. 2010; 30(14) 4833-44.

[90] Colciaghi F, Borroni B, Pastorino L, Marcello E, Zimmermann M, Cattabeni F, Padovani A, Di Luca M. [alpha]-Secretase ADAM10 as well as [alpha]APPs is reduced in platelets and CSF of Alzheimer disease patients. Mol Med. 2002; 8(2) 67-74.

[91] Manzine PR, de França Bram JM, Barham EJ, do Vale Fde A, Selistre-de-Araújo HS, Cominetti MR, Iost Pavarini SC. ADAM10 as a biomarker for Alzheimer's disease: a study with Brazilian elderly. Dement Geriatr Cogn Disord. 2013; 35(1-2) 58-66.

[92] Gorham P, Bark N, Björkhem I, Meaney S, Crisby M. Platelet alpha- and beta- secretase activities are not significantly affected by dementia or mild cognitive impairment in Swedish patients. Curr Alzheimer Res. 2010; 7(2) 134-139.

[93] Li QX, Fuller SJ, Beyreuther K, Masters CL. The amyloid precursor protein of Alzheimer disease in human brain and blood. J Leukoc Biol. 1999; 66(4) 567-574.

[94] Kokjohn TA, Van Vickle GD, Maarouf CL, Kalback WM, Hunter JM, Daugs ID, Luehrs DC, Lopez J, Brune D, Sue LI, Beach TG, Castaño EM, Roher AE. Chemical characterization of pro-inflammatory amyloid-beta peptides in human atherosclerotic lesions and platelets. Biochim Biophys Acta. 2011; 1812(11) 1508-1514.

[95] Skovronsky DM, Lee VM, Praticò D. Amyloid precursor protein and amyloid beta peptide in human platelets. Role of cyclooxygenase and protein kinase C. J Biol Chem. 2001; 276(20) 17036-17043.

[96] Casoli T, Di Stefano G, Giorgetti B, Grossi Y, Balietti M, Fattoretti P, Bertoni-Freddari C. Release of beta-amyloid from high-density platelets: implications for Alzheimer's disease pathology. Ann N Y Acad Sci. 2007; 1096 170-178.

[97] Casoli T, Di Stefano G, Giorgetti B, Balietti M, Recchioni R, Moroni F, Marcheselli F, Bernardini G, Fattoretti P, Bertoni-Freddari C. Platelet as a physiological model to investigate apoptotic mechanisms in Alzheimer beta-amyloid peptide production. Mech Ageing Dev. 2008; 129(3) 154-162.

[98] Corral-Debrinski M, Horton T, Lott MT, Shoffner JM, McKee AC, Beal MF, Graham BH, Wallace DC. Marked changes in mitochondrial DNA deletion levels in Alzheimer brains. Genomics. 1994; 23(2) 471-476.

[99] Hirai K, Aliev G, Nunomura A, Fujioka H, Russell RL, Atwood CS, Johnson AB, Kress Y, Vinters HV, Tabaton M, Shimohama S, Cash AD, Siedlak SL, Harris PL, Jones PK, Petersen RB, Perry G, Smith MA. Mitochondrial abnormalities in Alzheimer's disease. J Neurosci. 2001; 21(9) 3017-3023.

[100] Yan MH, Wang X, Zhu X. Mitochondrial defects and oxidative stress in Alzheimer disease and Parkinson disease. Free Radic Biol Med. 2013; 62 90-101.

[101] Wang X, Su B, Lee HG, Li X, Perry G, Smith MA, Zhu X. Impaired balance of mitochondrial fission and fusion in Alzheimer's disease. J Neurosci. 2009; 29(28) 9090-9103.

[102] Parker WD Jr, Filley CM, Parks JK. Cytochrome oxidase deficiency in Alzheimer's disease. Neurology. 1990; 40(8) 1302-1303.

[103] Parker WD Jr, Mahr NJ, Filley CM, Parks JK, Hughes D, Young DA, Cullum CM. Reduced platelet cytochrome c oxidase activity in Alzheimer's disease. Neurology. 1994; 44(6) 1086-1090.

[104] Bosetti F, Brizzi F, Barogi S, Mancuso M, Siciliano G, Tendi EA, Murri L, Rapoport SI, Solaini G. Cytochrome c oxidase and mitochondrial F1F0-ATPase (ATP synthase) activities in platelets and brain from patients with Alzheimer's disease. Neurobiol Aging. 2002; 23(3) 371-376.

[105] Valla J, Schneider L, Niedzielko T, Coon KD, Caselli R, Sabbagh MN, Ahern GL, Baxter L, Alexander G, Walker DG, Reiman EM. Impaired platelet mitochondrial activity in Alzheimer's disease and mild cognitive impairment. Mitochondrion. 2006; 6(6) 323-330.

[106] Crouch PJ, Blake R, Duce JA, Ciccotosto GD, Li QX, Barnham KJ, Curtain CC, Cherny RA, Cappai R, Dyrks T, Masters CL, Trounce IA. Copper-dependent inhibition of human cytochrome c oxidase by a dimeric conformer of amyloid-beta1-42. J Neurosci. 2005; 25(3) 672-9.

[107] Kawamoto EM, Munhoz CD, Glezer I, Bahia VS, Caramelli P, Nitrini R, Gorjão R, Curi R, Scavone C, Marcourakis T. Oxidative state in platelets and erythrocytes in aging and Alzheimer's disease. Neurobiol Aging. 2005; 26(6) 857-864.

[108] Vignini A, Nanetti L, Moroni C, Tanase L, Bartolini M, Luzzi S, Provinciali L, Mazzanti L. Modifications of platelet from Alzheimer disease patients: a possible relation between membrane properties and NO metabolites. Neurobiol Aging. 2007; 28(7) 987-994.

[109] Marcourakis T, Bahia VS, Kawamoto EM, Munhoz CD, Gorjão R, Artes R, Kok F, Caramelli P, Nitrini R, Curi R, Scavone C. Apolipoprotein E genotype is related to nitric oxide production in platelets. Cell Biochem Funct. 2008; 26(8) 852-858.

[110] Yu J, Jia JP. [Platelet function in patients with Alzheimer disease: analysis of 40 cases]. Zhonghua Yi Xue Za Zhi. 2009; 89(3) 183-186.

[111] Silva DF, Santana I, Esteves AR, Baldeiras I, Arduino DM, Oliveira CR, Cardoso SM. Prodromal metabolic phenotype in MCI cybrids: implications for Alzheimer's disease. Curr Alzheimer Res. 2013; 10(2) 180-190.

[112] Burbaeva GSh, Boksha IS, Savushkina OK, Turishcheva MS, Tereshkina EB, Starodubtseva LI, Gavrilova SI, Fedorova IaB, Zhuravin IA. [Platelet cytochrome c-oxidase and glutamine synthetase-like protein in patients with mild cognitive impairment]. Zh Nevrol Psikhiatr Im S S Korsakova. 2012; 112(2) 55-58.

[113] Parker WD Jr. Cytochrome oxidase deficiency in Alzheimer's disease. Ann N Y Acad Sci. 1991; 640 59-64.

[114] Mosconi L, de Leon M, Murray J, E L, Lu J, Javier E, McHugh P, Swerdlow RH. Reduced mitochondria cytochrome oxidase activity in adult children of mothers with Alzheimer's disease. J Alzheimers Dis. 2011; 27(3) 483-490.

[115] Van Zuylen AJ, Bosman GJ, Ruitenbeek W, Van Kalmthout PJ, De Grip WJ. No evidence for reduced thrombocyte cytochrome oxidase activity in Alzheimer's disease. Neurology. 1992; 42(6) 1246-1247.

[116] Adolfsson R, Gottfries CG, Oreland L, Wiberg A, Winblad B. Increased activity of brain and platelet monoamine oxidase in dementia of Alzheimer type. Life Sci. 1980; 27(12) 1029-1034.

[117] Götz ME, Fischer P, Gsell W, Riederer P, Streifler M, Simanyi M, Müller F, Danielczyk W. Platelet monoamine oxidase B activity in dementia. A 4-year follow-up. Dement Geriatr Cogn Disord. 1998; 9(2) 74-77.

[118] Bonuccelli U, Piccini P, Marazziti D, Cassano GB, Muratorio A. Increased platelet 3H-imipramine binding and monoamine oxidase B activity in Alzheimer's disease. J Neural Transm Park Dis Dement Sect. 1990; 2(2) 139-147.

[119] Parnetti L, Reboldi GP, Santucci C, Santucci A, Gaiti A, Brunetti M, Cecchetti R, Senin U. Platelet MAO-B activity as a marker of behavioural characteristics in dementia disorders. Aging (Milano). 1994; 6(3) 201-207.

[120] Zellner M, Baureder M, Rappold E, Bugert P, Kotzailias N, Babeluk R, Baumgartner R, Attems J, Gerner C, Jellinger K, Roth E, Oehler R, Umlauf E. Comparative platelet proteome analysis reveals an increase of monoamine oxidase-B protein expression in

Alzheimer's disease but not in non-demented Parkinson's disease patients. J Proteomics. 2012; 75(7) 2080-2092.

[121] Regland B, Gottfries CG, Oreland L. Vitamin B12-induced reduction of platelet monoamine oxidase activity in patients with dementia and pernicious anaemia. Eur Arch Psychiatry Clin Neurosci. 1991; 240(4-5) 288-291.

[122] Alexopoulos GS, Young RC, Lieberman KW, Shamoian CA. Platelet MAO activity in geriatric patients with depression and dementia. Am J Psychiatry. 1987; 144(11) 1480-1483.

[123] Soto J, Ulibarri I, Jauregui JV, Ballesteros J, Meana JJ. Dissociation between I2-imidazoline receptors and MAO-B activity in platelets of patients with Alzheimer's type dementia. J Psychiatr Res. 1999; 33(3) 251-257.

[124] Bongioanni P, Gemignani F, Boccardi B, Borgna M, Rossi B. Platelet monoamine oxidase molecular activity in demented patients. Ital J Neurol Sci. 1997; 18(3) 151-6.

[125] Danielczyk W, Streifler M, Konradi C, Riederer P, Moll G. Platelet MAO-B activity and the psychopathology of Parkinson's disease, senile dementia and multi-infarct dementia. Acta Psychiatr Scand. 1988; 78(6) 730-736.

[126] Schneider LS, Severson JA, Chui HC, Pollock VE, Sloane RB, Fredrickson ER. Platelet tritiated imipramine binding and MAO activity in Alzheimer's disease patients with agitation and delusions. Psychiatry Res. 1988; 25(3) 311-322.

[127] Konings CH, Scheltens P, Kuiper MA, Wolters EC. No evidence for abnormalities in kinetics of platelet monoamine oxidase in Alzheimer's disease. Clin Chim Acta. 1995; 240(1) 99-102.

[128] Ahlskog JE, Uitti RJ, Tyce GM, O'Brien JF, Petersen RC, Kokmen E. Plasma catechols and monoamine oxidase metabolites in untreated Parkinson's and Alzheimer's diseases. J Neurol Sci. 1996; 136(1-2) 162-168.

[129] Embi N, Rylatt DB, Cohen P. Glycogen synthase kinase-3 from rabbit skeletal muscle. Separation from cyclic-AMP-dependent protein kinase and phosphorylase kinase. Eur J Biochem. 1980; 107(2) 519-527.

[130] Chin PC, Majdzadeh N, D'Mello SR. Inhibition of GSK3beta is a common event in neuroprotection by different survival factors. Brain Res Mol Brain Res. 2005; 137(1-2) 193-201.

[131] Jope RS, Yuskaitis CJ, Beurel E. Glycogen synthase kinase-3 (GSK3): inflammation, diseases, and therapeutics. Neurochem Res. 2007; 32(4-5) 577-595.

[132] Grimes CA, Jope RS. The multifaceted roles of glycogen synthase kinase 3beta in cellular signaling. Prog Neurobiol. 2001; 65(4) 391-426.

[133] Muyllaert D, Kremer A, Jaworski T, Borghgraef P, Devijver H, Croes S, Dewachter I, Van Leuven F. Glycogen synthase kinase-3beta, or a link between amyloid and tau pathology? Genes Brain Behav. 2008; 7 Suppl 1 57-66.

[134] Barry FA, Graham GJ, Fry MJ, Gibbins JM. Regulation of glycogen synthase kinase 3 in human platelets: a possible role in platelet function? FEBS Lett. 2003; 553(1-2) 173-178.

[135] Forlenza OV, Torres CA, Talib LL, de Paula VJ, Joaquim HP, Diniz BS, Gattaz WF. Increased platelet GSK3B activity in patients with mild cognitive impairment and Alzheimer's disease. J Psychiatr Res. 2011; 45(2) 220-224.

[136] Matsushima H, Shimohama S, Fujimoto S, Takenawa T, Kimura J. Changes in platelet phospholipase C protein level and activity in Alzheimer's disease. Neurobiol Aging. 1995; 16(6) 895-900.

[137] Gattaz WF, Cairns NJ, Levy R, Förstl H, Braus DF, Maras A. Decreased phospholipase A2 activity in the brain and in platelets of patients with Alzheimer's disease. Eur Arch Psychiatry Clin Neurosci. 1996; 246(3) 129-131.

[138] Gattaz WF, Forlenza OV, Talib LL, Barbosa NR, Bottino CM. Platelet phospholipase A(2) activity in Alzheimer's disease and mild cognitive impairment. J Neural Transm. 2004; 111(5) 591-601.

[139] Talib LL, Yassuda MS, Diniz BS, Forlenza OV, Gattaz WF. Cognitive training increases platelet PLA2 activity in healthy elderly subjects. Prostaglandins Leukot Essent Fatty Acids. 2008; 78(4-5) 265-269.

[140] Krzystanek E, Krzystanek M, Opala G, Trzeciak HI, Siuda J, Małecki A. Platelet phospholipase A2 activity in patients with Alzheimer's disease, vascular dementia and ischemic stroke. J Neural Transm. 2007; 114(8) 1033-1039.

[141] Straface E, Matarrese P, Gambardella L, Vona R, Sgadari A, Silveri MC, Malorni W. Oxidative imbalance and cathepsin D changes as peripheral blood biomarkers of Alzheimer disease: a pilot study. FEBS Lett. 2005; 579(13) 2759-2766.

[142] Bongioanni P, Gemignani F, Boccardi B, Borgna M, Rossi B. Platelet monoamine oxidase molecular activity in demented patients. Ital J Neurol Sci. 1997 Jun;18(3): 151-156.

[143] Bongioanni P, Donato M, Castagna M, Gemignani F. Platelet phenolsulphotransferase activity, monoamine oxidase activity and peripheral-type benzodiazepine binding in demented patients. J Neural Transm. 1996; 103(4) 491-501.

[144] Humpel C. Identifying and validating biomarkers for Alzheimer's disease. Trends Biotechnol. 2011; 29(1) 26-32.

[145] Blennow K. CSF biomarkers for Alzheimer's disease: use in early diagnosis and evaluation of drug treatment. Expert Rev Mol Diagn. 2005; 5(5) 661-672.

[146] Marksteiner J, Hinterhuber H, Humpel C. Cerebrospinal fluid biomarkers for diagnosis of Alzheimer's disease: beta-amyloid(1-42), tau, phospho-tau-181 and total protein. Drugs Today (Barc). 2007; 43(6) 423-431.

[147] El Haouari M, Rosado JA. Platelet function in hypertension. Blood Cells Mol Dis. 2009; 42(1) 38-43.

[148] Li QX, Berndt MC, Bush AI, Rumble B, Mackenzie I, Friedhuber A, Beyreuther K, Masters CL. Membrane-associated forms of the beta A4 amyloid protein precursor of Alzheimer's disease in human platelet and brain: surface expression on the activated human platelet. Blood. 1994; 84(1) 133-142.

[149] Padovani A, Pastorino L, Borroni B, Colciaghi F, Rozzini L, Monastero R, Perez J, Pettenati C, Mussi M, Parrinello G, Cottini E, Lenzi GL, Trabucchi M, Cattabeni F, Di Luca M. Amyloid precursor protein in platelets: a peripheral marker for the diagnosis of sporadic AD. Neurology. 2001; 57(12) 2243-2248.

[150] Holmsen H. Signal transducing mechanisms in platelets. Proc Natl Sci Counc Repub China B. 1991; 15(3) 147-152.

Section 4

# Platelets in Tissue Regeneration and Wound Repair

Chapter 11

# Platelets in Tissue Regeneration

Ronaldo J. F. C. do Amaral and Alex Balduino

Additional information is available at the end of the chapter

http://dx.doi.org/10.5772/61184

## 1. Introduction

Platelets are especially well known for their thrombotic role. However, besides their role on stopping bleeding, platelets contribute for several mechanisms and steps in wound healing and tissue repair, such as inflammation, angiogenesis, cells proliferation, and differentiation. The potential of platelets to be used therapeutically to assist in wound repair led researchers around the world to look at platelet-based products and their capacity to promote tissue regeneration, *in vitro* and *in vivo*. In this chapter, we will discuss the main growth factors present in platelet granules that affect tissue regeneration. In addition, we will consider how platelet-derived products, such as those obtained from platelet-rich plasma (PRP), can be used to enhance tissue regeneration. We will review the applications of this knowledge in clinical trials, and *in vivo* models, as well as discussing the capacity for platelet products to substitute for classical components of media for *in vitro* cell culture.

## 2. Tissue repair related growth factors in platelets granules

Approximately, one trillion platelets circulate in the bloodstream of a human adult (4 liters of blood at $3X10^8$ platelets / ml). Platelets have a lifespan of approximately 10 days. They are synthesized by megakaryocytic cells in the bone marrow of long bones and approximately 10% are replenished daily. "Old" and damaged platelets are cleared from the blood by phagocytes in the liver and the spleen [1]. While in the circulation, platelets survey the vasculature for evidence of damage. If damage is perceived, they participate in hemostatic events. When platelets are activated upon vascular injury, they change their discoid form to a more spherical morphology with pseudopods, and they release their granular content [2]. Those are not only related to the coagulation process and hemostasis, but also to tissue repair. The granules are of 3 different types: $\alpha$-granules, dense granules, and lysosymes. $\alpha$-granules are the most abundant granule-type in human platelets (50-80 per platelet) and contain a diverse protein repertoire [3] including a variety of molecules with biological activity (Table 1). These molecules are released following platelet activation and play important functional roles at sites of vascular damage.

| CATEGORY | MOLECULE |
|---|---|
| GROWTH FACTORS | TGF-β (transforming growth factor beta)<br>PDGF (platelet-derived growth factor)<br>FGF (fibroblast growth factor)<br>EGF (epidermal growth fator)<br>VEGF (vascular endothelial growth factor) |
| ADHESION PROTEINS | Fibrinogen<br>Fibronectin<br>Vitronectin<br>Trombospondin-1 |
| COAGULATION FACTORS | Factor V<br>Factor IX<br>Protein S<br>Anti-thrombin |
| FIBRINOLYTIC FATORS | Plasminogen<br>Plasminogen activatior inhibitor<br>α-2 antiplasmin |
| PROTEASES AND ANTIPROTEASES | TIMP-4(*tissue inhibitor of metalloprotease-4)*<br>Metaloprotease-4<br>α-1-antitripsin |
| MEMBRANE GLYCOPROTEINS | CD40-L<br>P-selectin |
| OTHER PROTEINS | PF-4 (*platelet factor 4*)<br>Endostatins<br>β-tromboglobulins |

**Table 1.** Main bioactive molecules present in platelets alpha granules Adapted from [4].

Many platelet-derived bioactive proteins play critical roles in inflammation, angiogenesis and wound healing. For example, TGF-β1, the most abundant isoform of TGF-β present in platelets, has an important role in all wound healing phases. It coordinates multiple pathophysiological events including the initial recruitment of inflammatory cells to a site of injury, angiogenesis, re-epitheliazation following damage, and the induction of extracellular matrix production by fibroblasts [5]. PDGF is a chemoattractant molecule for fibroblasts and smooth muscle cells, as well as an inducer of proliferation of mesenchymal cells [6]. FGF-2, the main FGF isoform present in platelets, promotes angiogenesis by supporting

http://dx.doi.org/10.5772/61184

endothelial cell growth [7]. It is also a potent fibroblast mitogen and induces hyaluronic acid synthesis to facilitate a scarless wound healing [8]. EGF enables mesenchymal cells proliferation, chemotaxis and cytoprotection [9]. VEGF is a pro-angiogenic biomolecule that stimulates blood vessel formation [10], and expression of adhesion proteins that enhance leukocyte adhesion [11]. In fact, a total of more than 300 bioactive agents have been identified that are released from activated platelets [12]. These agents differ in their origin with some components being synthesized in the parent megakaryocyte while others are scavenged from plasma and concentrated in platelet granules [13].

Dense granules contain factors related to platelet activation, such as $Ca^{2+}$ and ADP, serotonin, histamine, dopamine, and catecolamines. Local release of these components, in response to platelet activation or thrombotic events, results in altered recruitment of inflammatory cell types and altered vascular permeability [14]. Finally, lysosomes contain hydrolytic enzymes and catalases [15]. The nature of the contents of the platelet granules are summarised in MItrugno et al (2015) in this publication.

Platelet activation, with concomitant release of granular contents, happens in parallel with coagulation or thrombosis. The natural participation of platelets and in hemostasis and tissue repair has led to the development of products that could help in those processes.

Due to the variety of possible uses and number of studies, PRP is perhaps the main platelet based product investigated for tissue regeneration purposes. PRP is a platelet concentrate in a small volume of plasma obtained after a centrifugal spin of whole blood to remove red cells and while cells. Regular platelet concentration in peripheral blood is 150-350 x $10^6$ per milliliter. In the context of tissue engineering and wound repair, the term PRP refers to a platelet concentration in plasma above this regular range, that can be injected into a wound site to affect or accelerate repair. The clinical use of PRP, mainly in the cases of bone and soft tissue regeneration, presents a platelet concentration of at least $10^9$ per milliliter, which is around 5 times higher than physiological levels [16]. For peri-implant bone regeneration, for example, the recommended platelet concentration is approximately $10^9$ per milliliter. In lower concentrations the effect is suboptimal and in higher it is inhibitory [17].

The therapeutic action of platelet concentrates derives from the release of factors involved in tissue repair upon platelet activation. The clot that is formed during that activation may also play a role of a temporary extracellular matrix which will allow cells proliferation and differentiation [16]. In that case, an elevated platelet concentration would be expected to generate an elevated local concentration of released bioactive factors. However the correlation between the platelet concentration and the concentration of released bioactive agents may not be exact, due to variations between blood donors [18], or between platelet preparation methods [19]. Moreover, some growth factors that act in tissue repair are also present in plasma. Such growth factors include HGF and IGF-1. Consequently, the concentrations of these factors at sites of wounds may only be slightly altered according to the platelet concentration [20]. Generally, it is considered that a platelet concentration 5 times higher than in peripheral blood can lead to an enhanced local concentration of growth factors that varies from 3 to 5 times in excess of normal pathophysiological levels [4]. Thus, by serving as a reservoir of concentrated growth factors involved in cell proliferation and differentiation, platelet concentrates can contribute to tissue growth and repair. In a similar manner, platelet-derived bioactive products may find use in cell culture protocols.

## 3. How platelet products can improve cell culture

Since the beginning of cell culture techniques, many innovations were designed to optimize the process of cell expansion *in vitro*, analyzing their differentiation capacity, as well as their response to chemicals and promising pharmaceutical molecules. With time, the field improved. Plastics, glasses, bioreactors and engineering technology evolved a lot, at the same time that the biological field also evolved.

Methods to grow cells *in vitro* try to reproduce appropriately all physiological conditions that are observed *in vivo*, and try to mimic it *in vitro*. The culture medium is the source of soluble factors that will enable cell growth and survival. Classical cell culture media are comprised of a basal balanced salt solution such as MEM (Eagle's minimal essential medium), DMEM (Dulbecco's modified Eagle's medium), IMDM (Iscove's modified DMEM), RPMI (Roswell Park Memorial Institute medium), Medium-199, HamF12 and McCoy's medium. Although they provide inorganic salts, amino acids, vitamins and glucose, a protein-rich supplement is required to provide growth factors. Traditionally, Fetal Bovine Serum (FBS) is added to the basal medium [21] as the main source of growth factors to stimulate cell proliferation; FBS contains transport proteins carrying hormones (e.g. transcortin), minerals, trace elements (e.g. transferrin), and lipids (e.g. lipoproteins). In addition, FBS contain attachment and spreading factors, acting as germination points for cell attachment; and stabilizing and detoxifying factors needed to maintain pH or to inhibit proteases either directly, such as $\alpha$-antitrypsin or $\alpha$2-macroglobulin, or indirectly, by acting as an unspecific sink for proteases and other (toxic) molecules [22]. FBS is obtained by cardiac puncture of bovine fetuses without anaesthesia. Jochems strongly discussed the ethical issues on the use of FBS. The use of cell culture is strongly recommended as an alternative to animal experimentation. However, the requirement for FBS, obtained from animal sources, end up making the concept of cell culture as an alternative to animal experimentation somewhat unethical [23].

Besides the ethical issues, scientific issues are also pointed on the use of FBS. Firstly, lot-to-lot variations make it necessary to test samples before purchase, as its molecular composition of FBS may vary [24]. FBS might interfere with cells genotype and phenotype, influencing experimental outcome. For example, it can promote cell proliferation in fibroblasts, whilst inhibiting it in epithelial cells [25]. It can be contaminated with viruses, bacteria, mycoplasmas, yeast, fungi, immunoglobulins, endotoxins, and possibly prions [26], contraindicating it for use for cells that would be further transplanted into humans. FBS is not totally chemically defined, as many substances present in it have not yet been characterized [27], some don't have their function fully elucidated, and others may even be toxic [28].

Serum, obtained from clotted whole blood, is known to be more suitable to cell culture than plasma from the same organism; despite the difficulty in obtaining it in large quantities. This is likely to be due to the release of proteins and growth factors from activated platelets during the clotting process [29], [30].Therefore, PRP, platelet lysates and other platelet-derived products can substitute FBS in cell culture. As the platelets are present in an elevated concentration, the growth factors important for cell culture are also more concentrated, as already discussed in this chapter. Finally, platelets can be easily obtained from human sources and therefore better mimic the effects of serum in human cells. Thinking of cell therapy, it can be used for growing cells that would be later transplanted into humans, especially when in an autologous approach.

## 4. How platelets can be used to improve tissue repair

Platelet concentrates, with the concentration of 5 $x10^{10}$ platelets / unit are usually used for the treatment and prevention of severe hemorrhage [31]. The use of blood products for wound closure and stimulation of repair, such as fibrin glues, was first described in the 1970s [32]. The platelet gel emerged in the 1990s as a cheaper and autologous alternative compared to fibrin glues [33]. In 1987, PRP emerged as a product of autologous transfusion after open heart surgery, to prevent the need for a homologous product [34]. In 1998, Marx et al. described the use of platelets as an accelerator of tissue repair/regeneration, in that case bone formation in bone grafts for maxillofacial surgery [35].

Since then, most of the studies have shown an increase in bone repair, musculoskeletal tissues (muscles, tendons, and cartilage) and other "soft" tissues when platelet concentrates are used [36]. In the case of bone repair in maxillofacial surgery, the use of a platelet product efficacy and safety have been proven. In that case, only 9 out of 1,287 maxillae and mandible short implants (<8,5mm) from 661 patients between 2001 and 2008 had been lost. All implants had been embedded in liquid PRGF (plasma-rich in growth fators). Briefly, PRGF is obtained by centrifugation of whole blood collected in 9ml tubes containing sodium citrate at 580 x g for 8 minutes. Next, the 1ml fraction above red cell fraction is collected and activated with calcium chloride [37]. Although platelet products lack osteoinductive factors as BMPs, they can enhance bone formation. When PRP is added to human autogenous bone grafts, the bone density is higher, higher the proportion of mature bone and lesser osteoclast resorption, compared to size and age-matched grafts without PRP after 4 months of surgery [36]. Human PRP with the presence of peripheral blood mononucleated cells had its angiogenic properties proven in a nude animal model of critical size calvarial defect. Moreover, when it has been used synergistically with BMP-2, the effect on bone healing was augmented, as observed by histology, bone mineral density and bone mineral content after 8 weeks of implantation [38]. As said before, the induction of bone regeneration is more effective when PRP is used with approximately 1 million platelets per microliter. This was shown in a study where femurs of New Zealand white rabbits receiving an titanium implant where treated or not with autologous PRP. Lower concentrations than 1 million platelets per microliter resulted in suboptimal peri-implant bone formation, whereas higher concentrations caused an inhibitory effect [17]. In addition, mesenchymal cells treated with PRP are also able to promote better repair and bone maturation in mandibular bone defects models, being pointed as an alternative to autogenous grafts. This has been shown when bone defects of canine mandible were filled with autologous PRP gel, autologous PRP gel with bone-marrow MSCs or autogenous particulate cancellous bone and marrow (PCBM). Briefly, PRP was obtained by 50mL blood collection in heparin, followed by two centrifugation steps which resulted in platelet concentration 438% above baseline. PRP activation was performed by adding thrombin/calcium solution. Increased bone formation and neovascularization was observed in the PRP plus MSC group. [39].

In muscle injuries, some factors present in PRP such as IGF-1 and bFGF can accelerate tissue repair. In contrast, TGF-β may lead to a fibrotic repair, increasing the possibility of the recurrence of new lesions [40]. Although mice with muscular injuries have demonstrated functional improvement when treated with high-frequency ultrasound-treated PRP, in order to lyse platelets and release of growth factor [41]. A preliminary study on muscle strain injuries in professional sportsman showed significant increase in the recovery time from injury when treated with autologous conditioned serum (ACS). ACS was obtained by blood collection without anti-coagulants followed by incubation and centrifugation for the retrieving of the serum [42]. Nonetheless, the action of PRP in muscle injuries still requires further investigation [43]. The first double-blinded, randomized, placebo controlled PRP clinical study on acute muscle injury, did not confirm the benefits for the use of PRP to enable the return to sports activities by athletes. In this case, PRP was prepared using a commercially available system (Arthrex double syringe ACP system) according to the manufacturer's instructions, and apparently was not activated prior to injection [44]. However, the methodology used in this work has been questioned, due to delayed administration and low dosage of PRP injections. The authors replied that there is no consensus on time of PRP injections, as well as that their PRP preparation method was in accordance with the literature [45].

Animal studies [46], [47] and human trials in tendon injuries show positive results through the use of PRP [48]–[50]. Although clinical trials with appropriate methodologies have not yet proven the effectiveness of PRP in this type of injury [51], localized platelet delivery can induce mobilization of circulating cells to sites of rat tendon injuries with concomitant increase in collagen synthesis [52]. *In vitro*, platelets can induce proliferation, collagen synthesis [53] and release of angiogenic factors in human tenocytes [54].A systematic review stated there were strong evidence against PRP injection for chronic lateral epicondylar tendinopathy. In a total of 6 studies, 5 showed no significant benefit at the final follow-up, while 1 presented benefits for PRP injections compared to corticosteroid injection [55]. However, the results presented in that review have been questioned [56]. Surprisingly, another systematic review, selecting 9 studies, concluded there was limited but evolving evidence to support PRP injections in lateral epicondylitis, suggesting that further studies regarding the preparation of PRP as well as the timing of the interventions are needed [57].

Cartilage, as an avascular tissue, and so injuries are usually critical and difficult to repair. Consequently, there is a need for new regenerative methods to address the specific demands imposed by cartilaginous injuries [58]. In 2003, PRGF was first used in a case of cartilaginous avulsion in a football player, causing an accelerated and rapid repair, which enabled the athlete's earlier return to sport activities [59]. Intra-articular PRP injections in patients with chronic cartilage degeneration also demonstrated positive results evaluated by clinical score methods as IKDC and EQ-VAS. In those studies, PRP was prepared by two-centrifugation steps which increased platelet concentration of 600% comparing to whole blood counting, and was activated by calcium solution prior to injection [60], [61]. On the other hand, *in vitro* analyses on chondrocytes proliferation and chondrogenic induction generated controversial results in the literature: In general, PRP induced chondrocyte proliferation [62]. Regarding chondrogenic induction, PRP appeared as an inducer [63], [64], while contradictory results showing the promotion of fibrogenic phenotype have also been observed [65], [66]. These antitheses may be related to different methodologies for PRP production, and therefore requires a better assessment of the PRP effect on chondrogenic cells.

PRP has also shown to induce mesenchymal stem cells (MSCs) proliferation. Regarding induction of osteogenesis on MSCs, mouse MSCs were treated with activated by thrombin/ calcium solution human PRP or washed platelets (WPLT), where the platelets had been suspended in phosphate saline rather than plasma, with equal platelets concentration, 4 times above the baseline. Interestingly, both stimulated cells proliferation in earlier time points, while WPLT induced higher proliferation than PRP in later time points. Alternatively, ALP activity and collagen type I expression, those indicatives of osteogenic differentiation, were increased in PRP rather than WPLT [67]. In others studies, PRP gel could induce osteocalcin and collagen type 1 expression in rat MSC [68], as well as activated PRP, with platelet concentration 4 times higher the baseline, induced greater human MSC mineralization [69]. Interestingly, when the growth factors present in PRP are released in a controlled manner, through the association of PRP with alginate hydrogel, human MSCs alkaline phosphatase activity is induced [70]. As for chondrogenic induction *in vitro*, mRNA levels for aggrecan, Sox-9, and Runx2 were increased in buffered, i.e. inactivated, PRP treated human MSCs [71]. Subchondral bone MSCs cultured in a 3D model also showed chondrogenic potential induced by PRP (activated by freezing and thawing process), but not osteogenic or adipogenic [72]. Moreover, PRP associated with MSCs was able to induce chondrogenesis *in vitro* and *in vivo* in full-thickness rabbit articular cartilage injury model [73]. Recently, a systematic review selected 27 articles analyzing the role of PRP on MSCs in vitro proliferation and differentiation, in comparison to FBS. It has been seen that PRP stimulates cells proliferation, preserves their immunomodulatory capacity and may delay the acquirement of a senescent phenotype. The majority of the studies also showed that PRP maintains cells adipogenic, osteogenic and chondrogenic differentiation capacity, in fewer cases enhanced it, while in rare cases diminished the adipogenic differentiation capacity [74].

Platelets have been shown to play an important role in the repair of many different tissues such as skin [75], nervous tissue [76], corneal [77], myocardial [78], and vascular [79]. In addition, platelet-derived products demonstrate distinct antimicrobial effects [80], and contribute to orthopedic repair [81] and plastic surgery applications [82]. It is worth noting the potential for therapeutic effects in sports medicine, as the need for elite athletes to recover quickly from injuries and achieve their regular level of efficiency is huge. PRP use is currently allowed by the global anti-doping agency [83].

There have been no reports of serious health problems arising after the therapeutic use of PRP so far, but despite evidence demonstrating its positive effects, especially in repair of musculoskeletal injuries, there are few published clinical studies, and even smaller the number of works with sufficient methodological quality to ensure evidence-based decision-making use of PRP [43]. Likewise, there is still a need for basic studies to better understand some still open issues, such as the optimal concentration of platelets, the harm or the benefits of the presence of leukocytes, a possible combination of recombinant proteins with PRP [15] and analysis of its action at the cellular level.

## 5. The need of standardization

Due to the variety of protocols, many classifications are used to characterize platelet preparations for tissue engineering purposes. Many groups refer generically to platelets used in tissue engineering applications as Platelet-Rich Plasma (PRP). However, this can cause confusion, since many biomedical researchers use the PRP abbreviation to refer to a simple enrichment by centrifugation of whole blood to remove red blood cells and leukocytes. Nonetheless, tissue engineers have adopted the term PRP to refer to platelet concentrates that can be re-injected to a site of tissue injury with or without modification or activation. Moreover, additional acronyms are used to sub classify the platelet preparations used in tissue injury-studies. Among these classifications, we can find: PDWHF (platelet derived wound healing factors) [84], L- PRP (leukocyte and platelet - rich plasma) [85], PRFM (plasma rich fibrin matrix) [86], PRGF (plasma rich in growth factors) [87], among others.

Likewise, the PRP gel preparation used in tissue engineering applications cannot be referred to as a " fibrin glue", as the clot formed in the PRP activation contain the same components and at similar concentrations to that found in a native blood clot and consists primarily of fibrin, fibronectin and vitronectin, besides the bioactive molecules. The fibrin glue is only considered a concentrate of fibrinogen, which is polymerized by thrombin and calcium [16]. This platelet gel was originally used as a substitute to fibrin glue in oral and maxillofacial surgery [33]. It was also used in cutaneous chronic wounds [88], including diabetic ulcers [89], degenerative disorders of the knee [90], gynecologic, cardiac, and general surgical procedures [91].

Various commercial systems for the preparation of autologous platelet products for local injection into wound sites have been developed. Among the main ones are: SmartPrep ® 2APC +TM (Harvest Technologies), Biomet GPS III ® (Biomet Manufacturing Corp.), Arthrex ACP ® (Arthrex Inc), Cascade ® platelet - rich fibrin matrix (Musculoskeletal Trasnplant Foundation), Cascade ® platelet - rich plasma therapy (Musculoskeletal Trasnplant Foundation), BTI plasma rich in growth factors (PRGF) (Biotechnology Institute) and Magellan ® Autologous Platelet Separator System (Arteriocyte) [92]. Despite such variety, the basic formulation of PRP consists of primarily autologous blood collection in the presence of anticoagulants. After collection, the blood is centrifuged once or twice in order to separate the plasma with platelets from erythrocytes and leukocytes and concentrate them. After the second centrifugation, part of the plasma is used to resuspend the platelet concentrate, formulating the final PRP. The portion of the plasma that is not used in this ressupension is commonly described as platelet-

http://dx.doi.org/10.5772/61184

poor plasma (PPP). The release of growth factors contained in platelets granules occurs following activation of the PRP with exogenous thrombin, collagen, or calcium chloride, forming a clot. Some methodologies also may use freeze-thawing cycles or sonication by ultrasound treatment in order to disrupt platelets membrane and release of the growth factors. In other cases, platelets may not be activated at all. Calcium chloride is important to enable fibrin polymerization and thrombin generation by the endogenous coagulation cascade. The final product, i.e. the supernatant liquid without the clot, is actually a serum derived from PRP [4]. Both commercial and non-commercial forms may vary on the speed and number of centrifugation steps to concentrate the platelets, the usage or not of anticoagulant, the type of anticoagulant, the presence of leukocytes, which may release matrix metalloproteinase and reactive oxygen species that can increase tissue damage, and the substance that will induce platelet activation. In the end, these variations generate diversity in types, concentration and speed of the release of growth factors, which may explain different results among papers [93]. In order to normalize and standardize platelets products for tissue engineering purposes, mainly by the platelet concentration, activation (whether it occurs or not an how), and presence of white blood cells, some classification systems have been proposed [83], [94].In summary, platelets act as reservoirs of growth factors and bioactive agents. The localized application of concentrated preparations of these reagents from autologous platelet donations appears to facilitate and accelerate wound healing and tissue repair. Some controversy exists as to the effectiveness of this treatment. However, significant variations in the platelet preparations, mainly platelet concentration and activation, may explain some or all of the variations.

## Author details

Ronaldo J. F. C. do Amaral[1,2] and Alex Balduino[2,3*]

*Address all correspondence to: alex.balduino@excellion.com.br

1 Universidade Federal do Rio de Janeiro, RJ, Brazil

2 Excellion Labs AMIL/UnitedHealth Group, RJ, Brazil

3 Laboratório de Biologia e Tecnologia Celular, Universidade Veiga de Almeida, RJ, Brazil

## References

[1] J. E. Kaplan and T. M. Saba, "Platelet removal from the circulation by the liver and spleen.," *Am. J. Physiol.*, vol. 235, no. 3, pp. H314–20, Sep. 1978.

[2] J. W. M. Heemskerk, E. M. Bevers, and T. Lindhout, "Platelet activation and blood coagulation.," *Thromb. Haemost.*, vol. 88, no. 2, pp. 186–93, Aug. 2002.

[3] A. Zufferey, D. Schvartz, S. Nolli, J.-L. Reny, J.-C. Sanchez, and P. Fontana, "Characterization of the platelet granule proteome: evidence of the presence of MHC1 in alpha-granules.," *J. Proteomics*, vol. 101, pp. 130–40, Apr. 2014.

[4] T. E. Foster, B. L. Puskas, B. R. Mandelbaum, M. B. Gerhardt, and S. a Rodeo, "Platelet-rich plasma: from basic science to clinical applications.," *Am. J. Sports Med.*, vol. 37, no. 11, pp. 2259–72, Nov. 2009.

[5] M. Pakyari, A. Farrokhi, M. K. Maharlooei, and A. Ghahary, "Critical Role of Transforming Growth Factor Beta in Different Phases of Wound Healing.," *Adv. wound care*, vol. 2, no. 5, pp. 215–224, Jul. 2013.

[6] J. Donovan, D. Abraham, and J. Norman, "Platelet-derived growth factor signaling in mesenchymal cells.," *Front. Biosci. (Landmark Ed.*, vol. 18, pp. 106–19, Jan. 2013.

[7] A. Sahni, O. D. Altland, and C. W. Francis, "FGF-2 but not FGF-1 binds fibrin and supports prolonged endothelial cell growth.," *J. Thromb. Haemost.*, vol. 1, no. 6, pp. 1304–10, Jun. 2003.

[8] S. Akita, K. Akino, and A. Hirano, "Basic Fibroblast Growth Factor in Scarless Wound Healing.," *Adv. wound care*, vol. 2, no. 2, pp. 44–49, Mar. 2013.

[9] J. Berlanga-Acosta, J. Gavilondo-Cowley, P. López-Saura, T. González-López, M. D. Castro-Santana, E. López-Mola, G. Guillén-Nieto, and L. Herrera-Martinez, "Epidermal growth factor in clinical practice - a review of its biological actions, clinical indications and safety implications.," *Int. Wound J.*, vol. 6, no. 5, pp. 331–46, Oct. 2009.

[10] D. I. R. Holmes and I. Zachary, "The vascular endothelial growth factor (VEGF) family: angiogenic factors in health and disease.," *Genome Biol.*, vol. 6, no. 2, p. 209, Jan. 2005.

[11] J.-K. Min, Y.-M. Lee, J. H. Kim, Y.-M. Kim, S. W. Kim, S.-Y. Lee, Y. S. Gho, G. T. Oh, and Y.-G. Kwon, "Hepatocyte growth factor suppresses vascular endothelial growth factor-induced expression of endothelial ICAM-1 and VCAM-1 by inhibiting the nuclear factor-kappaB pathway.," *Circ. Res.*, vol. 96, no. 3, pp. 300–7, Feb. 2005.

[12] J. A. Coppinger, G. Cagney, S. Toomey, T. Kislinger, O. Belton, J. P. McRedmond, D. J. Cahill, A. Emili, D. J. Fitzgerald, and P. B. Maguire, "Characterization of the proteins released from activated platelets leads to localization of novel platelet proteins in human atherosclerotic lesions.," *Blood*, vol. 103, no. 6, pp. 2096–104, Mar. 2004.

[13] S. W. Whiteheart, "Platelet granules: surprise packages.," *Blood*, vol. 118, no. 5, pp. 1190–1, Aug. 2011.

[14] D. Schumacher, B. Strilic, K. K. Sivaraj, N. Wettschureck, and S. Offermanns, "Platelet-derived nucleotides promote tumor-cell transendothelial migration and metastasis via P2Y2 receptor.," *Cancer Cell*, vol. 24, no. 1, pp. 130–7, Jul. 2013.

[15] A. T. Nurden, P. Nurden, M. Sanchez, I. Andia, and E. Anitua, "Platelets and wound healing.," *Front. Biosci.*, vol. 13, pp. 3532–48, Jan. 2008.

[16] R. E. Marx, "Platelet-rich plasma (PRP): what is PRP and what is not PRP?," *Implant Dent.*, vol. 10, no. 4, pp. 225–8, Jan. 2001.

[17] G. Weibrich, T. Hansen, W. Kleis, R. Buch, and W. E. Hitzler, "Effect of platelet concentration in platelet-rich plasma on peri-implant bone regeneration.," *Bone*, vol. 34, no. 4, pp. 665–71, Apr. 2004.

[18] B. L. Eppley, J. E. Woodell, and J. Higgins, "Platelet Quantification and Growth Factor Analysis from Platelet-Rich Plasma: Implications for Wound Healing," *Plast. Reconstr. Surg.*, pp. 1502–1508, Nov. 2004.

[19] R. Zimmermann, R. Jakubietz, M. Jakubietz, E. Strasser, A. Schlegel, J. Wiltfang, and R. Eckstein, "Different preparation methods to obtain platelet components as a source of growth factors for local application.," *Transfusion*, vol. 41, no. 10, pp. 1217–24, Oct. 2001.

[20] E. Anitua, M. Sánchez, M. M. Zalduendo, M. de la Fuente, R. Prado, G. Orive, and I. Andía, "Fibroblastic response to treatment with different preparations rich in growth factors.," *Cell Prolif.*, vol. 42, no. 2, pp. 162–70, Apr. 2009.

[21] Z. Yang and H. Xiong, "Culture Conditions and Types of Growth Media for Mammalian Cells," *Biomed. Tissue Cult.*, pp. 3–18, 2012.

[22] D. Brunner, J. Frank, H. Appl, H. Schöffl, W. Pfaller, and G. Gstraunthaler, "Serum-free cell culture: the serum-free media interactive online database.," *ALTEX*, vol. 27, no. 1, pp. 53–62, Jan. 2010.

[23] C. E. a Jochems, J. B. F. van der Valk, F. R. Stafleu, and V. Baumans, "The use of fetal bovine serum: ethical or scientific problem?," *Altern. Lab. Anim.*, vol. 30, no. 2, pp. 219–27, 2002.

[24] K. V. Honn, J. A. Singley, and W. Chavin, "Fetal Bovine Serum: A Multivariate Standard," *Exp. Biol. Med.*, vol. 149, no. 2, pp. 344–347, Jun. 1975.

[25] P. A. Knepper, C. S. Mayanil, W. Goossens, D. C. McLone, and E. Hayes, "The presence of transcription factors in fetal bovine sera.," *In Vitro Cell. Dev. Biol. Anim.*, vol. 34, no. 2, pp. 170–3, Feb. 1998.

[26] J. Hodgson, "Fetal Bovine Serum Revisited," *Bio/Technology*, vol. 11, no. 1, pp. 49–53, Jan. 1993.

[27] Y. Pan, P. K. Bender, R. M. Akers, and K. E. Webb, "One or more serum factors promote peptide utilization in cultured animal cells.," *J. Nutr.*, vol. 128, no. 4, pp. 744–50, Apr. 1998.

[28] D. Barnes and G. Sato, "Serum-free cell culture: a unifying approach," *Cell*, vol. 22, no. 3, pp. 649–655, Dec. 1980.

[29] S. D. Balk, S. P. Levine, L. L. Young, M. M. LaFleur, and N. M. Raymond, "Mitogenic factors present in serum but not in plasma.," *Proc. Natl. Acad. Sci. U. S. A.*, vol. 78, no. 9, pp. 5656–60, Sep. 1981.

[30] D. Gospodarowicz and C. R. Ill, "Do plasma and serum have different abilities to promote cell growth?," *Proc. Natl. Acad. Sci. U. S. A.*, vol. 77, no. 5, pp. 2726–30, May 1980.

[31] D. M. Dohan Ehrenfest, L. Rasmusson, and T. Albrektsson, "Classification of platelet concentrates: from pure platelet-rich plasma (P-PRP) to leucocyte- and platelet-rich fibrin (L-PRF).," *Trends Biotechnol.*, vol. 27, no. 3, pp. 158–67, Mar. 2009.

[32] H. Matras, "Fibrin seal: the state of the art.," *J. Oral Maxillofac. Surg.*, vol. 43, no. 8, pp. 605–11, Aug. 1985.

[33] D. H. Whitman, R. L. Berry, and D. M. Green, "Platelet gel: an autologous alternative to fibrin glue with applications in oral and maxillofacial surgery.," *J. Oral Maxillofac. Surg.*, vol. 55, no. 11, pp. 1294–9, Nov. 1997.

[34] M. Ferrari, S. Zia, M. Valbonesi, F. Henriquet, G. Venere, S. Spagnolo, M. A. Grasso, and I. Panzani, "A new technique for hemodilution, preparation of autologous platelet-rich plasma and intraoperative blood salvage in cardiac surgery.," *Int. J. Artif. Organs*, vol. 10, no. 1, pp. 47–50, Jan. 1987.

[35] R. E. Marx, E. R. Carlson, R. M. Eichstaedt, S. R. Schimmele, J. E. Strauss, and K. R. Georgeff, "Platelet-rich plasma: Growth factor enhancement for bone grafts.," *Oral Surg. Oral Med. Oral Pathol. Oral Radiol. Endod.*, vol. 85, no. 6, pp. 638–46, Jun. 1998.

[36] R. E. Marx, "Platelet-rich plasma: evidence to support its use," *J. Oral Maxillofac. Surg.*, vol. 62, no. 4, pp. 489–496, Apr. 2004.

[37] E. Anitua and G. Orive, "Short Implants in Maxillae and Mandibles: A Retrospective Study With 1 to 8 Years of Follow-Up," *J. Periodontol.*, vol. 81, no. 6, pp. 819–826, Jun. 2010.

[38] E.-J. Park, E.-S. Kim, H.-P. Weber, R. F. Wright, and D. J. Mooney, "Improved bone healing by angiogenic factor-enriched platelet-rich plasma and its synergistic enhancement by bone morphogenetic protein-2.," *Int. J. Oral Maxillofac. Implants*, vol. 23, no. 5, pp. 818–26, Jan. 2008.

[39] Y. Yamada, M. Ueda, T. Naiki, M. Takahashi, K.-I. Hata, and T. Nagasaka, "Autogenous injectable bone for regeneration with mesenchymal stem cells and platelet-rich plasma: tissue-engineered bone regeneration.," *Tissue Eng.*, vol. 10, no. 5–6, pp. 955–964, 2004.

[40] J. Menetrey, C. Kasemkijwattana, C. S. Day, P. Bosch, M. Vogt, F. H. Fu, M. S. Moreland, and J. Huard, "Growth factors improve muscle healing in vivo.," *J. Bone Joint Surg. Br.*, vol. 82, no. 1, pp. 131–7, Jan. 2000.

[41] J. W. Hammond, R. Y. Hinton, L. A. Curl, J. M. Muriel, and R. M. Lovering, "Use of autologous platelet-rich plasma to treat muscle strain injuries.," *Am. J. Sports Med.*, vol. 37, no. 6, pp. 1135–42, Jun. 2009.

[42] T. Wright-Carpenter, P. Klein, P. Schäferhoff, H. J. Appell, L. M. Mir, and P. Wehling, "Treatment of muscle injuries by local administration of autologous conditioned serum: a pilot study on sportsmen with muscle strains.," *Int. J. Sports Med.*, vol. 25, no. 8, pp. 588–93, Nov. 2004.

[43] L. Engebretsen, K. Steffen, J. Alsousou, E. Anitua, N. Bachl, R. Devilee, P. Everts, B. Hamilton, J. Huard, P. Jenoure, F. Kelberine, E. Kon, N. Maffulli, G. Matheson, O. Mei-Dan, J. Menetrey, M. Philippon, P. Randelli, P. Schamasch, M. Schwellnus, A. Vernec, and G. Verrall, "IOC consensus paper on the use of platelet-rich plasma in sports medicine.," *Br. J. Sports Med.*, vol. 44, no. 15, pp. 1072–81, Dec. 2010.

[44] G. Reurink, G. J. Goudswaard, M. H. Moen, A. Weir, J. A. N. Verhaar, S. M. A. Bierma-Zeinstra, M. Maas, and J. L. Tol, "Platelet-rich plasma injections in acute muscle injury.," *N. Engl. J. Med.*, vol. 370, no. 26, pp. 2546–7, Jun. 2014.

[45] E. Anitua, M. Sánchez, and S. Padilla, "More on platelet-rich plasma injections in acute muscle injury.," *N. Engl. J. Med.*, vol. 371, no. 13, p. 1264, Sep. 2014.

[46] P. Aspenberg and O. Virchenko, "Platelet concentrate injection improves Achilles tendon repair in rats.," *Acta Orthop. Scand.*, vol. 75, no. 1, pp. 93–9, Feb. 2004.

[47] L. V Schnabel, H. O. Mohammed, B. J. Miller, W. G. McDermott, M. S. Jacobson, K. S. Santangelo, and L. A. Fortier, "Platelet rich plasma (PRP) enhances anabolic gene expression patterns in flexor digitorum superficialis tendons.," *J. Orthop. Res.*, vol. 25, no. 2, pp. 230–40, Feb. 2007.

[48] K. Gaweda, M. Tarczynska, and W. Krzyzanowski, "Treatment of Achilles tendinopathy with platelet-rich plasma.," *Int. J. Sports Med.*, vol. 31, no. 8, pp. 577–83, Aug. 2010.

[49] A. Mishra and T. Pavelko, "Treatment of chronic elbow tendinosis with buffered platelet-rich plasma.," *Am. J. Sports Med.*, vol. 34, no. 11, pp. 1774–8, Nov. 2006.

[50] P. S. Randelli, P. Arrigoni, P. Cabitza, P. Volpi, and N. Maffulli, "Autologous platelet rich plasma for arthroscopic rotator cuff repair. A pilot study.," *Disabil. Rehabil.*, vol. 30, no. 20–22, pp. 1584–9, Jan. 2008.

[51] R. J. de Vos, P. L. J. van Veldhoven, M. H. Moen, A. Weir, J. L. Tol, and N. Maffulli, "Autologous growth factor injections in chronic tendinopathy: a systematic review.," *Br. Med. Bull.*, vol. 95, pp. 63–77, Jan. 2010.

[52] Y. Kajikawa, T. Morihara, H. Sakamoto, K. Matsuda, Y. Oshima, A. Yoshida, M. Nagae, Y. Arai, M. Kawata, and T. Kubo, "Platelet-rich plasma enhances the initial mobilization of circulation-derived cells for tendon healing.," *J. Cell. Physiol.*, vol. 215, no. 3, pp. 837–45, Jun. 2008.

[53] M. de Mos, A. E. van der Windt, H. Jahr, H. T. M. van Schie, H. Weinans, J. a N. Verhaar, and G. J. V. M. van Osch, "Can platelet-rich plasma enhance tendon repair? A cell culture study.," *Am. J. Sports Med.*, vol. 36, no. 6, pp. 1171–8, Jun. 2008.

[54] E. Anitua, I. Andía, M. Sanchez, J. Azofra, M. del Mar Zalduendo, M. de la Fuente, P. Nurden, and A. T. Nurden, "Autologous preparations rich in growth factors promote proliferation and induce VEGF and HGF production by human tendon cells in culture.," *J. Orthop. Res.*, vol. 23, no. 2, pp. 281–6, Mar. 2005.

[55] R.-J. de Vos, J. Windt, and A. Weir, "Strong evidence against platelet-rich plasma injections for chronic lateral epicondylar tendinopathy: a systematic review.," *Br. J. Sports Med.*, pp. 952–956, 2014.

[56] T. Gosens and A. K. Mishra, "Editorial in response to the systematic review by de Vos et al: 'Strong evidence against platelet-rich plasma injections for chronic lateral epicondylar tendinopathy: a systematic review,'" *Br J Sport. Med*, vol. 48, no. 12, pp. 945–946, 2014.

[57] Z. Ahmad, R. Brooks, S.-N. Kang, H. Weaver, I. Nunney, G. Tytherleigh-Strong, and N. Rushton, "The effect of platelet-rich plasma on clinical outcomes in lateral epicondylitis.," *Arthroscopy*, vol. 29, no. 11, pp. 1851–62, Nov. 2013.

[58] L. Nelson, J. Fairclough, and C. W. Archer, "Use of stem cells in the biological repair of articular cartilage.," *Expert Opin. Biol. Ther.*, vol. 10, no. 1, pp. 43–55, Jan. 2010.

[59] M. Sánchez, J. Azofra, E. Anitua, I. Andía, S. Padilla, J. Santisteban, and I. Mujika, "Plasma rich in growth factors to treat an articular cartilage avulsion: a case report.," *Med. Sci. Sports Exerc.*, vol. 35, no. 10, pp. 1648–52, Oct. 2003.

[60] E. Kon, R. Buda, G. Filardo, A. Di Martino, A. Timoncini, A. Cenacchi, P. M. Fornasari, S. Giannini, and M. Marcacci, "Platelet-rich plasma: intra-articular knee injections produced favorable results on degenerative cartilage lesions.," *Knee Surg. Sports Traumatol. Arthrosc.*, vol. 18, no. 4, pp. 472–9, Apr. 2010.

[61] G. Filardo, E. Kon, R. Buda, A. Timoncini, A. Di Martino, A. Cenacchi, P. M. Fornasari, S. Giannini, and M. Marcacci, "Platelet-rich plasma intra-articular knee injections for the treatment of degenerative cartilage lesions and osteoarthritis.," *Knee Surg. Sports Traumatol. Arthrosc.*, vol. 19, no. 4, pp. 528–35, Apr. 2011.

[62] A. Drengk, A. Zapf, E. K. Stürmer, K. M. Stürmer, and K.-H. Frosch, "Influence of platelet-rich plasma on chondrogenic differentiation and proliferation of chondrocytes and mesenchymal stem cells.," *Cells. Tissues. Organs*, vol. 189, no. 5, pp. 317–26, Jan. 2009.

[63] K. Akeda, H. S. An, M. Okuma, M. Attawia, K. Miyamoto, E. J.-M. a Thonar, M. E. Lenz, R. L. Sah, and K. Masuda, "Platelet-rich plasma stimulates porcine articular chondrocyte proliferation and matrix biosynthesis.," *Osteoarthritis Cartilage*, vol. 14, no. 12, pp. 1272–80, Dec. 2006.

[64] A. Spreafico, F. Chellini, B. Frediani, G. Bernardini, S. Niccolini, T. Serchi, G. Collodel, A. Paffetti, V. Fossombroni, M. Galeazzi, R. Marcolongo, and A. Santucci, "Biochemical investigation of the effects of human platelet releasates on human articular chondrocytes.," *J. Cell. Biochem.*, vol. 108, no. 5, pp. 1153–65, Dec. 2009.

[65] C. Kaps, a Loch, a Haisch, H. Smolian, G. R. Burmester, T. Häupl, and M. Sittinger, "Human platelet supernatant promotes proliferation but not differentiation of articular chondrocytes.," *Med. Biol. Eng. Comput.*, vol. 40, no. 4, pp. 485–90, Jul. 2002.

[66] C. Gaissmaier, J. Fritz, T. Krackhardt, I. Flesch, W. K. Aicher, and N. Ashammakhi, "Effect of human platelet supernatant on proliferation and matrix synthesis of human articular chondrocytes in monolayer and three-dimensional alginate cultures.," *Biomaterials*, vol. 26, no. 14, pp. 1953–60, May 2005.

[67] J. Duan, W. Kuang, J. Tan, H. Li, Y. Zhang, K. Hirotaka, and K. Tadashi, "Differential effects of platelet rich plasma and washed platelets on the proliferation of mouse MSC cells.," *Mol. Biol. Rep.*, vol. 38, no. 4, pp. 2485–90, Apr. 2011.

[68] J. van den Dolder, R. Mooren, A. P. G. Vloon, P. J. W. Stoelinga, and J. a Jansen, "Platelet-rich plasma: quantification of growth factor levels and the effect on growth and differentiation of rat bone marrow cells.," Tissue Eng., vol. 12, no. 11, pp. 3067–73, Nov. 2006.

[69] O. Kilian, I. Flesch, S. Wenisch, B. Taborski, A. Jork, R. Schnettler, and T. Jonuleit, "Effects of platelet growth factors on human mesenchymal stem cells and human endothelial cells in vitro.," *Eur. J. Med. Res.*, vol. 9, no. 7, pp. 337–344, 2004.

[70] S. S. Lin, R. Landesberg, H. S. Chin, J. Lin, S. B. Eisig, and H. H. Lu, "Controlled release of PRP-derived growth factors promotes osteogenic differentiation of human mesenchymal stem cells.," *Conf. Proc. IEEE Eng. Med. Biol. Soc.*, vol. 1, pp. 4358–61, Jan. 2006.

[71] A. Mishra, P. Tummala, A. King, B. Lee, M. Kraus, V. Tse, and C. R. Jacobs, "Buffered platelet-rich plasma enhances mesenchymal stem cell proliferation and chondrogenic differentiation.," *Tissue Eng. Part C. Methods*, vol. 15, no. 3, pp. 431–5, Sep. 2009.

[72] J. P. Krüger, S. Hondke, M. Endres, A. Pruss, A. Siclari, and C. Kaps, "Human platelet-rich plasma stimulates migration and chondrogenic differentiation of human subchondral progenitor cells.," *J. Orthop. Res.*, vol. 30, no. 6, pp. 845–52, Jun. 2012.

[73] X. Xie, Y. Wang, C. Zhao, S. Guo, S. Liu, W. Jia, R. S. Tuan, and C. Zhang, "Comparative evaluation of MSCs from bone marrow and adipose tissue seeded in PRP-derived scaffold for cartilage regeneration.," *Biomaterials*, vol. 33, no. 29, pp. 7008–18, Oct. 2012.

[74] E. Rubio-Azpeitia and I. Andia, "Partnership between platelet-rich plasma and mesenchymal stem cells: in vitro experience," *Muscle, Ligaments Tendons J.*, vol. 4, no. 1, pp. 52–62, 2014.

[75] E. Anitua, J. J. Aguirre, J. Algorta, E. Ayerdi, A. I. Cabezas, G. Orive, and I. Andia, "Effectiveness of autologous preparation rich in growth factors for the treatment of chronic cutaneous ulcers.," *J. Biomed. Mater. Res. B. Appl. Biomater.*, vol. 84, no. 2, pp. 415–21, Feb. 2008.

[76] M. Takeuchi, N. Kamei, R. Shinomiya, T. Sunagawa, O. Suzuki, H. Kamoda, S. Ohtori, and M. Ochi, "Human platelet-rich plasma promotes axon growth in brain-spinal cord coculture.," *Neuroreport*, vol. 23, no. 12, pp. 712–6, Aug. 2012.

[77] J. L. Alio, F. Arnalich-Montiel, and A. E. Rodriguez, "The role of 'eye platelet rich plasma' (E-PRP) for wound healing in ophthalmology.," *Curr. Pharm. Biotechnol.*, vol. 13, no. 7, pp. 1257–65, Jun. 2012.

[78] X.-H. Li, X. Zhou, S. Zeng, F. Ye, J.-L. Yun, T.-G. Huang, H. Li, and Y.-M. Li, "Effects of intramyocardial injection of platelet-rich plasma on the healing process after myocardial infarction.," *Coron. Artery Dis.*, vol. 19, no. 5, pp. 363–70, Aug. 2008.

[79] Z. Dong, B. Li, B. Liu, S. Bai, G. Li, A. Ding, J. Zhao, and Y. Liu, "Platelet-rich plasma promotes angiogenesis of prefabricated vascularized bone graft.," *J. Oral Maxillofac. Surg.*, vol. 70, no. 9, pp. 2191–7, Sep. 2012.

[80] T. M. Bielecki, T. S. Gazdzik, J. Arendt, T. Szczepanski, W. Król, and T. Wielkoszynski, "Antibacterial effect of autologous platelet gel enriched with growth factors and other active substances: an in vitro study.," *J. Bone Joint Surg. Br.*, vol. 89, no. 3, pp. 417–20, Mar. 2007.

[81] M. A. Smith and W. T. Smith, "Emerging techniques in orthopaedics: platelet-rich plasma.," *Orthop. Nurs.*, vol. 30, no. 4, pp. 260–3; quiz 264–5, Jan. 2011.

[82] B. L. Eppley, W. S. Pietrzak, and M. Blanton, "Platelet-rich plasma: a review of biology and applications in plastic surgery.," *Plast. Reconstr. Surg.*, vol. 118, no. 6, p. 147e–159e, Nov. 2006.

[83] A. Mishra, K. Harmon, J. Woodall, and A. Vieira, "Sports medicine applications of platelet rich plasma.," *Curr. Pharm. Biotechnol.*, vol. 13, no. 7, pp. 1185–95, Jun. 2012.

[84] L. E. Loss, G. A. Deitrick, and R. G. Duff, "A prospective randomized trial of autologous platelet-derived wound healing factors for treatment of chronic nonhealing wounds: a preliminary report.," *J. Vasc. Surg.*, vol. 16, no. 1, pp. 125–6; author reply 126–8, Jul. 1992.

[85] T. Yuan, S.-C. Guo, P. Han, C.-Q. Zhang, and B.-F. Zeng, "Applications of leukocyte- and platelet-rich plasma (L-PRP) in trauma surgery.," *Curr. Pharm. Biotechnol.*, vol. 13, no. 7, pp. 1173–84, Jun. 2012.

[86] A. P. Sclafani, "Applications of Platelet-Rich Fibrin Matrix in Facial Plastic Surgery," 2009.

[87] A. Wang-Saegusa, R. Cugat, O. Ares, R. Seijas, X. Cuscó, and M. Garcia-Balletbó, "Infiltration of plasma rich in growth factors for osteoarthritis of the knee short-term ef-

fects on function and quality of life.," *Arch. Orthop. Trauma Surg.*, vol. 131, no. 3, pp. 311–7, Mar. 2011.

[88] G. Crovetti, G. Martinelli, M. Issi, M. Barone, M. Guizzardi, B. Campanati, M. Moroni, and A. Carabelli, "Platelet gel for healing cutaneous chronic wounds.," *Transfus. Apher. Sci.*, vol. 30, no. 2, pp. 145–51, Apr. 2004.

[89] A. A. Akingboye, S. Giddins, P. Gamston, A. Tucker, H. Navsaria, and C. Kyriakides, "Application of autologous derived-platelet rich plasma gel in the treatment of chronic wound ulcer: diabetic foot ulcer.," *J. Extra. Corpor. Technol.*, vol. 42, no. 1, pp. 20–9, Mar. 2010.

[90] M. Napolitano, S. Matera, M. Bossio, A. Crescibene, E. Costabile, J. Almolla, H. Almolla, F. Togo, C. Giannuzzi, and G. Guido, "Autologous platelet gel for tissue regeneration in degenerative disorders of the knee.," *Blood Transfus.*, vol. 10, no. 1, pp. 72–7, Jan. 2012.

[91] P. A. M. Everts, M. M. Hoogbergen, T. A. Weber, R. J. J. Devilee, G. van Monftort, and I. H. J. T. de Hingh, "Is the use of autologous platelet-rich plasma gels in gynecologic, cardiac, and general, reconstructive surgery beneficial?," *Curr. Pharm. Biotechnol.*, vol. 13, no. 7, pp. 1163–72, Jun. 2012.

[92] L. H. Redler, S. a Thompson, S. H. Hsu, C. S. Ahmad, and W. N. Levine, "Platelet-rich plasma therapy: a systematic literature review and evidence for clinical use.," *Phys. Sportsmed.*, vol. 39, no. 1, pp. 42–51, Feb. 2011.

[93] E. Lopez-Vidriero, K. a. Goulding, D. a. Simon, D. H. Johnson, and M. Sanchez, "Poor standardization in Platelet-rich Therapies Hampers Advancement," *Arthrosc. J. Arthrosc. Relat. Surg.*, vol. 26, no. 6, pp. 724–725, Jun. 2010.

[94] J. M. Delong, R. P. Russell, and A. D. Mazzocca, "Platelet-rich plasma: The PAW classification system," Arthrosc. - J. Arthrosc. Relat. Surg., vol. 28, no. 7, pp. 998–1009, 2012.